Neuromechanical Basis of Kinesiology

Roger M. Enoka, PhD
University of Arizona

Human Kinetics Books
Champaign, Illinois

Library of Congress Cataloging-in-Publication Data

Enoka, Roger M., 1949–
  Neuromechanical basis of kinesiology.

  Bibliography: p.
  Includes index.
  1. Kinesiology. 2. Human mechanics. I. Title.
[DNLM: 1. Biomechanics. 2. Movement. 3. Musculo-
skeletal System—physiology. WE 103 E59n]
QP303.E56 1988   612′.7   87-29745
ISBN 0-87322-179-6

Developmental Editor: Jan Progen, EdD
Production Director: Ernie Noa
Projects Manager: Lezli Harris
Assistant Editor: Phaedra Hise
Copy Editor: Claire Mount
Proofreader: Bruce Owens
Typesetter: Sandra Meier
Text Design: Keith Blomberg
Text Layout: Cathy Romans
Cover Design: Hunter Graphics
Printed By: R.R. Donnelly

ISBN: 0-87322-179-6

The following figures are reprinted with permission of Macmillan Publishing Company from *Biomechanics*, Second Edition by Ellen Kreighbaum and Katharine M. Barthels. Copyright © 1981, 1985 by Macmillan Publishing Company: Figure 2.20A; Figure 5.17 (human figure only); Figure 7.5 (human figure only); Problem 7.5 (human figure only); Problem 7.6 (human figure only); Figure 8.5A; Figure 8.6A.

Printed in the United States of America

10 9 8 7 6 5 4 3 2

Human Kinetics Books
A Division of Human Kinetics Publishers, Inc.
Box 5076, Champaign, IL 61825-5076
1-800-747-4HKP

Contents

Preface

The term *kinesiology* is derived from two Greek verbs, *kinein* and *logos*, which translate as to move and to discourse, respectively. Literally, therefore, kinesiology refers to discourse on movement, or as in current usage, the study of motion. It is generally agreed that the Greek philosopher Aristotle (384-322 BC) be attributed the title *Father of Kinesiology*, since several of his treatises were the first to describe the actions of muscles and to subject them to geometrical analysis. Although the system Aristotle devised for explaining motion did contain some contradictions, his pioneering efforts laid the foundations for the work of people like Galileo and Newton. The work of these philosophers and scientists has led us to view human motion as the consequence of the interaction between muscles and the external forces imposed by the environment on the system. For as Aristotle wrote, ''The animal that moves makes its change of position by pressing against that which is beneath it'' (Aristotle, 1968; E. Forster, Trans., p. 489). This seemingly simple statement contains the two elements that provide the basis for this text: (a) the interaction between an animal, including man, and its environment; and (b) the way in which the animal organizes the pressing. Within this framework, the events we call movements can be regarded as the consequences of an interaction between a biological system and its surrounding environment. Several factors, including the following, influence this interaction (see also Higgins, 1985):

1. The structure of the environment—shape and stability.
2. The field of external forces—orientation relative to gravity, movement speed.
3. The structure of the system—bony arrangement, net muscle activity, segmental organization of the body, scale or size, motor integration (e.g., the need to provide postural support).
4. The role of the psychological state—degree of attentiveness, motivation.
5. The task or motor event to be achieved—the task represents the driving force behind the organization of the movement.

This perspective is well captured by Higgins (1985): ''Movement is inseparable from the structure supporting it and the environment defining it'' (p. 144).

To realize this theme, a course in kinesiology generally will include a consideration of the principles of mechanics as they pertain to the description and production of motion, an identification of the various components of the musculoskeletal system necessary for the production of movement, and an examination of the interaction of the biological model with its surroundings. With a restriction to human movement, such a focus describes the context of this text. Because such a focus does not represent the area of kinesiology in its totality, however, the text has been titled the *Neuromechanical Basis of Kinesiology* to reflect appropriately the included material.

The intent of this text is to provide a scientific basis for the study of human motion, so the various ideas and principles are discussed in scientific terms. This means that more attention is paid to precise definitions and measurements than we commonly use in everyday conversation. In addition to emphasizing the correct definitions of scientific terms, this approach involves the use of metric units of measurement. Metric units (Appendix A) are preferred over those we commonly use because they are used by the majority of the Earth's population and because they are more precisely defined. Consider, for example, the definitions of the units *mile*, *yard*, and *foot*: the mile was defined as the distance a Roman legion covered by marching 1,000 paces; the yard was defined as the distance from the tip of the nose of King Henry I of England to the end of his outstretched arm; and the foot was based upon the length of the human foot. In contrast, the metric system measures distance in meters with 1 m defined as the wavelength of an isotope of the element krypton. Multiples or fractions of meters are represented as decimal subdivisions (e.g., 10-km road race, 0.1-mm cell length). Obviously the latter measurements are more reliable and, therefore, more useful.

If we are to rise above the quagmire that is associated with many aspects of human movement (e.g., muscle-fiber types, flexibility training, warm-up, strength training), it is essential that we have as our basis a set of rigorously defined terms and concepts. The primary goal of this text is to provide such a foundation. This goal is well illustrated by the analogy from Sherlock Holmes on the following page: How could Holmes know of Watson's intentions? The answer, of course, is that he was able to use his well-known ability of deductive reasoning. In a similar vein, movement can be considered the conclusion of a process, and our task, based on rigorusly defined terms and concepts, is to appreciate the intervening steps between the starting point and the conclusion.

Roger M. Enoka

THE STRAND MAGAZINE.

Vol. xxvi.   DECEMBER, 1903.   No. 156.

THE RETURN OF SHERLOCK HOLMES.

By A. CONAN DOYLE.

III.—*The Adventure of the Dancing Men.*

HOLMES had been seated for some hours in silence with his long, thin back curved over a chemical vessel in which he was brewing a particularly malodorous product. His head was sunk upon his breast, and he looked from my point of view like a strange, lank bird, with dull grey plumage and a black top-knot.

"So, Watson," said he, suddenly, "you do not propose to invest in South African securities?"

I gave a start of astonishment. Accustomed as I was to Holmes's curious faculties, this sudden intrusion into my most intimate thoughts was utterly inexplicable.

"How on earth do you know that?" I asked.

He wheeled round upon his stool, with a steaming test-tube in his hand and a gleam of amusement in his deep-set eyes.

"Now, Watson, confess yourself utterly taken aback," said he.

"I am."

"I ought to make you sign a paper to that effect."

"Why?"

"Because in five minutes you will say that it is all so absurdly simple."

"I am sure that I shall say nothing of the kind."

"You see, my dear Watson"—he propped his test-tube in the rack and began to lecture with the air of a professor addressing his class—"it is not really difficult to construct a series of inferences, each dependent upon its predecessor and each simple in itself. If, after doing so, one simply knocks out all the central inferences and presents one's audience with the starting-point and the conclusion, one may produce a startling, though possibly a meretricious, effect. Now, it was not really difficult, by an inspection of the groove between your left forefinger and thumb, to feel sure that you did *not* propose to invest your small capital in the goldfields."

"I see no connection."

"Very likely not; but I can quickly show you a close connection. Here are the missing links of the very simple chain: 1. You had chalk between your left finger and thumb when you returned from the club last night. 2. You put chalk there when you play billiards to steady the cue. 3. You never play billiards except with Thurston. 4. You told me four weeks ago that Thurston had an option on some South African property which would expire in a month, and which he desired you to share with him. 5. Your cheque-book is locked in my drawer, and you have not asked for the key. 6. You do not propose to invest your money in this manner."

"How absurdly simple!" I cried.

"Quite so!" said he, a little nettled. "Every problem becomes very childish when once it is explained to you. Here is an unexplained one. See what you can make of that, friend Watson." He tossed a sheet of paper upon the table and turned once more to his chemical analysis.

Acknowledgments

Over the course of my education I have had the good fortune of being able to associate with many talented and insightful individuals. Among these persons, four deserve particular recognition for their contribution to many of the ideas and points of view that are included in this text. In this respect, I am most grateful to Drs. Ziaul Hasan, Robert S. Hutton, Doris I. Miller, and Douglas G. Stuart for their input, encouragement, and commitment to excellence.

It is one thing to have a conceptual framework with which to address a particular issue but another quite different capability to be able to convey this notion to others. Many students have assisted me in the development of this ability. The extent to which we have been successful is reflected in this text. I am indebted to those students who have assisted me in this endeavor.

Finally, I must express sincere gratitude to Marilyn Kramer, Chris Lamott, Becky Norris, and Dolores Sierra for their patient typing of the many versions of this material.

PART

I

The Force-Motion Relationship

Historically, movement has long been a source of fascination. Its various facets have intrigued inquirers from numerous disciplines. As the frontiers of science have expanded, however, it has become apparent that movement has as its basis rather complex biological and mechanical interactions. Many of us interested in movement have attempted to follow these developments closely and have been led to the study of movement from biomechanical and neurophysiological perspectives (e.g., Hasan, Enoka, & Stuart, 1985). The study of movement based on the interaction of biomechanics and neurophysiology can be quite complicated. The goal of this text is to examine some of the more fundamental aspects of this interaction and to emphasize how they can be used in the study of movement.

The approach used here adopts the Aristotlean point of view that "the animal that moves makes its change of position by pressing against that which is beneath it" (Aristotle, p. 489). The two key elements of this idea are the way in which we organize the pressing and the notion that movement involves an interaction between an animal

(including humans) and its environment. To consider these two aspects the text has been divided into three parts: Part I, "The Force-Motion Relationship," involves an examination of selected principles of physics as they relate to biomechanics and the study of movement; Part II, "The Simple Joint System," develop a biological model with which to emphasize various features of the interaction between the nervous system and skeletal muscle (i.e., the way in which we organize the pressing); and Part III, "Movement: A System-Surround Interaction," portrays movement as the interaction of a biological model (simple joint system) with the physical world. This approach is not limited to a biomechanical one but rather also includes selected features of neurophysiology. To emphasize this focus, the title of the text indicates that the contents pertain to the field of kinesiology. Although the distinction between biomechanics and kinesiology is sometimes cloudy (Atwater, 1980), it can be delineated as follows:

Biomechanics—The application of the principles of mechanics to the study of

1

biological systems (American Society of Biomechanics, 1986)

Kinesiology—The study of movement (Atwater, 1980)

On this basis, kinesiology represents a broader focus that encompasses both biomechanics and neurophysiology as they pertain to the study of movement.

The intent of Part I is to characterize mechanically the interaction between the world in which movement occurs and the body parts that are moved (biomechanics). This will involve the introduction of terms and concepts commonly used to describe motion, an examination of the notion of force and its relationship to movement, and the identification of general techniques that can be used to analyze motion. Although most of these aspects of the force-motion relationship are illustrated with a variety of numerical examples, it is important not to get lost in the mathematics but rather to try to focus on the concepts that are being developed. To assist in this effort, Appendix B provides a brief review of some elementary mathematics for those of you who might need it.

Objectives

The objective of this text is to describe movement as the interaction of a biological model (a simplified version of us) with the physical world in which we live. In this first part, the goal is to define the mechanical bases of movement. The specific objectives are

- to describe movement in precise, well-defined terms;
- to define force and its various forms;
- to consider the role of force in movement; and
- to analyze movement from three different mechanical perspectives.

CHAPTER

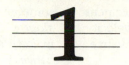

Motion

Position-Velocity-Acceleration

Although it is not difficult to appreciate the aesthetic qualities or the difficulty of a movement such as a triple-twisting backward 1 1/2 somersault dive, it is another matter to describe the movement in precise terms. The accurate and precise description of human movement is accomplished by the use of the terms *position*, *velocity*, and *acceleration*. Such a description of motion, one that ignores the causes of motion, is known as a **kinematic** description. Although these kinematic terms are often used in our everyday language, their precise meanings are usually ignored or abandoned. As in any scientific endeavor, the observations and principles that are elaborated are only as good as the concepts and definitions on which they are based. Due to the complexity of movement, it is important, indeed crucial, that our analyses rely on the rigorous definitions of the motion descriptors (position, velocity, and acceleration).

Definition

The **position** of an object refers to its location in space relative to some baseline value or axis. For example, the term *3-m diving board* indicates the position of the diving board above the water level of the pool. Similarly, the height of the high-jump bar is specified relative to the ground, the position of the finish line in a running race is indicated with respect to the start, the third and fifth positions in ballet refer to the position of one foot relative to the other, and so on. When an object experiences a change in position, it has been displaced and **motion** has occurred. Motion cannot be detected instantaneously because for motion to exist it is necessary to compare the position of the object at one instant in time with its position at another instant. *Motion, therefore, is an event that occurs in **space** and **time**.*

When an object is described as experiencing a **displacement**, the reference is to the spatial (space) element of motion, that is, the change in location of the body. Alternatively, an account of both the spatial and temporal (time) elements of motion involves the term *speed* or *velocity*. (The distinction between speed and velocity concerns scalar and vector quantities, respectively, as outlined in Appendix B. Specifically, speed is simply the magnitude of the velocity vector and as such has no regard for the change in direction.) Speed defines, How fast?, whereas velocity answers, How fast and in what direction? **Velocity** is defined as the rate of change in position with respect to time. In other words, how rapidly did the change in position occur and in what direction? Since displacement refers to a change in position, then velocity can be described as the time rate (derivative) of displacement.

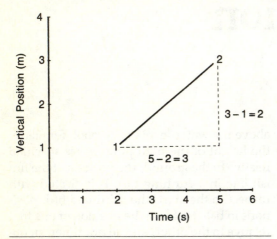

Figure 1.1. Relationship between velocity and a position-time graph.

Figure 1.1 represents two observations, separated in time by 3 s, of the vertical position of an object above some baseline value. The change in vertical position over this 3-s period was 2 m; therefore, the rate of change in position was 2 m in 3 s, that is, 2 m/3 s or 0.67 m•s⁻¹. Thus the average velocity of the object in moving from Position 1 to 2 was 0.67 m•s⁻¹, where m•s⁻¹ refers to meters per second (i.e., m/s). Stated more explicitly,

$$\text{velocity} = \frac{\Delta \text{ position}}{\Delta \text{ time}} \quad (1.1)$$

where Δ (delta) indicates a *change in* some parameter. Graphically, therefore, velocity refers to the slope of the position-time graph. Because a line graph, such as Figure 1.3,

depicts the relationship between two (or sometimes more) variables, *a change in the slope of the line as it becomes more or less steep indicates a change in the relationship between the variables*. The slope of the line, therefore, is determined numerically by subtracting an initial-position value from some final value (Δ position) and dividing the change in position by the amount of time it took for the change to occur (Δ time). Slope, therefore, refers to the rate of change in a variable such that the steeper the slope, the greater the rate of change, and vice versa.

Vertical displacement can vary not only in **magnitude** (i.e., size) but also in **direction** (i.e., up-down). Figure 1.2 illustrates some of these alternatives by noting the position of an object at five instances in time. Use of Equation 1.1 produces velocities 0.75, 1.50, 0, and −1.00 m•s⁻¹ for movement of the object from Positions 1 to 2, 2 to 3, 3 to 4, and 4 to 5, respectively. The steeper the slope of the position-time graph (e.g., Position 2 to 3 = 1.50 m•s⁻¹ vs. Position 1 to 2 = 0.75 m•s⁻¹),

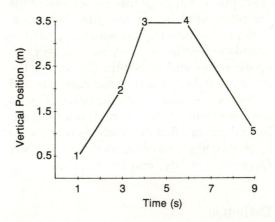

Figure 1.2. The variation in velocity associated with unequal changes in magnitude and direction in a position-time graph.

the greater the velocity. Conversely, a downward slope (e.g., Position 4 to 5) indicates a negative velocity. No change in position (e.g., Position 3 to 4) represents a zero velocity.

It is not sufficient, however, to describe motion only in terms of the occurrence and rate of a displacement. For example, a ball held 1.23 m above the ground and dropped will reach the ground 0.5 s later. The change in position is 1.23 m and the average velocity is 2.46 m•s^{-1} (i.e., 1.23 m/0.5 s). However, the ball does not travel with a constant velocity, but rather the velocity changes over time. Starting with a zero velocity at release, the speed of the ball increases to a value of 4.91 m•s^{-1} just prior to contact with the ground. This rate of change in velocity with respect to time is referred to as **acceleration**. The acceleration that the ball experiences while it falls is constant and has a value of 9.81 m•s^{-2}. If the velocity of an object is measured in meters per second (m•s^{-1}), then acceleration indicates the change in meters per second per second (m•s^{-2}). Consequently,

$$\text{acceleration} = \frac{\Delta \text{ velocity}}{\Delta \text{ time}} \qquad (1.2)$$

Acceleration, therefore, represents the change in velocity with respect to time or the change in the rate of change of position with respect to time. A running back in football who is described as having good acceleration has the ability to change velocity (speed and direction) quickly.

Previously, it was indicated that, because velocity is defined as the rate of change in position with respect to time, velocity can be represented graphically as the slope of the position-time graph. Similarly, with acceleration defined as the rate of change in velocity with respect to time, acceleration can be

indicated as the slope of the velocity-time graph. Thus, Figure 1.2 could be relabeled from a vertical position-time graph to a vertical velocity-time graph, and the relationships identified between the position-time curve and velocity could similarly apply to the velocity-time profile and acceleration. That is, acceleration refers to the slope of the velocity-time graph. For example, suppose Figure 1.2 was relabeled as a vertical velocity-time graph, and Point 2 had the coordinates of 2.0 m/s and 3 s whereas Point 3 had the coordinates of 3.5 m/s and 4 s. The rate of change from Point 2 to 3 would be the acceleration and would be calculated using Equation 1.2.

$$\text{acceleration} = \frac{3.5 - 2.0}{4 - 3} \quad \frac{\text{m•s}^{-1}}{\text{s}}$$
$$= 1.5 \text{ m/s/s (or m•s}^{-2})$$

Similarly, the acceleration from Points 1 to 2, 3 to 4, and 4 to 5 would be 0.75, 0, and −0.83 m•s^{-2}, respectively.

The acceleration experienced by the ball in the above example was due to the gravitational attraction between two masses, the planet Earth and the ball. The force of **gravity** produces a constant acceleration of approximately 9.81 m•s^{-2} at sea level. In general, *an object acted upon by a force will experience an acceleration.* A constant force (i.e., gravity) applied to an unsupported object produces a constant acceleration, and, conversely, the absence of a force means that the object is at rest or is traveling at a constant velocity (i.e., no acceleration). What would the velocity-time graph look like for these two conditions? Since acceleration can be depicted as the slope of a velocity-time graph, it should be possible to visualize the shape of a velocity-graph when an acceleration is present and when it is absent.

Equations of Motion

From these elementary definitions of velocity (Equation 1.1) and acceleration (Equation 1.2), it is possible to derive algebraic expressions involving time (t), position (**r**), velocity (**v**), and acceleration (**a**) that are often useful in the description of motion. Throughout the text, symbols representing vector terms (e.g., position, velocity, acceleration) are boldfaced. In deriving these equations of motion, $\mathbf{v}_i$ and $\mathbf{v}_f$ refer to initial and final velocity, respectively, and $\mathbf{r}_i$ and $\mathbf{r}_f$ similarly refer to initial and final position.

1. Express final velocity as a function of initial velocity, acceleration, and time.

$$\text{average acceleration} = \frac{\Delta \text{ velocity}}{\Delta \text{ time}}$$

$$\mathbf{a} = \frac{\mathbf{v}_f - \mathbf{v}_i}{t} \qquad (t = \Delta \text{ time})$$

$$\mathbf{v}_f = \mathbf{v}_i + \mathbf{a}t \tag{1.3}$$

For example, let us reconsider the ball-drop example that was mentioned previously. The ball was dropped from a height of 1.23 m, and 0.5 s later it reached the ground with a final velocity of 4.9 m•s⁻¹. According to Equation 1.3, the variables that affected final velocity were the initial velocity ($\mathbf{v}_i$) of the ball, its acceleration (**a**), and the duration of fall (t) that the ball experienced. In this example, $\mathbf{v}_i$ was zero, **a** was that due to gravity (9.81 m•s⁻²), and t was 0.5 s. You should insert these values into Equation 1.3 and verify the final velocity. Suppose you were interested in determining the final velocity of a pitched baseball as it crossed the plate. What would you need to know? As before, you would need to know $\mathbf{v}_i$, **a**, and t. The major difficulty would be in coming up with a value for **a**, because other forces in addition to gravity will be acting on the ball.

2. Derive an expression for position in terms of initial and final velocity, acceleration, and time.

$$\text{average velocity} = \frac{\Delta \text{ position}}{\Delta \text{ time}}$$

$$\frac{\mathbf{v}_f + \mathbf{v}_i}{2} = \frac{\mathbf{r}_f - \mathbf{r}_i}{t}$$

Substitute Equation 1.3 for $\mathbf{v}_f$,

$$\mathbf{r}_f - \mathbf{r}_i = \frac{\mathbf{v}_i + \mathbf{a}t + \mathbf{v}_i}{2} t$$

$$\mathbf{r}_f - \mathbf{r}_i = \frac{2\,\mathbf{v}_i + \mathbf{a}t}{2} t$$

$$\mathbf{r}_f - \mathbf{r}_i = \mathbf{v}_i t + 1/2\ \mathbf{a}t^2 \tag{1.4}$$

Equation 1.4 indicates that the change in position of an object (or the distance that the object travels from one point in time to another) depends on three things: its initial velocity (v_i), the acceleration (a) it experiences, and time (t). Another way of saying this is that the object's position will be different if any of these three variables changes. One use of this relationship is to determine how the position of an object changes as time varies. For example, consider an individual who is diving off a 10-m tower (Problem 1.9); by varying the value of t from 0 to 1.5 s in 0.1-s increments we can determine the trajectory (position-time graph) of the diver during the performance. That is, in Problem 1.9 the initial velocity of the diver is zero so that Equation 1.4 reduces to

$$r_f - r_i = 1/2 \, at^2$$

for this problem. If we assume that the effects of air resistance are so small that we can ignore them, then the acceleration is simply that which is due to gravity. The set of position-time data (as in Table 1.1) can then be determined by doing a number of calculations using the above equation in which the value of t is incremented each time by 0.1 s.

3. Relate final velocity to initial velocity, acceleration, and position.

$$\text{average velocity} = \frac{\Delta \text{ position}}{\Delta \text{ time}}$$

$$\frac{v_f + v_i}{2} = \frac{r_f - r_i}{t}$$

In this condition, however, t is unknown, so we rearrange Equation 1.3 to express t as the dependent variable [$t = (v_f - v_i)/a$] and substitute in the above expression.

$$\frac{v_f + v_i}{2} = \frac{r_f - r_i}{(v_f - v_i)/a}$$

$$\frac{v_f + v_i}{2} = (r_f - r_i) \frac{a}{v_f - v_i}$$

$$2a(r_f - r_i) = (v_f + v_i)(v_f - v_i)$$

$$2a(r_f - r_i) = v_f^2 - v_i^2$$

$$v_f^2 = v_i^2 + 2a(r_f - r_i) \tag{1.5}$$

As with both Equations 1.3 and 1.4, Equation 1.5 illustrates that a kinematic variable (final velocity in this case) can be determined from three other parameters. For example, the speed of a bullet at some known distance from a gun (e.g., 10 m) depends on the velocity of the bullet as it left the gun (initial velocity), the acceleration experienced by the bullet (i.e., due to air resistance), and the specified distance (10 m in this example).

When initial velocity is zero (e.g., the object experiencing the motion began at rest), the equations are further simplified:

$$\mathbf{v}_f = \mathbf{a}t$$
$$\mathbf{r}_f - \mathbf{r}_i = 1/2\ \mathbf{a}t^2$$
$$\mathbf{v}_f^2 = 2\mathbf{a}(\mathbf{r}_f - \mathbf{r}_i)$$

Table 1.1 Calculation of Velocity and Acceleration From a Set of Position-Time Data

	Position (m)	Time (s)	Velocity (Δ position/Δ time) (m·s⁻¹)		Acceleration (Δ velocity/Δ time) (m·s⁻²)	
1	0.00	0.000				
		0.050	(0.59−0.00)/(0.100−0.000)	= 5.9		
2	0.59	0.100			(3.6−5.9)/(0.150−0.050)	= −23.0
		0.150	(0.95−0.59)/(0.200−0.100)	= 3.6		
3	0.95	0.200			(1.0−3.6)/(0.225−0.150)	= −34.7
		0.225	(1.00−0.95)/(0.250−0.200)	= 1.0		
4	1.00	0.250			(−1.0−1.0)/(0.275−0.225)	= −40.0
		0.275	(0.95−1.00)/(0.300−0.250)	= −1.0		
5	0.95	0.300			(−3.6−[−1.0])/(0.350−0.275)	= −34.7
		0.350	(0.59−0.95)/(0.400−0.300)	= −3.6		
6	0.59	0.400			(−5.9−[−3.6])/(0.450−0.350)	= −23.0
		0.450	(0.00−0.59)/(0.500−0.400)	= −5.9		
7	0.00	0.500			(−5.9−[−5.9])/(0.550−0.450)	= 0.0
		0.550	(−5.9−0.00)/(0.600−0.500)	= −5.9		
8	−0.59	0.600			(−3.6−[−5.9])/(0.650−0.550)	= 23.0
		0.650	(−0.95−[−0.59])/(0.700−0.600)	= −3.6		
9	−0.95	0.700			(−1.0−[−3.6])/(0.725−0.650)	= 34.7
		0.725	(−1.00−[−0.95])/(0.750−0.700)	= −1.0		
10	−1.00	0.750			(1.0−[−1.0])/(0.775−0.725)	= 40.0
		0.775	(−0.95−[−1.00])/(0.800−0.750)	= 1.0		
11	−0.95	0.800			(3.6−1.0)/(0.850−0.775)	= 34.7
		0.850	(−0.59−[−0.95])/(0.900−0.800)	= 3.6		
12	−0.59	0.900			(5.9−3.6)/(0.950−0.850)	= 23.0
		0.950	(0.00−[−0.59])/(1.000−0.900)	= 5.9		
13	0.00	1.000				

Numerical Calculation

Table 1.1 represents a set of data with which to further examine the relationships between position, velocity, and acceleration. The 13 position values, each recorded at a different instant in time, represent the vertical path that an object travels over a 1-s epoch. The object first rises above an initial position (0.0 m) to a height of 1.0 m before being displaced by an equal amount (−1.0 m) below the original position and finally returning to 0.0 m. The velocity of the object during this motion is calculated by applying Equation 1.1 to selected intervals of time for which position information is available. For example, from Table 1.1 we could select the intervals of 0.0 to 1.0 s, 0.0 to 0.25 s, or 0.0 to 0.1 s. If we applied Equation 1.1, the average velocity for these three intervals would be

$$0.0 - 1.0 \text{ s} = \frac{0.0 - 0.0}{1.0 - 0.0}$$
$$= 0 \text{ m/s}$$

$$0.0 - 0.25 = \frac{1.0 - 0.0}{0.25 - 0.0}$$
$$= 4 \text{ m/s}$$

$$0.0 - 0.1 = \frac{0.59 - 0.0}{0.1 - 0.0}$$
$$= 5.9 \text{ m/s}$$

The smaller the intervals of time, the closer the calculated velocity will match that experienced by the object. That is, as Δ becomes smaller, the error in the calculation diminishes; in fact, as Δ approaches zero and becomes infinitesimal, then Δ is replaced with d and such expressions as $\Delta r/\Delta t$ become dr/dt. In Table 1.1, velocity has been determined for each interval over which position data is recorded. For example, the displacement during the first interval (0.59 − 0.0 = 0.59 m) is divided by the time elapsed during the interval (0.1 − 0.0 = 0.1 s) to produce

the velocity for that interval (0.59/0.1 = 5.9 m•s⁻¹). The calculated value (5.9 m•s⁻¹) represents the *average* velocity over that interval and consequently is recorded at the midpoint in time of the interval (0.05 s). Similarly, the first acceleration value (−23.0 m • s⁻²), which is determined with Equation 1.2, is listed at the midpoint in time (0.10 s) of the first velocity interval (0.05 to 0.15). By this procedure *the average value of velocity is determined for each position interval and the average acceleration is calculated for each velocity interval.* Thus, from a set of 13 position-time observations are calculated 12 velocity-time and 11 acceleration-time values.

The graphical relationship between a motion descriptor (e.g., position, velocity) and its rate of change has already been mentioned. Specifically, we have emphasized that the slopes of the position- and velocity-time graphs represent velocity and acceleration, respectively. Further evidence of these relationships is provided in Table 1.1 in that, when position increases (Positions 1 to 4 and 10 to 13) velocity is positive and when position decreases (Positions 4 to 10) velocity is negative. A similar dependency, which you should verify, exists between the slope (increase or decrease) of velocity and the sign of the acceleration values.

Graphical Relationship

On the basis of these associations, it is possible to estimate the rate of change in a kinematic variable from the shape of the kinematic variable-time graph. Figure 1.3 illustrates this process based on the changes in thigh angle of a skilled runner for one stride (defined as one complete cycle, from left foot takeoff to left foot takeoff in this example). The thigh angle is measured with respect to the right horizontal, and its measurement is indicated in the upper panel of

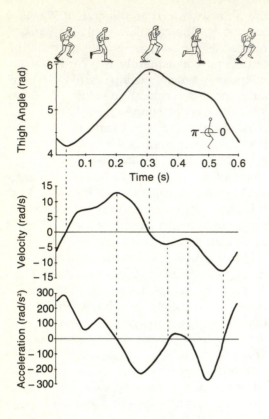

Figure 1.3. The graphic derivation of angular velocity-time and angular acceleration-time profiles from angular position-time and angular velocity-time graphs, respectively. The measured angle is for the limb with the filled-in shoe.

the figure. The angle is measured in radians (1 rad = 57.3 degrees), the SI unit (Appendix A) for angle.

The first step in this procedure of deriving the velocity-time graph from the position-time graph is to identify the relative **minima** and **maxima**. This means to note any—and there may be several—peaks and valleys that exist in the curve. The reason for identifying these points is that they denote instants at which the rate of change has a value of zero.

That is, the slope of the graph is neither upward (positive) nor downward (negative) but zero. In Figure 1.3, the thigh angle-time function has one minimum and one maximum. From these points of zero slope and thus zero velocity, a perpendicular line is extended to the time axis of the velocity-time graph to mark the locations in time of zero velocity. In Figure 1.3 these occur at about 0.03 and 0.30 s, respectively.

The second step is to determine the slope of the position-time graph between these minima and maxima. The slope of the graph will be the same (i.e., positive or negative) between these points because, as points of zero velocity, they identify the location in time at which the position-time curve changes its slope (i.e., changes direction). In each of these intervals between the minima and maxima the slope may become more or less steep, but it will remain either upward (positive) or downward (negative). In the thigh angle-time figure there is one minimum and one maximum and, therefore, three such intervals (i.e., from the beginning of the movement to the minimum, from the minimum to the maximum, and from the maximum to the end of the movement). The slopes of the position-time graph associated with these intervals are negative, positive, and negative, respectively. Thus the velocity-time graph has values (positive or negative) similar to the slope of the thigh angle-time function for each interval. For example, for the first interval, from the beginning of the movement to the minimum, both the position slope and the velocity values are negative. Since a negative velocity value is associated with a downward position-time slope, then negative velocities in Figure 1.3 indicate a backward rotation of the thigh (i.e., a reduction in the measured angle). In total, the velocity-time graph of Figure 1.3 indicates two intervals of backward thigh rotation separated in time by an interval of forward thigh rotation. The variation in the magnitude of the velocity over time indicates how the speed of this rotation varies, whereas the sign (positive or negative) indicates the direction (forward or backward) of rotation.

The derivation of the acceleration-time relationship from the velocity-time graph is accomplished by the same two-stage procedure: (a) identification of the relative minima and maxima, and (b) determination of the slope during the identified intervals. From Figure 1.3, the velocity-time curve contained four minima and maxima and thus there were four instances at which the acceleration-time graph had to cross through zero. The resulting acceleration-time relationship was a five-interval alternating positive-negative curve. The interpretation of an acceleration-time graph is generally more complicated than position- and velocity-time graphs. In Figure 1.3, a positive acceleration indicates an acceleration in the direction of forward rotation; during the first acceleration interval, the thigh rotated first backward then forward (seen from the velocity-time graph) but throughout the interval experienced an acceleration in the forward direction (recall the proportionality between acceleration and force). This concept is important and we will return to it several more times; in general, an object (or body segment) may be moving in one direction (positive or negative velocity) yet it may be experiencing an acceleration in the opposite direction. *It is not possible to tell the direction of acceleration from the direction of a movement.*

We are unable to know the precise magnitude of the rate of change by this **qualitative** process outlined in Figure 1.3; it merely gives a positive or negative sign for the rate of change and possibly its approximate value. On the other hand, Table 1.1 indicates a **quantitative** approach by which the values of the derivatives can be more accurately determined. A qualitative analysis tells us,

What type or kind? whereas quantitative analysis answers, How much?

Linear and Angular Motion

In the preceding discussion, the careful reader will have noted that the magnitude of displacement has been indicated with either of two units of measurement, meters (m) or radians (rad), the distinction between the two, of course, being that of **linear** and **angular** motion, respectively. Linear motion refers to an equivalent displacement in space of all parts of the object. Conversely, when all the parts of the object do not experience the same displacement, the object has rotated and hence we describe its motion as angular. A combination of linear (**translation**) and angular (**rotation**) motion in a single plane is called **planar** motion. It is rotation about a point, which is itself moving. When this occurs in more than one plane, we talk of general motion (three dimensional). In most human movement, body segments undergo both linear and angular motion.

A **meter**, the unit of measurement for linear motion, is defined as the wavelength of one line in an isotope of the element krypton. Conversely, a **radian** is the ratio of a distance on the circumference of the circle to the radius of the circle. When this distance on the circumference equals the radius, the ratio has a value of 1 and the object has rotated 1 rad (57.3 degrees). For example, consider the discus event in which the length of the thrower's arm from the shoulder joint to the discus has a value of 63 cm. As the arm rotates about the shoulder joint, the discus moves in a circular path. When the discus has moved along this path 63 cm (equal to the length of the arm and thus equal to the radius of the circle), the arm and discus have been rotated through the angle of 1 rad (Appendix B).

If the intent of a measurement is to describe rotary motion, then angular units are appropriate; otherwise use linear terms. The commonly used symbols and associated units of measurement for linear and angular position, velocity, and acceleration are outlined in Table 1.2. As indicated, the symbols are usually Latin letters for linear terms and Greek for angular.

Table 1.2 Linear and Angular Symbols and the SI Units of Measurement

	Linear		Angular	
	Symbol	Unit	Symbol	Unit
Position	$\mathbf{r}$	m	θ (theta)	rad
Displacement	$\Delta\mathbf{r}$	m	$\Delta\theta$ (theta)	rad
Velocity	$\mathbf{v}$	$m \cdot s^{-1}$	ω (omega)	$rad \cdot s^{-1}$
Acceleration	$\mathbf{a}$	$m \cdot s^{-2}$	α (alpha)	$rad \cdot s^{-2}$

Human movement is angular in nature, being due to the rotation of body segments about one another. For example, walking translates an individual from one location to another, in a linear sense. Yet for this movement to occur, the foot rotates about the ankle joint, the leg (or shank) rotates about the knee joint, the thigh rotates about the hip joint, and so on. In the analysis of movement, this seemingly minor observation assumes considerable significance.

In the measurement of human movement we graph some variable (e.g., thigh angle, ball height) against time. Due to the rotary nature of human movement, however, it is often more revealing to examine the relationship between two angles during an activity. Such graphs, called **angle-angle diagrams** (Cavanagh & Grieve, 1973), usually plot a relative angle (i.e., the angle between two adjacent body segments) against the absolute angle of a body segment (i.e., the angle relative to a reference in the environment).

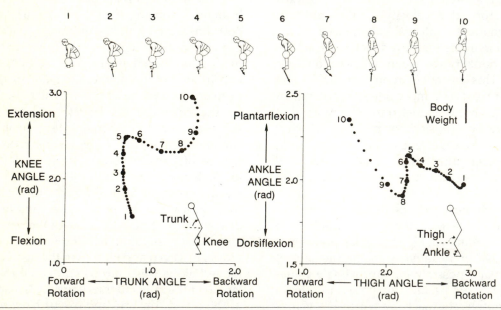

Figure 1.4. Angle-angle relationships during the first part of an Olympic weight-lifting event, the clean and jerk. The numbers associated with the knee-trunk and ankle-thigh diagrams correspond to the positions of the lifter indicated at the top of the figure.

Figure 1.4 illustrates this point by showing two angle-angle diagrams during part of a weight-lifting movement in which the barbell was lifted from Position 1 through Position 10. The knee-trunk diagram illustrates that the movement comprises three distinct phases: (a) Position 1 to 5, extension of the knee joint and slight forward rotation of the trunk; (b) Position 5 to 8, backward rotation of the trunk and flexion of the knees; and (c) Position 8 to 10, knee-joint extension and some backward-forward trunk rotation. Similarly, the ankle-thigh angle-angle diagram comprises three phases: (a) forward thigh rotation-ankle plantarflexion, (b) constant thigh angle-ankle dorsiflexion, and (c) forward thigh rotation-ankle plantarflexion. An interesting feature of Figure 1.4 is the extent to which the three phases for the two angle-angle diagrams coincide, thus emphasizing that the movement is accomplished by co-ordinated displacements about the lower extremity joints. A further feature of these

graphs is that, since the dots are about 10 ms apart, the further apart the dots, the greater the velocity of the movement.

Acceleration and Muscle Activity

To pursue further the relationship between acceleration and force, consider the following example of an elbow extension-flexion movement in a horizontal plane passing through the shoulder joint (Figure 1.5A).

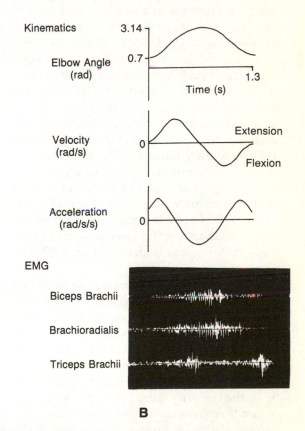

A	**B**

Figure 1.5. A simple extension-flexion movement of the forearm-hand segment about the elbow joint. (A) Photograph of the subject with the arm in the initial position. (B) Position- (elbow angle), velocity-, acceleration-, and electromyogram- (EMG) time records associated with the movement in the horizontal plane. The EMG records are for two elbow flexor muscles (biceps brachii and brachioradialis) and one extensor muscle (triceps brachii). The kinematic features of the movement (position, velocity, and acceleration) are largely determined by the net muscle activity (viz., the resultant EMG activity). Photos by Peter B. Worden.

Suppose the movement began with the upper arm raised straight out to the side (an angle of 1.57 rad [90 degrees] from the torso) and with an angle of 0.70 rad (40 degrees) between the upper arm and forearm. In one continuous movement of moderate speed, the upper arm is held stationary while the elbow joint is extended horizontally to 3.14 rad (180 degrees) and flexed back to the starting position (0.70 rad). In general, flexion at a joint results in a decrease of the angle between the two body segments that meet at the joint (upper arm and forearm in this example), whereas extension refers to an increase in the angle. What would be the shape of an appropriate position-time graph associated with such a movement? In the movement, the upper arm remains stationary and the forearm rotates about the elbow joint; a plot of elbow angle over time should provide an adequate description of the event. Due to the elementary nature of the movement, in which the minimum angle (0.70 rad) occurred at the beginning and end of the movement and the maximum angle was at complete extension (3.14 rad), it is not difficult to anticipate the shape of the position-time graph. Indeed, the upper panel of Figure 1.5B confirms this expectation.

Without regard to the previously described relationships between position, velocity, and acceleration, answer two questions about the movement; focus only on the elbow joint rotation: Where was the velocity zero? and, Where was the acceleration zero? First, at which point in the extension-flexion event was the velocity zero? Velocity was zero when there was no displacement, which occurred at the beginning and the end of the movement and for an instant when the direction of the movement changed from extension to flexion. For now, focus on the zero velocity at the direction change. The velocity-time graph in Figure 1.5B does indicate that angular velocity was zero and hence that the change in direction occurred at the maximum displacement (3.14 rad). However, this could have been deduced graphically from the previous comments on the equivalency between velocity and the slope of the position-time function. As the graph illustrates, when the value of velocity was positive (above zero) the elbow was extending, and when the velocity was negative the elbow was flexing. Thus a change in the sign of velocity (e.g., positive to negative) indicates a change in the direction of the movement.

Now consider the acceleration question. Apart from the start and the end of the movement, when was the acceleration zero? An intuitive response to this question is more difficult, as the criteria for declaring a zero acceleration is not that obvious. With velocity the decision was more straightforward and merely involved locating instances of no displacement. The parallel approach for acceleration is to identify intervals in which the change in velocity is zero.

The answer to this question is most easily obtained with reference to a velocity-time graph. Given the graphic relationship between a variable and its derivative, the angular acceleration-time curve in Figure 1.5B indicates the acceleration was zero when the value of velocity was at its maximum (0.3 s) and minimum (1.0 s). That is, acceleration was zero when the slope of the velocity-time graph was zero. The acceleration-time graph could be described as triphasic as it comprises three epochs of acceleration: (a) from the beginning until about 0.3 s, the movement consisted of an acceleration in the extension direction; (b) subsequently, acceleration experienced a sign change, and for most of the movement (0.3 to 1.0 s) the acceleration was in the direction of elbow flexion; and (c) the movement concluded with another epoch of extension-directed acceleration. Note that the acceleration-time profile cannot be predicted directly from the position-time graph.

Could this acceleration-time profile have been determined by any means other than the velocity-time graph? In other words, is it possible to identify the instances of zero acceleration without knowledge of the velocity-time function? As an answer to this question, consider the pattern of muscular activity necessary to produce the movement. Often in kinesiology it is more useful to describe movements in terms of muscle groups rather than specific muscles. In this elbow extension-flexion example, the movement involves the muscle groups indentified as elbow extensors and elbow flexors (i.e., muscle groups that provide the movement of interest). From a knowledge of anatomy it is possible to identify the individual muscles included in each group. The group elbow flexors, for example, includes biceps brachii, brachialis, and brachioradialis as the major muscles (prime movers) contributing to elbow flexion. Thus the question can be restated: What was the pattern of elbow-extensor and elbow-flexor activity during the movement under consideration?

One of the aspects of Part II of the text (''The Simple Joint System'') will be to examine the manner in which the nervous system activates muscle. For now, suffice it to say that this communication is an electrochemical process in which the final stage is electrical in nature. Therefore, to determine whether or not a muscle is active, it is only necessary to monitor the electrical activity of the muscle. This technique is known as **electromyography** (**EMG**) and involves the use of electrodes placed on the surface of or within (intramuscular) the muscle to monitor the electrical input (voltage) to the muscle. Figure 1.5 includes an EMG record of the activity of the elbow extensors and flexors during the elbow extension-flexion move-

ment. Although both muscle groups were active throughout portions of the movement (a phenomenon known as **cocontraction**), there is a high correlation between the *net* muscle activity (EMG) and the acceleration-time profile. Later on we will consider in more detail the mechanical effect of muscle activity on body segments. One basic feature of muscle activity is that it exerts a force and can cause body segments to rotate. In this particular horizontal elbow extension-flexion movement there are no other significant horizontal forces so that the acceleration about the elbow joint is largely determined by the activity of the muscles about the joint. Thus, in response to the zero-acceleration question, it is possible to identify the instances of zero acceleration if the pattern of net muscular activity is known.

Given this relationship between force and acceleration, then the acceleration-time graph shown in Figure 1.5B must also represent the pattern of net muscle activity about the elbow joint. However, it often seems difficult to understand, at least initially, why a simple elbow extension-flexion movement would involve a triphasic pattern of net muscle activity. To move a limb at moderate speed in *one direction* toward a target involves a burst of muscle activity by the **agonist** (the muscle[s] primarily responsible for producing the movement) to accelerate the limb toward the target, a burst by the **antagonist** (the muscle[s] whose actions oppose the agonist) to slow down (brake) the limb and control its approach to the target, and some final activity by the agonist to arrive at the target. This sequence of muscle activity for a unidirectional movement is referred to as the **three-burst pattern**. In a movement that involves a *change in direction* (e.g., extension to flexion), the latter component of this activity pattern (i.e., the second agonist burst) is usually absent.

This elbow extension-flexion movement

comprises two parts, one extension and the other flexion. Each part of the movement is controlled by two bursts of muscle activity, one to accelerate the limb toward the target and the other to slow the limb down. *The acceleration toward the target is accomplished by the activity of the agonists, and the slowing down is done by the antagonists.* For the extension part of the movement the target is 3.14 rad, the agonist is the elbow-extensor muscle group, and the antagonist is the elbow flexors. For the flexion part of the movement, the target is the return to the starting position (0.70 rad), the agonist is the elbow flexors, and the antagonist is the elbow extensors. Functionally, therefore, the total movement needs four bursts of muscle activity: (a) agonist extensor, (b) antagonist flexor, (c) agonist flexor, and (d) antagonist extensor. Since the acceleration caused by the elbow flexors, whether the muscle group is serving an agonist or antagonist role, is in the direction of elbow flexion (negative acceleration in Figure 1.5B), the pattern of net muscle activity appears as a triphasic profile, that is, elbow extensors, elbow flexors, and elbow extensors.

In general, however, the relationship exhibited in this elbow extension-flexion example between the activity of the muscles about a joint and the acceleration of the body segment is a rather special case. The acceleration that a body segment experiences is a reflection of *all* the forces acting on the segment. For example, if the elbow extension-flexion movement was performed in a vertical plane, gravity would exert an influence on the movement and the acceleration-time graph would be different to that depicted in Figure 1.5B. When the movement is performed in a horizontal plane, the muscles exert the only significant force on the forearm in this plane and thus produce the special illustrated relationship between muscle activity and acceleration of the forearm.

Kinematics of Gait

As an example of the use of these motion descriptors (position, velocity, and acceleration) in the analysis of human movement, let us consider some kinematic characteristics of gait. Human gait simply involves alternating sequences in which the body is supported first by one limb, which is contacting the ground, and then by the other limb. Although this sounds quite straightforward, its control is sufficiently complex that, despite our technological advances, no machine has yet been built that mimics our gait.

Human gait has two modes, walking and running. The distinction between the two modes lies in the percentage of each cycle that the body is supported by foot contact with the ground. During walking there is always at least one foot on the ground, and for a brief period of each cycle both feet are on the ground; walking can be characterized as an alternating sequence of single- and double-support. In contrast, running involves alternating sequences of support and nonsupport, with the proportion of the cycle spent in support varying with speed; as speed increases, the time of support decreases. During a single cycle, however, whether walking or running, each limb experiences a sequence of support and nonsupport. The period of support is referred to as the **stance** phase, and nonsupport is known as the **swing** phase. These intervals are separated by two events, the instant at which the foot contacts the ground (footstrike, FS) and the instant at which the foot leaves the ground (takeoff, TO). Gait cycles are usually defined relative to these events. For example, one complete cycle, from left foot takeoff to left foot takeoff, is defined as a **stride**.

Figure 1.6 summarizes these relationships, depicting the stride as containing two steps, where a **step** is defined as the part of the cycle from the takeoff (or footstrike) of one foot to the takeoff (or footstrike) of the other foot. Within a stride four events of footstrike and takeoff occur, two for the reference (ipsilateral) limb and two for the other (contralateral) limb. These are shown in Figure 1.6 as ipsilateral takeoff (ITO), contralateral footstrike (CFS), contralateral takeoff (CTO), and ipsilateral footstrike (IFS). The swing phase exists between the events of ITO and IFS

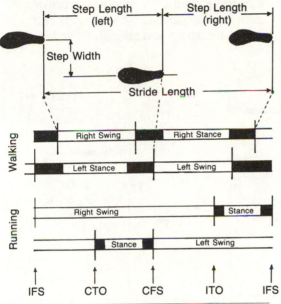

Figure 1.6. The events and phases characterizing walking and running gaits. The events indicated at the bottom of the figure refer to the right leg during a running stride: IFS = ipsilateral footstrike, ITO = ipsilateral takeoff, CFS = contralateral footstrike, CTO = contralateral takeoff; in this example, ipsilateral = right, and contralateral = left. During walking there is always at least one foot on the ground whereas during running there are alternating periods of support (stance) and nonsupport (swing). *Note.* From ''Biomechanics of the Human Gait'' by E.Y.S. Chao, 1986, in G.W. Schmid-Schonbein et al. (Eds.), *Frontiers in Biomechanics* (p. 226), New York: Springer. Copyright 1986 by Springer-Verlag, Inc. Adapted by permission.

whereas stance occurs from IFS to ITO. The contralateral limb is taken through a similar sequence of swing and stance. The analysis of gait includes at least two concerns, intra- and interlimb considerations. Intralimb analyses address the details of a single limb (e.g., Figure 1.8), whereas interlimb analyses concern the relationships between the different limbs.

Running speed is the result of the interaction of two variables, stride length and stride rate (Vaughan, 1985). If stride length remains constant, then as stride time decreases (i.e., stride rate increases) running speed will increase. If stride rate remains constant, speed increases as stride length increases. These effects of stride rate and length are indicated in Figure 1.7. Within certain limits there are a number of length-rate combinations that will produce a desired speed.

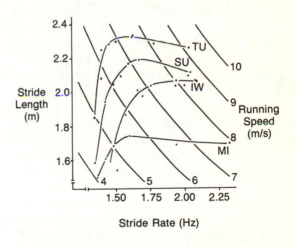

Figure 1.7. The relationships among stride rate, stride length, and running speed. *Note.* From ''Temporal Patterns in Running'' by M. Saito, K. Kobayashi, M. Miyashita, and T. Hoshikawa, 1974, in R.C. Nelson and C.A. Morehouse (Eds.), *Biomechanics IV* (p. 107), Baltimore: University Park Press. Copyright 1974 by University Park Press. Adapted by permission.

For example, according to Figure 1.7 an individual could run at 6 m•s⁻¹ (speed is shown by the lines that run from top left- to bottom right-hand sides of the figure) with a stride length-rate combination of about 1.73 m and 1.75 Hz or 2.05 m and 1.50 Hz.

Figure 1.7 indicates that as we change running speed we change stride rate and stride length in combination rather than individually. The strategy adopted by four runners is depicted in Figure 1.7. The data were obtained by filming the individuals as they ran at different speeds and then measuring stride length and rate from the film. Consider the results obtained for Subject SU, whose change in speed from 4.3 to 8.5 m/s seemed to be accomplished in two phases: (a) initial changes in speed (4.3 to 7.0 m/s) were due to a combined increase in stride length (1.6 to 2.2 m) and stride rate (1.4 to 1.7 Hz); (b) subsequent speed increases (7.0 to 8.5 m/s) were achieved by a slight decrease in stride length (about 10 cm) but a sustained increase in stride rate (1.7 to 2.0 Hz). In general, the trained runners (Subjects TU, SU, and IW) increased stride length up to 7.0 m•s⁻¹ whereas the untrained runner (MI) did so only up to 5.5 m•s⁻¹. All four runners, however, achieved initial increases in speed (up to 6.0 m/s for the trained runners) mainly by increasing stride length. The typical explanation given for this strategy (i.e., change stride length rather than rate) is that it requires less energy to lengthen the stride within reasonable limits than to increase the rate.

Cyclical activities, such as walking and running, are ideal movements to represent in angle-angle diagrams because the beginning and end of the event are located at about the same point on the diagram. This type of graphic display has proven useful in comparing movement forms (Hershler & Milner, 1980a, 1980b; Miller, 1978). For example, the knee-thigh diagram of a normal subject during running can be compared to that of

a lower extremity amputee to evaluate the effectiveness of various protheses in restoring normal-looking gait. In this type of analysis, emphasis is placed on comparing the shape of the respective angle-angle diagrams (e.g., Figure 1.8 vs. 1.9).

The interpretation of Figure 1.8 involves following the curve around in a counterclockwise direction. This diagram illustrates the angle-angle relationship for one limb during a running stride. As mentioned previously, each limb experiences two events during a stride, footstrike and takeoff. From footstrike

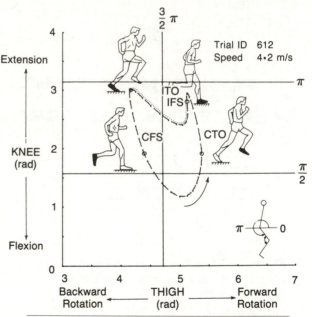

Figure 1.8. Knee-thigh diagram of the left limb of a skilled runner during a running stride. The designations IFS, ITO, CFS, and CTO indicate ipsilateral (left) footstrike, ipsilateral takeoff, contralateral (right) footstrike, and contralateral takeoff, respectively. These events are indicated by the illustrations of the runner. *Note.* From ''Below-Knee Amputee Running Gait'' by R.M. Enoka, D.I. Miller, and E.M. Burgess, 1982, *American Journal of Physical Medicine,* **61**, p. 70. Copyright 1982 by Williams and Wilkins. Reprinted by permission.

to takeoff (stance phase), the foot is in contact with the ground. Conversely, from takeoff to footstrike, the foot of the illustrated (ipsilateral) limb is not in contact with the ground (swing phase). In addition, during the swing phase (ITO to IFS), the other (contralateral) limb first contacts and then leaves the ground (CFS and CTO, respectively). Accordingly, Figure 1.8 reveals (a) after ITO, the thigh rotates forward about the hip joint and the knee flexes to a minimum value; (b) following the minimum angle, the knee extends until just before IFS while the thigh continues to rotate forward and then begins rotating backward; and (c) during stance (IFS to ITO), the knee first flexes then extends, and the thigh rotates backward.

When the topic of angle-angle diagrams was first introduced in this chapter, several features were emphasized, and these are again apparent in Figure 1.8. A relative angle (knee) is plotted against an absolute angle (thigh). The graph illustrates the combined actions of knee flexion-extension and thigh forward-backward rotation. In addition, three reference axes are shown with which to evaluate the range of motion of the movement: (a) the $3/2 \pi$ axis indicates a thigh angle at which the thigh would be in a vertical position, (b) the π axis (3.14 rad) represents a knee angle of complete extension, and (c) the $\pi/2$ axis shows a right angle (1.57 rad) for the knee joint. According to Figure 1.8, therefore, the thigh passes in front of and behind vertical, the knee joint is never fully extended, and the smallest knee angle is less than a right angle during a normal running stride at 4.2 m/s.

In comparison to this normal knee-thigh diagram, the three below-knee amputee graphs depicted in Figure 1.9 indicate a substantial difference during the stance phase (i.e., the region from IFS to ITO). Specifically, the amputee knee-thigh diagrams reveal a knee-joint pattern of a constant angle followed by flexion rather than the normal

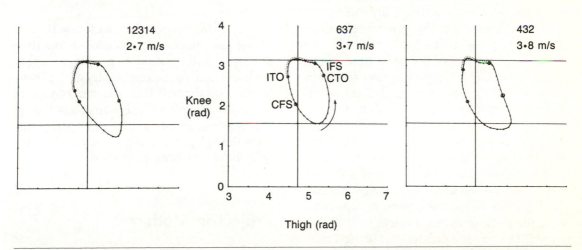

Figure 1.9 Knee-thigh diagrams for three below-knee amputees running at speeds from 2.7 to 3.8 m•s⁻¹. The diagrams illustrate that the amputees did not flex their knee joints at the beginning of stance, as is the normal sequence of events. *Note.* From ''Below-Knee Amputee Running Gait'' by R.M. Enoka et al., 1982, *American Journal of Physical Medicine,* **61**, p. 78. Copyright 1982 by Williams and Wilkins. Reprinted by permission.

flexion-extension sequence. Since Figure 1.9 shows the knee-thigh diagrams for the prosthetic limbs of the below-knee amputees, it is perhaps not surprising that the graphs appeared as they did. This failure to flex the knee during stance means that the amputees just used their limb as a rigid lever about which to rotate while the prosthetic foot was on the ground. This type of graphic display could be used in a clinical setting to monitor a rehabilitation program aimed at correcting this strategy so that the gait would appear more normal.

Another useful feature of these cyclic angle-angle diagrams is that, in addition to shape comparisons, the size of the diagram indicates the range of motion experienced at each joint during the event. For example, we would expect that increases in stride length as a runner increases speed are due to changes in the range of motion (amount of motion) at various lower extremity joints. Figure 1.10 indeed confirms this expectation by noting that, as speed increases (3.88 and 7.56 m•s⁻¹ for the two diagrams), the amount of rotation both of the thigh and about the knee joint increases; the larger angle-angle diagram represents the greater speed.

At this point a good exercise to test your grasp of the angle-angle diagram approach is to sketch a knee-thigh diagram as a runner goes uphill and then downhill. The key to this exercise is to think of how the movement would change relative to the three reference axes. For example, it seems reasonable to expect that a runner going downhill would extend the knee less than on the flat, flex the knee less at the minimum angle, and have the thigh remain in front of vertical (forward rotation) for a greater part of the stride. Try sketching this relationship.

The angle-angle diagram format, first proposed by Cavanagh and Grieve (1973), has largely been confined to representing position information. Some investigators (e.g.,

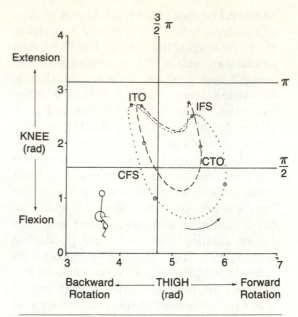

Figure 1.10. Knee-thigh angle-angle diagram as a function of running speed. The smaller (dashed) and larger (dotted) diagrams were for speeds of 3.88 and 7.56 m•s⁻¹, respectively. (Adapted from Miller, Enoka, McCulloch, Burgess, Hutton, and Frankel, 1979).

Miller, 1978) have experimented with plots of angular velocity and acceleration, but these attempts have not been readily accepted, probably due to the complexity of the waveforms. Similarly, given current computer-graphics capabilities, it is surprising that no three-dimensional angle-angle diagrams, with time (e.g., running speed) as the third axis, have yet been published.

Projectile Motion

These relationships between position, velocity, and acceleration can also be used to provide many of the details about the trajectory that a projected (thrown) object will travel. The simplest case is one in which we assume that the effect of air resistance is so small (e.g., due to the size of the object or the absence of wind) that we can neglect it. Given this condition, there are a number of facts that we can use to help us explore the motion of a projectile:

- The path that the object travels while it is in the air is parabolic.
- The time that the object spends in the air depends on the magnitude of its velocity at release.
- The only force that the projectile experiences will be that due to gravity, and this will cause a vertical acceleration of -9.81 m/s^2.
- Because there is no force acting in the horizontal direction, the horizontal acceleration of the object will be zero, which means its horizontal velocity will be constant.
- At the peak of its trajectory, the object changes its vertical direction of motion, which means that its vertical velocity will be zero at this point.

On the basis of these facts, the velocity-time profile of a projectile at five selected instances throughout its trajectory is shown in Figure 1.11.

From the definitions of velocity (Equation 1.1) and acceleration (Equation 1.2), let us consider an example of projectile-motion analysis. A ball is released from a throw at an angle of 1.05 rad with respect to the horizontal, 2.5 m above the ground with a resultant velocity along the line of projection of 6 m/s.

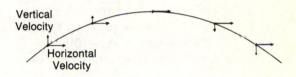

Vertical Velocity

Horizontal Velocity

Figure 1.11. The parabolic trajectory experienced by projectiles: such as the center of gravity of a basketball player shooting a jump shot or a trampolinist performing tricks, and the flight of a discus, shot, or javelin. If the effects of air resistance are small, the horizontal component of the velocity vector remains unchanged throughout the flight. The vertical component, however, changes throughout the event, being greatest at the beginning and the end and zero at the peak.

1. How long does the ball take to reach its highest point? The trajectory is parabolic, so the ball will continue going up until the vertical velocity has a value of zero.

$$\bar{a} = \frac{\Delta v}{\Delta t}$$
$$= (v_f - v_i)/t$$

$$-9.81 = (0 - 5.2)/t$$
$$t = -5.2/-9.81$$
$$t = 0.53 \text{ s}$$

($\bar{a}$ = average acceleration)

$$v_i = 6 \sin 1.05$$
$$= 5.2 \text{ m/s}$$

2. How high (vertically) does the ball get? The height reached is that due to its release velocity plus the height above the ground at which it was released.

$$\bar{\mathbf{v}} = \frac{\Delta \mathbf{r}}{\Delta t} \qquad\qquad (\bar{\mathbf{v}} = \text{average velocity})$$

$$(5.2 + 0)/2 = \Delta \mathbf{r}/0.53$$
$$\Delta \mathbf{r} = 0.53\,(5.2 + 0)/2$$
$$= 1.38 \text{ m}$$
$$\text{Total height} = 1.38 + 2.5 \qquad\qquad (2.5 = \text{release height})$$
$$= 3.88 \text{ m}$$

3. What is the vertical velocity of the ball when it hits the ground?

$$\bar{\mathbf{a}} = \frac{\Delta \mathbf{v}}{\Delta t}$$

$$-9.81 = (\mathbf{v}_f - \mathbf{v}_i)/t$$
$$-9.81 = (\mathbf{v}_f - 0)/t \qquad\qquad (\mathbf{v}_i = \text{velocity at peak})$$
$$\mathbf{v}_f = -9.81\,t$$

Once we know how long it takes the ball to go from its peak to the ground, then we can determine its final velocity just prior to impact.

4. How long does it take the ball to reach the ground? We already know that the ball took 0.53 s to reach its peak, but to reach the ground the ball has to fall an additional 2.5 m (the release height).

$$\bar{\mathbf{v}} = \frac{\Delta \mathbf{r}}{\Delta t}$$

$$(\mathbf{v}_f + \mathbf{v}_i)/2 = -3.88/t \qquad\qquad (-3.88 \text{ because it falls}$$
$$(\mathbf{v}_f + 0)/2 = -3.88/t \qquad\qquad \text{that distance})$$

Substitute in the known relationship (from above) for $\mathbf{v}_f$.

$$-9.81\,t/2 = -3.88/t$$
$$t^2 = (-3.88 \times 2)/-9.81$$
$$t^2 = 0.79$$
$$t = 0.89 \text{ s}$$

Thus, for the above unknown of $\mathbf{v}_f$

$$\mathbf{v}_f = -9.81 \times 0.89$$
$$\mathbf{v}_f = -8.73 \text{ m/s} \qquad\qquad (\text{negative} = \text{downward})$$

5. How long did the ball spend in flight?

$$t = t_{up} + t_{down}$$
$$= 0.53 + 0.89$$
$$= 1.42 \text{ s}$$

6. What horizontal distance did the ball travel—that is, how far was it thrown? In contrast to the previous calculations, this one uses the horizontal, as opposed to the vertical, information.

$$\bar{\mathbf{v}} = \frac{\Delta \mathbf{r}}{\Delta t}$$

$$(\mathbf{v}_f + \mathbf{v}_i)/2 = \Delta \mathbf{r}/t$$

$$\mathbf{v}_i = 6 \cos 1.05$$
$$= 3 \text{ m/s}$$

Since the horizontal velocity component remains constant, $\mathbf{v}_f = \mathbf{v}_i$

$$(3 + 3)/2 = \Delta \mathbf{r}/1.42$$
$$\Delta \mathbf{r} = 1.42 \times 3$$
$$= 4.24 \text{ m}$$

The main feature of this example is that all of the details of the ball's trajectory were determined by the simple application of the definitions for velocity and acceleration. In particular, these details were determined without the need to resort to unwieldly, complicated-looking formulae. However, take note that this procedure applies to conditions when the effects of air resistance are so small that they can be ignored.

The predictability of the trajectory of a projectile (i.e., parabolic) can also be used to cast doubt on a common practice in sports. How many times have you heard a coach exhort, "Keep your eyes on the ball!"? Most athletes interpret this suggestion to mean that by watching the projectile *all the way* to the bat, racket, foot, and so forth, the performance can be adjusted to accommodate changes in the trajectory of the projectile. This is absurd! For example, suppose you are playing defense in a volleyball game, and an opponent hits (spikes) the ball at you at a speed of 100 mph (45 m/s). The shortest time with which we can react to a stimulus, the reaction time, is about 120 ms. In 120 ms, the volleyball will travel about 5.4 m. In other words, no matter what happens to the trajectory of the ball over the last 5.4 m, you will be unable to react fast enough to generate an appropriate change in performance—you may as well close your eyes for the last 5.4 m. Consequently, the key is not to watch the ball all the way to your hands, but rather to *predict* the trajectory of the ball so that you can initiate, in plenty of time, an appropriate response. In fact, there is probably a high correlation between success in sport (e.g., volleyball, tennis, soccer, football) and how quickly an athlete can predict the trajectory of the projectile.

Problems

1.1.   Determine the height of a 5-ft 8-in. person in appropriate SI units.

1.2. What would your height and weight be in SI units if you were 5 ft 5 in. and 150 lb?

    a. 1.65 cm 668 N
    b. 1.65 m 669 kg
    c. 1.65 cm 68 kg
    d. 1.65 m 669 N
    e. 1.65 m 68 kg

1.3. Which is not one of the seven base units of the SI system?

    a. length
    b. force
    c. temperature
    d. time
    e. mass

1.4. According to the January, 1988 issue of *Track and Field News*, ''Records Section,'' the world-record performances for selected race distances appear as follows:

Distance	Women	Men
100 m	10.76 s	9.83 s
200 m	21.71 s	19.72 s
400 m	47.60 s	43.86 s
800 m	1 min 53.28 s	1 min 41.73 s
1,500 m	3 min 52.47 s	3 min 29.46 s
1 mi	4 min 16.71 s	3 min 46.32 s
3,000 m	8 min 22.62 s	7 min 32.10 s
5,000 m	14 min 37.33 s	12 min 58.39 s
10,000 m	30 min 13.74 s	27 min 13.81 s
Marathon	2 hr 25 min 17.00 s	2 hr 07 min 12.00 s

Calculate the average speed at which these performances were run.

1.5. Select the appropriate SI unit of measurement for each variable.

acceleration	_____	a.	$kg \cdot m \cdot s^{-1}$
		b.	$rad \cdot s^{-1}$
area	_____	c.	$J \cdot s$
		d.	N/m
force	_____	e.	$N \cdot s^{-1}$
		f.	N
impulse	_____	g.	$kg \cdot m/s^{2}$
		h.	$N \cdot m^{-1}$
mass	_____	i.	μm^{3}
		j.	kg
momentum	_____	k.	$rad \cdot s^{-2}$
		l.	lb

torque	_____	m.	N•s
		n.	cm²
work	_____	o.	J
		p.	N/s
		q.	N•m

1.6. A constant force (e.g., gravity) applied to an unsupported object produces a constant acceleration, and the absence of a force means that the object is at rest or traveling at a constant velocity (i.e., zero acceleration). Draw a velocity-time graph for these two conditions.

1.7. When velocity is at a maximum, acceleration will be
a. minimum
b. positive
c. negative
d. zero
e. maximum

1.8. With regard to Figure 1.2, identify the incorrect statements:
a. The object is going downward from Position 4 to 5.
b. The magnitude of the velocity from Position 2 to 3 is less than that for Position 1 to 2.
c. From Position 3 to 4, velocity is 0.
d. The units of measurement for velocity are m/s.
e. The graph gives information about the magnitude only and not the direction of the velocity vector.

1.9. A diver performs a dive from a handstand position off the 10-m tower. Assume that the effects of air resistance are negligible.
a. Use Equation 1.4 to calculate the time it takes for the diver to reach the water.
b. Determine the position (Equation 1.4) of the diver at 0.1-s intervals, and plot the results on a position-time graph.
c. What is the velocity of the diver at the time contact is made with the water?
d. What is the diver's acceleration at the 5-m mark?

1.10. Suppose that an athlete runs a 9.98-s 100-m race. What was the average horizontal acceleration of the athlete during the race, and what was his horizontal velocity when he crossed the finish line? Assume that the velocity of the athlete increased continuously from zero (initial) to some final value.

1.11. What is the magnitude of the average acceleration (in m/s²) required to slow a cyclist from 22 to 7 mph in 51 s?

1.12. A punted soccer ball reaches a peak height of 23 m in an indoor stadium. If we assume that the effects of air resistance are negligible, how fast is the ball going when it hits the ground?

1.13. Derive the acceleration-time graph from the velocity-time graph.

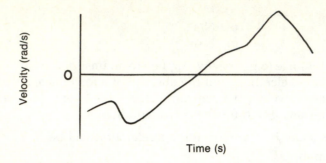

1.14. A ball is held 1.23 m above the ground and is dropped. It reaches the ground 0.5 s later.

a. What was the average velocity (direction, magnitude, and units) of the ball during the fall?

b. What was the average acceleration experienced by the ball while it was falling?

c. Suppose that the ball rebounds from the ground to a height of 1.0 m where it is caught. Qualitatively graph the position-time relationship of the ball from its release until it is caught. Label the axes with the appropriate variables and their units of measurement.

1.15. The following position-time data represent the angular motion of the leg during a punt. Calculate and graph the associated angular velocity and acceleration curves.

Angle (rad)	Time (s)
2.57	0.115
2.59	0.130
2.62	0.145
2.79	0.161
3.11	0.176
3.46	0.191
3.89	0.206
4.45	0.221 contact
5.06	0.236
5.49	0.252
5.83	0.267
5.90	0.282
5.93	0.297
5.93	0.312
6.02	0.327

1.16. The motions involved in an overarm throw are quite complex. For example, Atwater (1970) has reported the following velocity-time profile for the ball during a throw. From these data, qualitatively graph both the position- and acceleration-time curves.

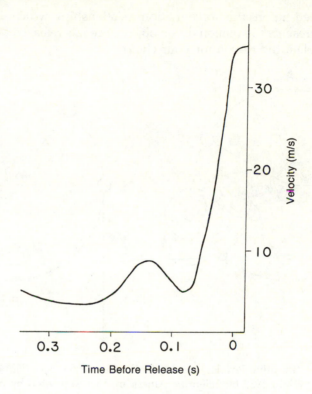

1.17. The following position-time data of a runner were obtained during a 50-m sprint.

Distance (m)	0	10	21	29	40
Time (s)	0	3.1	4.3	5.5	6.6

What was the runner's

a. average speed over 40 m?
b. acceleration at 21 m?
c. acceleration at 5.5 s?

1.18. Indicate (by circling the statement letter) the correct statements about the kinematics of gait.

a. A stride is defined as the interval from ipsilateral footstrike to contra-lateral footstrike.
b. Initial increases in running speed are produced solely by increases in stride rate.
c. Time was depicted on the angle-angle diagrams.

    d. Knee angle reaches 3.14 rad during a normal running gait (i.e., as seen on knee-thigh angle-angle diagrams).

    e. The size of an angle-angle diagram indicates the range of motion associated with a movement.

1.19. Based upon the force-motion relationship, which diagram correctly represents the motion of the object once it is released (McCloskey, 1983)? Explain the reason for your choice.

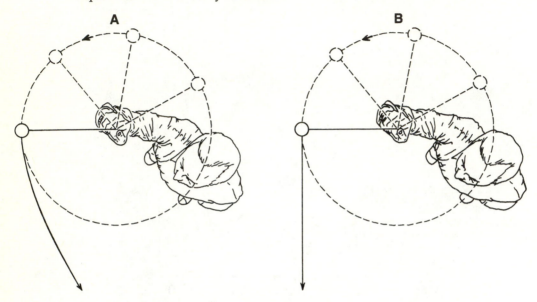

Note. From ''Intuitive Physics'' by M. McCloskey, 1983, *Scientific American,* **248,** p. 128. Copyright 1983 by Scientific American, Inc. Reprinted by permission.

1.20. The following data were obtained from a film of an individual who was running at about 5.6 m/s. The measured angles (rad) are for the thigh and leg relative to the right horizontal:

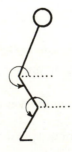

The time between each frame of film is 0.00667 s.

Frame	Thigh	Leg	Event
1	5.73	4.29	CTO
4	5.70	4.47	
7	5.65	4.75	
10	5.60	4.90	
13	5.51	4.95	
16	5.40	4.94	
19	5.30	4.81	IFS
22	5.24	4.59	
25	5.20	4.40	
28	5.12	4.24	
31	4.94	4.08	
34	4.71	3.96	
37	4.49	3.89	
40	4.25	3.90	
43	4.12	3.91	ITO
46	4.10	3.77	
49	4.12	3.53	
52	4.17	3.32	
55	4.27	3.08	
58	4.39	2.85	
61	4.49	2.72	CFS
64	4.65	2.67	
67	4.88	2.66	
70	5.09	2.81	
73	5.30	3.10	
76	5.53	3.39	
79	5.67	3.74	
82	5.70	4.10	
85	5.71	4.27	

Calculate the knee angle for each of these positions and then plot a knee-thigh angle-angle diagram.

1.21. A javelin is thrown at an angle of 0.78 rad to the horizontal with a release velocity directed along the line of projection of 22.5 m/s. What are the horizontal and vertical components of the release velocity?

1.22. An athlete is about to jump with an initial takeoff velocity of 2.9 m/s.
   a. How high can she raise her center of gravity if she jumps straight up?
   b. What height will she reach if her takeoff velocity is at an angle of 0.70 rad to the ground?

1.23. A basketball player drives in for a lay-up and leaves the ground at an angle of 0.72 rad to the horizontal with a velocity of 14.6 m/s. A defensive player goes straight up to block the shot with a velocity of 12.2 m/s.

a. Which player jumps higher?

b. How long is each player in the air, assuming they do not come into contact with each other?

1.24. A juggler performs in a room with a ceiling that is 2 m above the level of his hands. He throws a ball vertically so that it just reaches the ceiling.

a. With what initial vertical velocity does he throw the ball?

b. How long does it take for the ball to reach the ceiling?

c. He throws up a second ball with the same initial velocity at the instant that the first ball is at the ceiling. How long after the second ball is thrown do the two balls pass each other?

d. When the balls pass each other, how far are they above the juggler's hands?

1.25. A golf ball is driven horizontally from a point that is 3 m above a level fairway. If the ball lands (and stops) on the fairway at a point 150 m horizontally from the start, what was the velocity of the ball immediately after it was hit?

CHAPTER

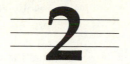

Force

Force is a concept that is used to describe the *interaction* of an object with its surroundings, including other objects. It can be defined as an agent that produces or tends to produce a change in the state of rest or motion of an object. For example, a ball sitting stationary (zero velocity) on a pool table will remain in that position unless it is acted upon by a force. Similarly, a person gliding on ice skates will maintain a constant velocity unless a force changes the motion, that is, the speed (magnitude) and/or the direction. The study of motion that includes consideration of force as the cause of movement is an area of mechanics known as **kinetics**.

The actions of forces can be divided into two groups (Brancazio, 1984): contact and noncontact forces. Contact forces refer to all pushes and pulls that are exerted by one object in direct contact with another object. These include such effects as air resistance, friction, muscle force, and ground reaction force. Noncontact forces refer to effects not due to contact and include such phenomena as gravity and the attraction and repulsion of nuclear charges. This classification, however, is somewhat arbitrary because all contact forces are in reality due to the resistance of one object's interatomic noncontact forces against another object's interatomic noncontact forces. For such reasons, physicists

argue that there are four fundamental forces in nature and that these are all noncontact forces. However, since our focus is the study of the effects of forces in movement, we shall use, for simplicity, the distinction between contact and noncontact forces.

As a vector, force has both magnitude and direction and can be treated graphically or trigonometrically to determine the resultant effect of several forces (**composition**) or alternatively to resolve a resultant effect into several components (**resolution**). These characteristics are useful in the analysis of human movement as they can be used to determine (a) the net effect of several forces acting upon an object or body segment, and (b) the functional effect (e.g., rotation vs. stabilization) of a single force acting upon a system. Figure 2.1 illustrates the former procedure (composition) by determining the resultant effect of coactivation of both the clavicular and sternal portions of the pectoralis major muscle. The graphic technique involves manipulating forces represented as arrows (vectors), where arrow length indicates force magnitude and the orientation of the arrow represents force direction. One feature of vectors that is useful in this procedure is that they can slide along their line of action and still have the same effect. The technique involves (a) careful measurement of

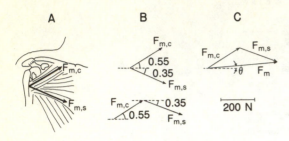

Figure 2.1. Graphical composition of the resultant force ($\mathbf{F}_m$) associated with the activation of both the clavicular ($\mathbf{F}_{m,c}$) and sternal ($\mathbf{F}_{m,s}$) components of the muscle pectoralis major. (A) Clavicular and sternal components at the muscle pectoralis major. (B) Head-to-tail addition of $\mathbf{F}_{m,c}$ and $\mathbf{F}_{m,s}$. (C) Resultant ($\mathbf{F}_m$) is determined by joining the tail of $\mathbf{F}_{m,c}$ to the head of $\mathbf{F}_{m,s}$. Angles are measured in radians (1 rad = 57.3 deg).

arrow lengths and angles, and (b) a scale factor with which length is related to force. Figure 2.1A indicates the direction and magnitude of the force exerted by each of the clavicular ($\mathbf{F}_{m,c}$) and sternal ($\mathbf{F}_{m,s}$) portions of the muscle pectoralis major: The clavicular component exerts a force of 224 N, which is directed at an angle of 0.55 rad above horizontal, and the sternal component has a magnitude of 251 N and acts 0.35 rad below horizontal. The process of graphically determining the net effect involves adding the components head to tail by sliding either one of the vectors along its line of action (Figure 2.1B) and then joining the open ends (open tail to open head) to produce the resultant (Figure 2.1C). The magnitude of the resultant is obtained by measuring the length of the arrow (4 cm), and then converting this measurement to newtons (400 N) with the indicated scale. Direction is obtained by measuring the angle with a protractor. The resultant effect ($\mathbf{F}_m$), therefore, has a magnitude of 400 N and a direction of 0.1 rad above horizontal.

Given a resultant force, it is possible to resolve it graphically into components. This procedure (Figure 2.2) simply involves constructing a parallelogram (Appendix B) such that the resultant represents the diagonal and thus the sides of the parallelogram indicate the magnitude and direction of the components. Again, the magnitude can be determined by use of a scale factor. In many instances, especially in focusing on muscle force, the parallelogram becomes a rectangle so that we can identify components that are oriented at right angles (1.57 rad, 90 degrees) to each other. In the analysis of muscle force, these **orthogonal** (perpendicular) components are referred to as the normal and tangential components, so defined because of their functional implications. The **normal** component represents the proportion of muscle force that acts perpendicular to the long bone of the segment and therefore produces the rotation of the body segment. The **tangential** component indicates the proportion directed along the bone toward the joint and thus contributes to joint stabilization or compression.

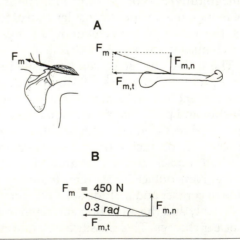

Figure 2.2. Graphic resolution of the resultant force ($\mathbf{F}_m$) produced by activation of middle deltoid muscle. (A) The normal ($\mathbf{F}_{m,n}$) and tangential ($\mathbf{F}_{m,t}$) components. (B) The trigonometric relations between $\mathbf{F}_{m,n}$ and $\mathbf{F}_{m,t}$.

These same procedures (composition and resolution) can be accomplished using trigonometry, the advantage being that less graphic precision is required. Suppose the resultant force in Figure 2.2 has a magnitude of 450 N and its line of action is 0.3 rad (17.2 degrees) with respect to the humerus; calculate the magnitude of the components. First, reconstruct the parallelogram and add the given data (Figure 2.2B), and use known trigonometry identities to solve for $F_{m,n}$ and $F_{m,t}$.

$$\sin 0.3 = \frac{F_{m,n}}{450}$$
$$F_{m,n} = 450 \times \sin 0.3$$
$$= 450 \times 0.2955$$
$$F_{m,n} = 133 \text{ N}$$

$$\cos 0.3 = \frac{F_{m,t}}{450}$$
$$F_{m,t} = 450 \times \cos 0.3$$
$$= 450 \times 0.9553$$
$$F_{m,t} = 430 \text{ N}$$

Thus the normal component has a magnitude of 133 N and the tangential component a magnitude of 430 N. Both of these values seem reasonable because (a) the angle of pull of most muscles is rather shallow and thus most of the resultant force is generated in the tangential direction, and (b) the resultant represents the diagonal of the parallelogram and therefore should be the largest of the three values.

To verify that the graphic and trigonometric procedures are comparable, you could graphically resolve the resultant in Figure 2.2 to determine the magnitude of the normal and tangential components. Redraw the resultant (F_m) on graph paper with a scale of 1 cm = 25 N and with the arrow directed 0.3 rad above horizontal. Next, draw the rectangle around the resultant so that the resultant appears as the diagonal. Measure the lengths of the two sides ($F_{m,n}$ and $F_{m,t}$) and use the scale factor to convert these distances to forces. How similar are the trigonometric ($F_{m,n}$ = 133 N and $F_{m,t}$ = 430 N) and graphic results?

Newton's Laws of Motion

Newton (1642-1727) addressed the relationship between force and motion and provided three statements, which are known collectively as the *laws of motion*. These laws are referred to as the laws of inertia, acceleration, and action-reaction.

I. The Law of Inertia

Every body continues in its state of rest or uniform motion in a straight line except when it is compelled by external forces to change its state.

More simply, *a force is required to stop, start, or alter motion*. The reality of this law is easily demonstrated by astronauts as they perform maneuvers in a weightless (zero gravity) environment (e.g., tossing objects to one another or performing gymnastic stunts). In a gravitational world, however, forces act continuously upon bodies, and a change in motion occurs when there is a *net imbalance* of forces. In this context, the term *body* can refer to the entire human body, just a part of (e.g., thigh, hand, torso) the human body, or even to some object (e.g., shot put, baseball bat, Frisbee).

To appreciate fully the implications of this law, it is necessary to understand what is meant by the term *inertia*. The concept of inertia relates to the difficulty with which an object's motion is altered, a property that depends on the mass of the object. **Mass**, expressed in grams (g), is a measure of the amount of matter comprising an object.

Inertia is related directly to mass and refers to the resistance an object offers to any change in its motion. Consider two objects of different mass but with the same amount of motion (similar velocities): It is more difficult to alter the motion of the more massive object, and hence it is described as having a greater inertia. Since motion is described in terms of velocity, the inertia of an object is a property of matter that is only revealed when the object is being accelerated, that is, when there is a change in velocity.

According to the law of inertia, an object in motion will continue in uniform motion (constant velocity) unless acted upon by a force. This means that the tendency of an object in motion is to travel in a straight line. For example, consider the situation in Problem 1.19. An individual swings a ball tied to a string over his head. When the string is released, will the ball follow the trajectory depicted in A or B? To answer this question we simply need to invoke Newton's law of inertia. If no force is acting on an object, then the object will, due to its inertia, travel in a straight line. Once the individual releases the string in Problem 1.19, there is no horizontal force acting on the ball; hence, it will travel in a straight line (B). But then how can a pitched ball in baseball or softball be made to vary from a straight line? Quite simply, according to the law of inertia, other forces (e.g., air resistance, gravity) must be acting on the ball once it has been released.

Since uniform motion is represented as a constant velocity, both in magnitude and direction, a force must be present when an object travels along a curved path. This force prevents the object from following its natural tendency of traveling in a straight line. This can be demonstrated by considering the motion of the ball in Problem 1.19 at two instances in time. For these two positions, the motion of the ball is indicated by a velocity vector (Figure 2.3).

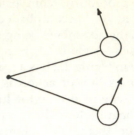

Figure 2.3. Ball on a string that is being displaced at a constant speed. The magnitude of the velocity vector remains constant, but its direction changes.

Since the length of the arrow (magnitude of the vector) is the same in the two positions, the ball is traveling at a constant velocity (magnitude). However, the direction of the vector is different in the two positions. This change in direction represents a change in one feature of motion and hence can only be caused by the presence of a force. This inwardly directed force that changes the direction but not the magnitude (speed) of velocity during angular motion is known as **centripetal** force. Without going into its derivation, centripetal force is defined as

$$\mathbf{F}_c = m\mathbf{v}^2/r \qquad (2.1)$$

where m = mass, $\mathbf{v}$ = velocity, and r = the radius of the curved path. In Problem 1.19, if the speed of the ball ($\mathbf{v}$) and the length of the string (r) stayed the same, then the centripetal force ($\mathbf{F}_c$) would have to increase to maintain this condition if the mass of the ball were increased; the force would be reduced if the mass of the ball were decreased. In contrast, for a constant ball mass (m) and velocity ($\mathbf{v}$) the centripetal force would decrease if the length of the string (r) increased. These points can be summarized by rearranging

Equation 2.1 so that velocity is on the left-hand side.

$$v = \sqrt{\frac{F_c r}{m}}$$

Thus velocity, and hence position, is directly related to F_c and r and inversely related to m; as F and r get smaller, so does v, but as m gets smaller, v gets larger.

II. The Law of Acceleration

The rate of change of momentum of a body is proportional to the applied force, and takes place in the direction in which the force acts.

The term **momentum** (p) describes the quantity of motion possessed by a body and is defined as the product of mass (m) and velocity (v). A runner with a mass of 60 kg moving at a horizontal speed of 8 m•s^{-1} possesses a momentum of 480 kg•m/s. Thus

$$p = mv \qquad (2.2)$$

and the rate of change of momentum can be written as

$$\frac{\Delta p}{\Delta t} = \frac{\Delta(mv)}{\Delta t}$$

The Δm is of negligible concern to human movement (i.e., mass is constant) and, therefore, according to the law of acceleration, the applied force (F) is proportional to the rate of change of momentum,

$$F = \frac{\Delta p}{\Delta t} = m\frac{\Delta v}{t}$$

Further, as $\Delta v/\Delta t$ represents the time rate of change of velocity, it is equivalent to acceleration (a), and

$$F = ma \qquad (2.3)$$

Thus Equation 2.3 is the algebraic expression of Newton's law of acceleration and states that force is equal to mass times acceleration. Conceptually this is a cause-and-effect relationship. The left side (F) can be regarded as the cause because it represents the interactions between a system and its environment. In contrast, the right side reveals the effect because it indicates the kinematic effects (ma) of the interactions on the system.

III. The Law of Action-Reaction

To every action there is an equal and opposite reaction.

This implies that every force that one body exerts on another is counteracted by a force that the second body exerts on the first. That is, two forces (the same magnitude but opposite direction) act simultaneously or not at all. This emphasizes the notion that *force represents an interaction between an object and its surroundings*. For example, consider a person performing a jump shot in basketball. During the act of jumping, the person exerts a force against the ground and, conversely, the ground responds with a reaction force (the ground reaction force) on the jumper. The law of action-reaction indicates that the forces provided by the jumper and the ground are equivalent in magnitude but opposite in direction. The consequence of these forces, as specified by the law of acceleration (F = ma), is an acceleration experienced by each body (i.e., the basketball player and the ground) that depends upon its mass. If the average force were 1,500 N and the person had a mass of 75 kg, then the person would be subjected to an average acceleration of 20 m•s^{-2}. Due to the large mass of the planet Earth, however, the acceleration experienced by the ground would be imperceptible. That is, the product of mass and acceleration in this example should equal 1,500. Since the mass of the ground is large (compared to the basketball player), then the acceleration of the ground will be small.

Free-Body Diagram

In the analysis of human motion it is readily apparent that there are many variables that influence a performance. The **free-body diagram** reduces the complexity of a chosen analysis and involves drawing a simplified diagram, usually a stick figure, of the system isolated from its surroundings and noting all the interactions between the system and its surroundings. The free-body diagram is an analytical technique; it defines the extent of the analysis. Since force is the concept used to denote the interactions between a system and its surroundings, *a free-body diagram is a simplified figure upon which all the external forces that influence the system are indicated with arrows* (i.e., force is represented as a vector). The term *system* is used to refer to parts of the human body and objects involved in the analysis and varies according to the problem being addressed. One of the greatest difficulties encountered by beginning students is defining the system for a particular analysis.

For example, suppose we wanted to determine the magnitude and direction of the ground reaction force experienced by a runner (Figure 2.4A). The first step is to specify and draw the system (Figure 2.4B). The next step is to identify all the external forces acting on the system with arrows of correct length (magnitude) and direction, and their appropriate labels (Figure 2.4C). In general, these will include the weight of the system and forces arising from contact with other bodies (e.g., ground reaction forces, and fluid or air resistance). *External* forces in a free-body diagram are those exerted from outside

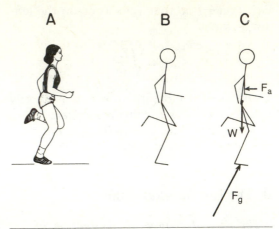

Figure 2.4. Derivation of a free-body diagram from (A) real-life figure to (B) the identification of the system and (C) the inclusion of the forces imposed on the system by the surroundings. The forces represent air resistance (F_a), weight (**W**), and ground reaction force (F_g).

the system, in contrast to those generated within the system (e.g., forces due to bone, ligament, and muscle). Internal forces are not included in a free-body diagram.

If the aim of the analysis is to examine the muscle activity across a joint during an activity, however, then a different system is required. If we want to consider a particular interaction, such as the muscle activity associated with a particular movement, then we must define the system so that the interaction becomes an external force. Another way of thinking of this procedure is to specify the system so that we can see the agent causing the interaction. In the case of determining muscle activity this involves figuratively cutting through the desired joint (e.g., knee joint). Around each joint there are a variety of tissues that include muscle, joint capsule, ligaments, and so forth. We usually mechanically distinguish the effects of muscle from those of the other tissues. Consequently, when we draw a free-body diagram that involves cutting through a joint, *we identify a net muscle force (the resultant muscle force) and a force that accounts mainly for the bone-on-bone contact (the joint reaction force) of adjacent body segments.* Let us return to the example outlined in Figure 2.4. To examine the effects of the muscles across the knee joint at the instant illustrated in Figure 2.4B, the appropriate free-body diagram would appear as shown in Figure 2.5.

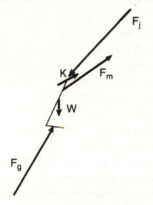

Figure 2.5. Free-body diagram of a system (leg + foot) upon which four external forces are acting. F_g = ground reaction force, F_j = joint reaction force, F_m = resultant muscle force, K = knee joint, W = system weight.

Suppose the situation arose in which a weight lifter, whose training program included power cleans (the barbell is lifted from about knee height to the chest in one continuous movement), began to develop back pains after several months of training. An appropriate analysis might include determining how much force the muscles that extend the back and hip exert during the movement. Because this force is greatest at the beginning of the movement, the analysis would focus on the weight lifter at this position (Figure 2.6A). Since the object of the analysis is to calculate a muscle force, the system must be defined so that the muscle effect is illustrated as an

external force. This involves figuratively cutting through the hip joint so that the system becomes either the part of the weight lifter above the hip joint plus barbell or the part of the weight lifter below the hip joint. In the former instance, the stick figure would simply include a circle for the head and a line for the trunk and arms (Figure 2.6B).

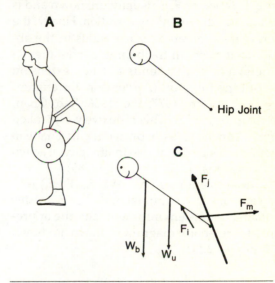

Figure 2.6. The derivation of a free-body diagram to analyze part of a weight-lifting movement: (A) Whole-body diagram of the weight lifter in the position chosen for analysis. (B) System used to expose the forces across the hip joint. (C) Free-body diagram showing the interactions between the system and its surroundings.

The next step would be to illustrate all the interactions, drawn as force vectors (arrows), between the system (upper body of the weight lifter plus the barbell) and the surroundings. First, one of the most obvious forces is that due to gravity, that is, the weight of the barbell (W_b) and the weight of the upper body of the lifter (W_u). The direction of the weight vectors is always vertically downward. Second, by cutting through a joint, two forces must be represented as external forces. These are the resultant (net) muscle force ($\mathbf{F}_m$) and the joint reaction force ($\mathbf{F}_j$), the latter representing the forces due to ligaments, joint capsules, and bone-on-bone contact. Although the direction of the $\mathbf{F}_m$ is reasonably straightforward in that it opposes the rotation produced by the weight vectors, the direction of $\mathbf{F}_j$ is usually unknown and is arbitrarily drawn in any direction. Finally, the pressure generated by the fluids in the abdominal cavity (intraabdominal pressure, $\mathbf{F}_i$) exerts a force that tends to cause extension about the hip joint (Andersson, Örtengren, & Nachemson, 1977; Eie, 1966; Rab, Chao, & Stauffer, 1977). This reflexively controlled force functions as a protective mechanism and has a significant role in lifting-type activities (Marras, Joynt, & King, 1985).

These five forces ($\mathbf{W}_b$, $\mathbf{W}_u$, $\mathbf{F}_m$, $\mathbf{F}_j$, $\mathbf{F}_i$) represent the major interactions between this system and its environment, and the appropriate free-body diagram is drawn as shown in Figure 2.6C.

Noncontact Forces

Once we define a system with a free-body diagram, we are able to consider the interactions (forces) that are likely to occur between a system and its surroundings. As previously indicated, we shall distinguish the actions of forces on the basis of whether or not the interaction involves contact between bodies. For our purposes, *the most prominent noncontact forces are those associated with the nuclear components of atoms and that due to gravity.* Later in the text we will consider the role of the interatomic forces in movement in the context of the electrical interaction between nerve and muscle. For now let us focus on gravity.

Newton has characterized **gravity** in a statement known as the **law of gravitation**:

All bodies attract one another with a force proportional to the product of their masses and inversely proportional to the square of the distance between them.

That is,

$$\mathbf{F} \propto \frac{m_1 m_2}{r^2} \qquad (2.4)$$

where m_1 and m_2 are the masses of two bodies and $\mathbf{r}$ is the distance between them.

These forces of attraction between objects are generally regarded as negligible in the study of human movement with the exception of the attraction between the Earth and various objects. The magnitude of this attraction, a force known as weight, depends on the mass of the objects involved and the distance between them. **Weight** is an expression of the amount of gravitational attraction between an object and Earth. As a force, it is measured in newtons (N). Of course, weight varies proportionately with mass—the greater the mass, the greater the attraction—but the two are separate quantities. Consider a shot used for the shot put at rest on a smooth floor. To pick it up requires a reasonable effort, yet to set it rolling along the floor requires a much smaller effort. This difference in effort hints at the distinction between weight and mass. As another example, consider the world-record performance in the long jump of Bob Beamon in the 1968 Olympics in Mexico City (Ward-Smith, 1983). Beamon's total body mass was about 75 kg at that time, but his weight was 736 N at sea level and 735 N in Mexico City (altitude, 2,250 m). In other words, his mass was unaffected by altitude, but his weight, due to the variation in gravity, depended on the altitude at which it was measured.

Weight represents the interaction between an object and Earth, and the magnitude of that interaction depends on their respective masses and the distance between them;

therefore, gravity decreases as altitude increases above sea level. This accounts for the advantage of performing at high altitude in events where the contestant must overcome gravity (e.g., long jump, shot put, weight lifting).

The *magnitude of the total-body weight vector* is determined quite readily as the value read off a bathroom scale. The validity of this procedure can be demonstrated with a simple analysis based on Newton's law of acceleration (Equation 2.3),

$$\sum \mathbf{F} = \mathbf{ma}$$

which states that the sum (Σ = sigma) of the external forces (**F**) produces an acceleration (**a**) of the system that depends on the mass (m) of the system. The quantities of force and acceleration are boldfaced to indicate that they are vectors. Since weight acts only in the vertical direction (z), the analysis can be confined to those components that act vertically: Weight (**W**) is directed downward and indicated as negative; and the reaction force (**R**$_z$), which is provided by the scale, is directed upward and indicated as positive. The decision to label **W** negative and **R**$_z$ positive is quite arbitrary; however, it is essential to distinguish between these differences in direction. To meet these needs, each free-body diagram should be accompanied by a reference axis that shows the positive directions of each component (Figure 2.7): positive vertical (z),

horizontal (x), and rotary. If the analysis is three-dimensional, then the third direction (y) is also indicated.

The appropriate free-body diagram is shown in Figure 2.7, and the analysis is as follows:

$$\sum \mathbf{F}_z = \mathbf{ma}_z$$
$$-\mathbf{W} + \mathbf{R}_z = \mathbf{ma}_z$$
$$\mathbf{W} = \mathbf{R}_z - \mathbf{ma}_z$$

But since the person is stationary, $\mathbf{a}_z = 0$:

$$\mathbf{W} = \mathbf{R}_z - 0$$
$$\mathbf{W} = \mathbf{R}_z$$

The *direction of the weight vector* is always vertically downward, toward the center of the Earth; the vector originates from a point referred to as the center of gravity. The **center of gravity** (CG) represents a balance point, a location about which all the particles of the object are evenly distributed. It is an abstract point that moves when the body segments are moved relative to one another. The CG is not confined to the physical limits of the object; for example, consider a donut, the CG for which is undoubtedly located within the inner hole. In fact, successful high jumpers have as a trademark an ability to project the CG outside their bodies or at least toward the outer limits. In Figure 2.8, the height that a jumper can clear comprises three components (Hay, 1975): (i) the height (H_1) of the CG above the ground at takeoff, (ii) the height (H_2) that the jumper can raise the CG above H_1, and (iii) the difference between the maximum height reached by the CG and the height of the bar (H_3). With regard to H_3, although a person may jump 2.28 m (7 ft 6 in.), this does not imply that the CG was raised to that height, but merely that the body passed over the bar—the two conditions are not synonymous. A somewhat similar rationale applies to pole vaulting (Fletcher & Lewis, 1960; Hubbard, 1980). The significance of this example is that once the jumper

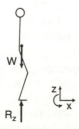

Figure 2.7. Free-body diagram of the whole body. **R**$_z$ = vertical component of the ground reaction force, **W** = weight.

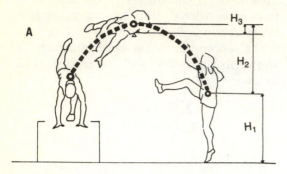

A

For a 2.13 m (7 ft) jump:
H_1 =   1.44 m
H_2 =   0.78 m
H_3 = − 0.09 m

─────────

2.13 m

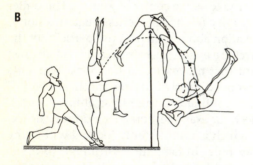

B

Figure 2.8. Contributions to the height recorded in the high jump. (A) Schematic high jump with some values for a 2.13-m jump. (B) Theoretical technique in which the jumper is able to project the center of gravity out of the body such that it does not pass over the bar. *Note.* From James G. Hay, *The Biomechanics of Sports Techniques*, 2/E, © 1978, pp. 426, 433. Reprinted by permission of Prentice-Hall, Inc., Englewood Cliffs, New Jersey.

has left the ground, the path that the CG will follow has been predetermined (recall the details of projectile motion in chapter 1). Consequently, the ability to project the CG out of the body (i.e., attain a positive H_3) serves as a means to acquire extra clearance height.

Since many human movement analyses require a segmental approach (i.e., analyzing one body segment at a time), it is often necessary to know something about the masses of the different body segments. Several investigators (e.g., Chandler, Clauser, McConville, Reynold, & Young, 1975; Dempster, 1955; Hanavan, 1964; Miller & Morrison, 1975) have derived simple mathematical expressions with which to estimate various **anthropometric** (measurements of the human body) dimensions based on measurements made on cadavers—the *cadaver-based approach*. For example, based upon measurements made on 6 cadavers, Chandler et al. (1975) have indicated that the mass of individual body segments can be estimated as a percentage of total-body weight (Table 2.1).

Table 2.1 Regression Equations Estimating Body-Segment Weights and Locations of Center of Gravity

Segment	Weight (N)	CG location (%)
Head	0.032 BW + 18.70	66.3
Trunk	0.532 BW − 6.93	52.2
Upper arm	0.022 BW + 4.76	50.7
Forearm	0.013 BW + 2.41	41.7
Hand	0.005 BW + 0.75	51.5
Thigh	0.127 BW − 14.82	39.8
Leg	0.044 BW − 1.75	41.3
Foot	0.009 BW + 2.48	40.0

Note. See Appendix D for the body-segment organization used by Chandler et al. (1975). Body-segment weights are expressed as a percentage of total-body weight (BW), and the segmental center of gravity (CG) locations are expressed as a percentage of segment length as measured from the proximal end of the segment.

The mathematical expressions that specify the relationships between total-body weight and segment weight are known as regression equations. In general, *regression equations allow us to estimate the value of one parameter based upon values for another parameter*. In Table 2.1, segment weight can be estimated from total-body weight, and the location of the CG for each segment can be estimated from the measurement of segment length. For example, suppose an individual weighed 750 N. According to Table 2.1,

trunk weight = 0.532 × 750 − 6.93
= 392 N

which accounts for 52% of total-body weight. Also according to Table 2.1,

hand weight = 0.005 × 750 + 0.75
= 4.5 N

which represents about 0.4% of total-body weight. Exactly what Chandler et al. meant by the designations of trunk, hand, and so forth is indicated in Appendix D. In a similar manner, if the length of an individual's thigh (hip to knee) was 36 cm, then according to Chandler et al. the CG for that thigh would be located at 39.8% of that distance from the hip joint.

CG location = 36 × 0.398
= 14.3 cm from the hip joint

Mathematical modeling is another common approach used to determine the anthropometric characteristics of human subjects by representing the human body as a set of geometric components, such as spheres, cylinders, and cones (Hall & DePauw, 1982; Hanavan, 1964, 1966; Hatze, 1980, 1981a, 1981b; Miller, 1979). One of the first to use this method was Hanavan (1964, 1966); Figure 2.9 shows the Hanavan model, which divides the human body into 15 simple geometric solids of uniform density. The advan-

tage of this model is that it requires only a few simple anthropometric measurements (e.g., segment lengths and circumferences) to predict the center of gravity and moment of inertia (the angular equivalent of mass) for each body segment.

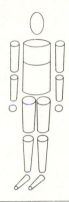

Figure 2.9. The Hanavan model of the human body.

A third approach to determining body segment parameters is the use of *radioisotopes*. With this approach, various properties of body segments are determined based on the measurement of the intensity of a gamma-radiation beam before and after it passes through a segment. The principle involves scanning a subject's body and obtaining the surface density and coordinates of the body segments affected by the radiation. Zatsiorsky and Seluyanov (1983) performed this on 100 male subjects (age = 23.8 ± 6.2 yr, height = 1.74 ± 0.06 cm, weight = 730 ± 91 N) and derived regression equations (Table 2.2) with which to estimate body segment parameters for other subjects.

As an example of the application of these procedures, let us briefly consider a segmental analysis of the weight lifter depicted previously in the "Free-Body Diagram" section. If we represent the weight lifter as a stick figure (Figure 2.10A), then the first question to consider is, How many segments should

Table 2.2   Regression Equations Estimating Body-Segment Masses and Locations of Centers of Gravity

Segment	Mass (kg)			CG location (%)		
	B_0	B_1	B_2	B_0	B_1	B_2
Foot	−0.8290	0.0077	0.0073	3.7670	0.0650	0.0330
Shank	−1.5920	0.0362	0.0121	−6.0500	−0.0390	0.1420
Thigh	−2.6490	0.1463	0.0137	−2.4200	0.0380	0.1350
Hand	−0.1165	0.0036	0.0017	4.1100	0.0260	0.0330
Forearm	0.3185	0.0144	−0.0011	0.1920	−0.0280	0.0930
Upper arm	0.2500	0.0301	−0.0027	1.6700	0.0300	0.0540
Head	1.2960	0.0170	0.0143	8.3570	−0.0025	0.0230
Upper torso	8.2144	0.1862	0.0584	3.3200	0.0076	0.0470
Middle torso	7.1810	0.2234	−0.0663	1.3980	0.0058	0.0450
Lower torso	−7.4980	0.0976	0.0490	1.1820	0.0018	0.0434

Note. The multiple regression equations are in the form $Y = B_0 + B_1X_1 + B_2X_2$, where Y = predicted segment mass or CG location, X_1 = total body mass (kg), X_2 = height (cm), B_0, B_1, B_2 = coefficients given in the table. Body-segment mass and segmental center of gravity (CG) locations are expressed as functions of body mass (measured in kilograms) and height (measured in centimeters). From "The Mass and Inertia Characteristics of the Main Segments of the Human Body" by V. Zatsiorsky and V. Seluyanov, 1983, in H. Matsui and K. Kobayashi (Eds.), *Biomechanics VIII-B* (p. 1156), Champaign, IL: Human Kinetics. Copyright 1983 by Human Kinetics. Adapted by permission.

we use to represent the lifter? If we analyze the movement shown at the top of Figure 1.4, then we can consider the arms as one segment because they do not bend at the elbow. In addition, since the movement is confined to the sagittal plane, we assume that the left and right sides of the body are more or less doing the same thing. As a result of these simplifications we can reduce our free-body diagram from the maximum of 15 segments (based on Hanavan's model) to 6 segments; the whole-body stick figure will become six separate systems (Figure 2.10B).

In such an analysis the object is often to determine the contribution of each body segment to the various parts of a movement (Miller, 1980). In the weight-lifting example above, suppose the object is to determine the

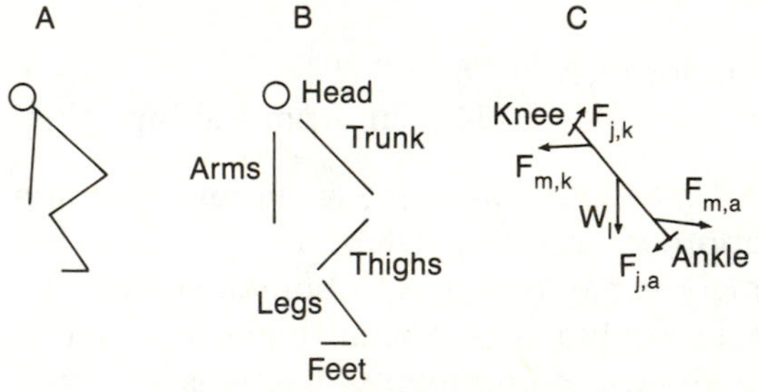

Figure 2.10. Free-body diagram of a weight lifter. (A) Whole-body stick figure. (B) Segmental components. (C) Free-body diagram of the leg. $F_{j,a}$ and $F_{j,k}$ = ankle and knee joint reaction forces, $F_{m,a}$ and $F_{m,k}$ = ankle and knee resultant muscle forces, W_l = weight of the leg.

role of the muscles crossing the knee joint. The first task is to draw the appropriate free-body diagram (Figure 2.10C).

Before the analysis can proceed, however, it is necessary to know the location of the CG and the magnitude of the weight vector (W_1) for the segment. Both of these quantities can be estimated from the data in Table 2.1. The CG is not located in the center of the segment because it represents a balance point about which the mass is evenly distributed; most body segments (e.g., forearm, thigh, leg) have more mass at the proximal end. As a consequence, the CG for most body segments is located closer to the proximal end (knee joint for one leg) of the segment. According to Table 2.1, the CG for the leg is located at 41.3% of leg length from the knee joint. If the leg of the weight lifter measured 36 cm then the CG would be situated 14.9 cm ($36 \times 0.413 = 14.9$) from the knee. Similarly, the magnitude of the weight vector is determined as a function of total-body weight. For an 800-N weight lifter, the weight of one leg would be 33.5 N ($0.044 \times 800 - 1.75 = 33.5$).

Contact Forces

In contrast to our discussion of noncontact forces, we typically identify a number of forces that affect movement due to contact between bodies. This characterization identifies not different types of forces, but merely differences in the agent causing the interaction. Six such forces are commonly encountered in the analysis of human movement: joint reaction force, ground reaction force, fluid resistance, elastic force, inertial force, and muscle force.

Joint Reaction Force

When a system is defined such that the muscles about a joint represent an external force, then the concept of a **joint reaction force** is invoked to *account for the net forces generated by bone-on-bone contact between adjacent body segments*. In most instances both the magnitude and the direction of the joint reaction force are unknown; consequently, the joint reaction force is represented in the free-body diagram as an arrow of arbitrary magnitude and direction through the joint. Given the appropriate data and analytical technique, however, it is possible to determine the joint reaction force. Examples of joint reaction forces are provided in Figures 2.5 and 7.3.

Ground Reaction Force

The ground reaction force is used to describe the *reaction force provided by the supporting horizontal surface*. It is derived from Newton's law of action-reaction. This effect may indeed refer to the ground or, just as easily, to a gymnasium floor. The ground reaction force is measured by a force platform that is a scale-like structure that is embedded in the ground so that its surface is at the same level as the ground. Researchers began using this technique in the 1930s (Elftman, 1938, 1939; Fenn, 1930; Manter, 1938), although the idea had been proposed some time before this (Amar, 1920; Marey, 1874).

As with the joint reaction force and, in fact, all forces and motion, the ground reaction force exists in three-dimensional space. The resultant ground reaction force is resolved into three components whose directions are functionally defined as vertical (upward-downward), forward-backward, and side to side. These components represent the proportions of the resultant ground reaction force that will produce an acceleration of the system in these respective directions. The horizontal components (forward-backward and side to side) represent the tangential component of a contact force and hence are known as **friction**. The magnitude of friction is equal to the resultant force acting along the surface in the plane of contact.

In this vein, Figure 2.11 illustrates the vertical component (R_z) of the ground reaction force that is associated with walking and with running (for a more elegant treatment of the differences between walking and running, consult Alexander, 1984b). These data indicate the manner in which R_z changed from the instant of foot contact with the ground (beginning of the time axis) until the instant that same foot left the ground (the time at which R_z returned to zero). In the analysis of locomotion, this epoch is known as the stance or support phase (e.g., Figure 1.6). R_z is nonzero only when the foot is in contact with the ground. It is important to note that R_z changes continuously throughout the period of support. In running, the duration of the support phase is shorter and the magnitude of R_z is greater. Why is there a difference in magnitude between walking and running? Consideration of Newton's law of acceleration (Equation 2.3) will provide an answer. Of course, the ground is capable of generating a much greater force than is indicated in Figure 2.11, but both the magnitude and direction are in response to the action exerted by the system (i.e., the person walking or running). Should the ground prove unable to match the system-produced force, then the system would crash through the ground, as for example in the case of a weight lifter dropping a barbell through a gymnasium floor.

To emphasize the three-dimensional nature of forces, particularly the ground reaction force, consider the foot's motion during the support phase of a running stride (see also Cavanagh et al., 1985; Cavanagh, Pollock, & Landa, 1977; Chao, 1986; Vaughan, 1985).

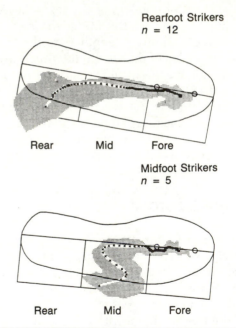

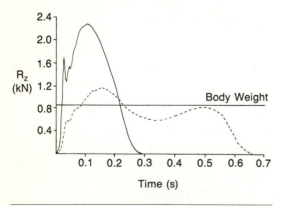

Figure 2.11. Vertical component of the ground reaction force (R_z) during the period of support in walking (dashed line) and running (solid line).

Figure 2.12. The displacement of the center of pressure (point of application of the ground reaction force vector) during the stance phase of a running stride. Runners tend to fall into categories, those who contact the ground initially with the midfoot region and those who contact with the rearfoot. *Note.* From ''Ground Reaction Forces in Distance Running'' by P.R. Cavanagh and M.A. Lafortune, 1980, *Journal of Biomechanics, 13*, p. 401. Copyright 1980 by Pergamon Press, Ltd. Reprinted by permission.

The initial part of the foot to contact the ground varies with speed but is generally the lateral border, between the midfoot and the heel, with the foot in a supinated position (rotated with the sole toward the midline of the body). After this initial footstrike, the foot is pronated (opposite direction of rotation to supination) and the ankle dorsiflexed (ankle flexion). As the runner's center of gravity passes over the foot, both the knee and ankle (plantar flexion) joints begin to extend. By the time the foot leaves the ground, the point of application (known as the *center of pressure*) of the ground reaction force vector has moved from the lateral border of the foot at footstrike to a point at or near the base of the big toe (Figure 2.12). These movements are

accomplished by the ground reaction force and its components as depicted in Figure 2.13; (a) the vertical component (R_z) is directed upward throughout support; (b) the forward-backward component (R_y) is first directed backward then forward—this change in direction occurs as the runner's center of gravity passes over the foot; and (c) the side-to-side component (R_x), which has a lesser magnitude and is more variable than R_z and R_y, largely reflects the foot pronation-supination motion (Figure 2.14) and is directed laterally throughout most of support (Figure 2.13).

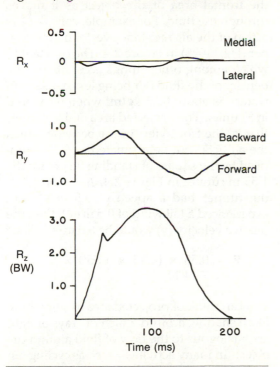

Figure 2.13. Generalized force-time curves for the three components of the ground reaction force during the support phase of a running stride. The forces are expressed relative to body weight (**BW**); R_z = vertical, R_y = forward-backward, R_x = side to side.

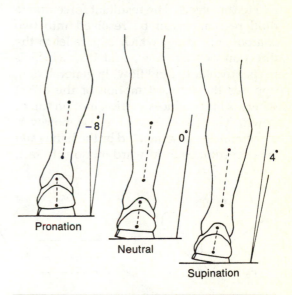

Figure 2.14. Rearfoot angle measurements of right leg during stance. The distinction between pronation (negative), neutral (zero), and supination (positive) has to do with the angle between the leg and the foot. *Note.* From "The Study of Rearfoot Movement in Running" by T.E. Clarke, E.C. Frederick, and C. Hamill, 1984, in E.C. Frederick (Ed.), *Sport Shoes and Playing Surfaces* (p. 170), Champaign, IL: Human Kinetics. Copyright 1984 by Human Kinetics. Reprinted by permission.

Fluid Resistance

Both human motion (e.g., ski jumping, cycling, swimming, skydiving) and projectile motion (e.g., discus, golf ball) can be profoundly influenced by the fluid (gaseous or liquid) medium in which they occur. As an object passes through a fluid, there is a transfer of energy from the object to the fluid. This phenomenon is referred to as **fluid resistance**. In essence, *this transfer depends upon the extent to which the fluid is being disturbed by the object.* As a consequence, the transfer (fluid resistance) increases as the speed of the object increases. Figure 2.15 is a typical schematization of this process in which the object is stationary and the fluid moves relative to the object. The resultant force due to fluid resistance can be resolved into two components: **drag**, which is parallel to the direction of fluid flow; and **lift**, which is perpendicular to fluid flow. In general, drag opposes the forward motion of the object whereas lift produces vertical motion (up or down). This is not always the case, however; in swimming, lift generated by the hands and legs contributes to forward motion. In fact,

the key to a successful swimming stroke is to move the hands through the water so that both the drag and the lift components contribute to the forward motion of the swimmer (Schleihauf, 1979). Although an object moving through a fluid always experiences drag, the lift component is present only if the object spins or lacks perfect symmetry.

The magnitude of the fluid resistance (F_f) vector can be determined from

$$F_f = kAv^2 \qquad (2.5)$$

where k is a constant, A represents the **projected area** of the object, and **v** refers to the velocity of the fluid relative to the object. Projected area refers to a silhouette view of the frontal area of the object as it moves through the fluid. For example, consider the action of the air-resistance vector on the runner (Hill, 1928) in Figure 2.4. The constant k, which among other things accounts for the density of the fluid (air being less dense than water), is about 0.55 kg/m^3 when measured in SI units. The projected area of the runner, that is, the front-view of the body on which the air acts, can be estimated as 0.15 multiplied by the square of standing height for the 1.55-m runner in Figure 2.4, A = 0.36 m^2. If the runner had a speed of 6.5 m•s⁻¹ and experienced a tail wind of 0.5 m•s⁻¹, then the relative velocity (**v**) would be 6.0 m•s⁻¹. Thus

$$F_f = 0.55 \times (0.15 \times 1.55^2) \times 6.0^2$$
$$= 7.14 \text{ N}$$

You can think of projected area as something like a shadow around which the rays of light are analogous to the flow of fluid around the object. In many activities, such as cycling, an athlete pays considerable attention to the size of the projected area (e.g., the bunched stance of a cyclist).

Calculations have indicated (Shanebrook & Jaszczak, 1976) that, at middle-distance running speeds (approx 6.0 m•s⁻¹), up to 8%

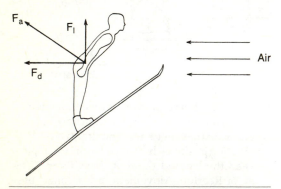

Figure 2.15. Air resistance encountered by a ski jumper. The air is shown moving relative to the jumper. The resultant air-resistance vector (F_a) is resolved into two components, drag (F_d) and lift (F_l).

of the energy expended by the runner is used in overcoming air resistance, whereas at sprinting speeds this value can be up to 16% of the total energy expenditure. Drafting (shielding) can abolish 80% of this cost. Ward-Smith (1985) has done some calculations along these lines to look at the effects of head and tail winds on performance times in a 100-m sprint:

Wind speed (m/s)	Head wind (s)	Tail wind (s)
1	+0.09	−0.10
3	+0.26	−0.34
5	+0.38	−0.62

With a 3-m/s head wind, 100-m time would be increased by 0.26 s, whereas a 3-m/s tail wind would decrease the time by 0.34 s. The effects of the head and tail 3-m/s winds are not symmetrical for 3 m/s and 5 m/s (i.e., there are not similar gains and losses) because the issue is not the *force* associated with the wind but rather the *work* done against it. Similarly, 80% of the power generated by a cyclist traveling on level ground at 8.05 m•s⁻¹ (18 mph) is used to overcome air resistance (Gross, Kyle, & Malewicki, 1983).

The magnitude of the fluid resistance vector depends on the extent to which the fluid is disturbed by the object. Equation 2.5 indicates that this disturbance is proportional to the size of the projected area and the speed of the object relative to the fluid. Since the projected area is a function of the orientation of the object to the fluid, variation in the orientation can be used to alter the lift and drag experienced by the object as it passes through the medium.

For example, consider a person water skiing behind a boat. The ability of the skier to remain on top of the water is due to the force exerted by the fluid on the skis. The lift component of this F_f force must be at least as great as the downward forces, the latter being due mainly to the weight of the skier. As the boat goes faster (i.e., as the speed of the skis relative to the water increases), the magnitude of the projected area can decrease to maintain the necessary lift. In fact, this trade-off between projected area and relative velocity occurs throughout the skiing run. At the start, the skier in the water points the skis almost vertical. In this position the projected area of the skis to the water is maximized. As the boat begins to move and tow the skier, the skis disturb the water and create a lift force. At the beginning of the run, the projected area must be great because it combines with a low relative speed to generate the F_f and raise the skier to the surface. Because a lesser projected area is necessary, the skis can be lowered as the speed of the boat increases. Once the skier releases the towrope, the lift force eventually becomes insufficient and the skier sinks into the water.

From these examples, it is apparent that the effects an object experiences as it moves through a fluid depends to a certain extent on the relative velocity of the object. A sky diver represents an interesting example of this phenomenon. After jumping from the plane, the speed of the sky diver will increase up to some terminal value. How do we determine the value of this terminal velocity? Once again, the analysis should begin with an appropriate free-body diagram (Figure 2.16).

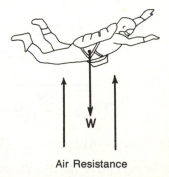

Figure 2.16. The forces experienced by a sky diver during free-fall.

When the sky diver jumps out of the airplane, the system (sky diver, parachute, and associated equipment) is accelerated, due to gravity, toward the ground. However, the downward acceleration of the system is only briefly equal to the value for gravity (9.81 m•s^{-2}), because as system speed increases, the opposing effect of air resistance increases. We know from Equation 2.5 that the magnitude of air resistance increases as the square of velocity; thus, as $\mathbf{v}$ increases, then so does the force due to air resistance. The speed of the system will continue to increase (i.e., acceleration will be nonzero) until the force due to air resistance is equal to the weight of the system (i.e., the acceleration due to gravity). When these two forces are equal, speed will remain constant and the system will have reached a terminal velocity. Because velocity remains constant (i.e., zero acceleration) and the system is in equilibrium at terminal velocity, the forces must be balanced; thus

$$\mathbf{W} = \mathbf{F}_f$$

Further, since we have defined $\mathbf{F}_f$ (Equation 2.5), then

$$\mathbf{W} = k A \mathbf{v}^2$$

We can rearrange this relationship to determine the terminal velocity:

$$\mathbf{v} = \sqrt{\frac{\mathbf{W}}{kA}}$$

If $k = 0.55$ kg•m^{-3}, $A = 0.36$ m^2, and $\mathbf{W} = 750$ N, then

$$\mathbf{v} = \sqrt{\frac{750}{0.55 \times 0.36}}$$

terminal velocity = 61.55 m•s^{-1} (137.7 mph)

Despite being in free-fall conditions, experienced sky divers are able to maneuver reasonably well, performing somersaults, cartwheels, and other sorts of movements. How can they do this? As we know from the free-body diagram (Figure 2.16), sky divers experience two forces as they fall. Both of these forces, weight and air resistance, are distributed forces; that is, they are distributed over the entire system but are drawn as acting at one or two points. The weight vector is always drawn acting at the CG. Similarly, the force due to air resistance has a central balance point—the center of air resistance. If the line of action of the air-resistance vector does not pass through the CG, then the air resistance will exert a torque about the CG and cause the sky diver to experience angular motion. The sky diver can accomplish this by moving the limbs, so altering the projected area and hence shifting the center of air resistance so that the vector does not pass through the CG.

Elastic Force

When a pulling force is applied to a material or tissue, its length can be increased. This stretch (i.e., the increase in length) is possible because of the atomic structure and organization of the material. The extent of the stretch depends on the nature of the material and the magnitude of the force. The relation between the applied force and the amount of stretch is given by the simple expression:

$$\mathbf{F} = kx \qquad (2.6)$$

where $\mathbf{F}$ = force, k = proportionality constant, and x = amount of stretch. Take, for example, a spring. The constant k refers to the stiffness of the spring, whether it is easy or difficult to stretch. A high value for k means the spring is stiff and difficult to stretch. In addition, Equation 2.6 shows that the further you stretch the spring the more force you have to apply. These same relations also apply to biological tissues. If the force causing the stretch is not substantial enough to damage the material, the material (or spring) will return to some semblance of its former length once the force is removed. If the material is able to return to its original length, then we say that the stretch was within its *elastic* limits. If the material is unable to recover its former length, the stretch extended into the material's *plastic* region, causing at least a partial reorganization of the structure of the material. This plasticity-induced reorganization causes a weakening of the material. The objective of flexibility exercises is, in fact, to induce plastic changes in biological tissues so that the range of motion about a joint is increased.

When a pushing or pulling force stretches a material, energy is stored in the material. As a consequence, once the disturbing force is removed, *the energy stored in the material will provide the fuel (a form of potential energy) for an **elastic force**, which tends to return the material to its original length*. For example, when a trampolinist bounces on a trampoline, the bed is stretched to an extent that depends on the magnitude of the pushing force provided by the trampolinist's body. Toward the bottom of the bounce, the pushing force is equal to the elastic force exerted by the bed. Thereafter, the elastic force becomes greater and the trampolinist is accelerated upward. The ability of biological tissue, particularly muscle, to store energy and subsequently utilize it by exerting an elastic force is thought to have significant effects in elite movement performance (we will examine this issue in chapter 7).

Inertial Force

Newton has told us that a moving object will continue to move in a straight line and at a constant speed unless it is acted on by a force (law of inertia). The object's resistance to any change in its motion is called its **inertia**. As a consequence, *an object in motion can, due to its inertia, exert a force on another object*. As a simple example of this effect, place one of your forearms in a vertical position (hand pointing upward) with the upper arm horizontal. Relax the muscles in your forearm that cross the wrist joint. Slowly begin to oscillate your forearm in a small arc in a forward-backward direction. As the movement becomes more vigorous, you should notice that your hand begins to flail, particularly if your hand is relaxed. You suspect, of course, that the motion of your hand has been caused by the forearm, and you are quite correct. Indeed, the forearm (due to its motion) has exerted an inertia force on the hand and caused the motion of the hand. This simple example emphasizes the mechanical coupling that exists between our body segments.

The hammer throw provides yet another example of the magnitude of inertia force in human movement. The distance an athlete can throw the hammer depends on the hammer's speed and the angle and height at which it is released. For the world-record performance of 86.33 m, the hammer travels at 29.1 m•s^{-1} (65 mph) at release if the angle of release is optimum (0.78 rad, 45 degrees). To achieve this release speed, an athlete often uses five revolutions while traveling across a 2.13-m diameter ring. During this procedure the athlete applies two forces to the hammer (Figure 2.17): (a) a pulling force that provides an angular acceleration to increase the speed of rotation, and (b) a centripetal force to maintain the angular nature of the motion. Brancazio (1984) estimated that to achieve a release speed of 29.1 m•s^{-1}, the athlete must provide an average pulling force of about 45 N throughout the event and a centripetal force of about 2.8 kN at release.

Since forces act in pairs (action-reaction), then the hammer must exert a force on the

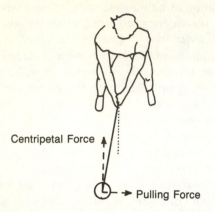

Figure 2.17. Forces exerted by the thrower on the hammer. *Note.* From *Sport Science: Physical Laws and Optimum Performance* (p. 296) by P.J. Brancazio, 1984, New York: Simon and Schuster. Copyright 1984 by Peter Brancazio. Adapted by permission.

thrower (centrifugal force) of 2.8 kN at release. The inertial effect due to the centrifugal force can be quite easily visualized by imagining that the athlete held on to rather than released the hammer. As soon as the centripetal force exerted by the thrower became less than 2.8 kN (i.e., due to a decrease in the friction force between the feet and the ground), the centrifugal force would cause the athlete to be dragged out of the throwing circle.

Although this hammer-throw example is perhaps an extreme account of inertial effects, such effects are significant in everyday events like running and kicking. In particular, the motion of one body segment (e.g., thigh) can quite readily affect the motion of another body segment (e.g., leg). For example, Figure 2.18 shows the changes that occur in knee angle and resultant muscle torque about the hip and knee joints during the swing phase of a running stride (Phillips & Roberts, 1980). The net muscle torque about the hip joint is essentially biphasic: flexor for the first half of swing and extensor

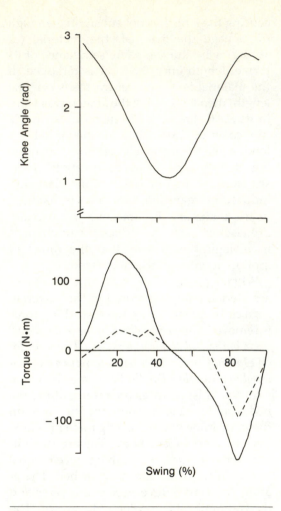

Figure 2.18. Knee angle and resultant muscle torques about the hip (solid line) and knee (dash line) joints during the swing phase of a running stride. The subject was a Masters runner who was running at 5.06 m/s. The data represent the part of the stride from ITO to IFS. Positive torque indicates the forward (counterclockwise) direction (i.e., hip flexor and knee extensor torques). (Adapted from Phillips & Roberts, 1980.) *Note.* From "Muscular and Non-Muscular Moments of Force in the Swing Limb of Masters Runners" by S.J. Phillips and E.M. Roberts, 1980, in J.M. Cooper and B. Haven (Eds.), *Proceedings of the Biomechanics Symposium* (pp. 265-266), Bloomington, IN: Indiana State Board of Health.

for the second half. The flexor hip torque rotates the thigh forward while the extensor torque slows down this forward rotation. Similarly, the resultant muscle torque about the knee joint appears biphasic with an intermediate period of a zero torque. However, the net knee torque is functionally opposite to the hip activity in that the extensor epoch preceded the flexor activity. Thus a net hip flexor torque is associated with a net knee extensor torque, and in the latter part of swing there is an association of the net hip extensor and the knee flexor torques. The role of the resultant muscle torque about the knee joint is made clearer when we consider the way in which knee angle changes during swing. During the period of knee extensor torque, the knee is flexing; this means that the knee extensor muscles are being lengthened (i.e., eccentric). Similarly, most of the knee flexor activity is eccentric. A *major role of this eccentric muscle activity*, for both the extensors and flexors, *is to control the effects of the thigh inertia force on the leg* (Phillips, Roberts, & Huang, 1983). Indeed, the control of movements involving more than one body segment must take into account the mechanical interactions between the segments (Bizzi & Abend, 1983).

Muscle Force

Previously, human movement was described as the consequence of the mechanical interaction between muscle and the environment. In this scheme the role of muscle is to exert a force that acts through the tendon onto the bone and causes the body segment (e.g., arm, thigh, torso) to rotate. However, the generalized concept of force (i.e., a push or a pull that alters or tends to alter an object's state of motion) cannot be extrapolated to muscle because a muscle cannot push, it can only pull. In mechanical terms, *muscle can exert a **tensile** (pulling) and not a **compressive***

(pushing) force. However, the effect of muscle activation can exert compressive forces (e.g., bone-on-bone contact at a joint).

Because of muscle's unidirectional capability of force exertion, movement about a joint is controlled by an opposing set of muscle groups. For example, elbow extension-flexion is controlled by one muscle group's causing extension (elbow extensors) and another group's generating flexion (elbow flexors). The resulting motion depends upon the net muscle activity across the joint and its relationship to the external load imposed on the system.

Since force is a vector, the quantity, muscle force, can be represented as an arrow and described in terms of the vector characteristics of direction and magnitude. In this context, the analysis of the human body and its interaction with its surroundings is based on the following four assumptions. *First*, most skeletal muscles exert forces across a joint and can cause body segments to rotate, which allows us to treat many of the human body functions as inanimate machines. Crowninshield & Brand (1981) attribute this assumption to Leonardo da Vinci (1452-1519). *Second*, the human body is a series of body segments that are rigid; the deformation of soft tissue and the movement of body fluids within the body segment will have a negligible effect on the movement (Braune & Fischer, 1889). *Third*, the direction of the muscle-force vector is a straight line between the proximal and distal attachments, with the application of force represented as a point (Brand et al., 1982). In reality, of course, the attachment of muscles is not at a single point but spread over a finite (i.e., measurable) area. Every force is applied across this finite area and is therefore described as **distributed**. However, when the size of the area is negligible compared to the other dimensions of the system, the force may be considered to be acting at a point. *Fourth*, as an extension of the idea that movement in a gravitational world is determined by the net imbalances of forces (law of inertia), mechanical analyses focus on the net effect of muscles crossing a joint, hence the terms **resultant muscle force** and its rotary equivalent **resultant muscle torque**. Although this assumption does not account for the complexity of the human body as a biological system, it does enable us to obtain mechanical solutions. Throughout this text we will deal continually with resultant muscle forces and torques, but we should remember that these terms refer to net effects, which are undoubtedly quite different from the extent of the absolute activity. Indeed, as indicated previously (Figure 1.5), many human movements involve the co-contraction of flexors and extensors, the net effect of which is due to the muscle group that is the most active.

The magnitude of the muscle force vector is a difficult quantity to measure in humans (because to do so requires a force transducer to be placed in series with the contractile tissue) and is generally *estimated* from a measurement of the **cross-sectional area** of the muscle (Fick, 1904), with the section made perpendicular to the orientation of the fibers. Cross-sectional area is a measurement of the end-on view of the area at the level that the section (cut) has been made. These measurements can be obtained from cadavers or, less accurately, from ultrasonic and computer tomography (CT) scans. For example, the cross-sectional area of the prime movers for elbow flexion and extension have been measured as follows (An, Hui, Morrey, Linscheid, & Chao, 1981):

Biceps brachii	
Long head	2.5 cm²
Short head	2.1 cm²
Brachialis	7.0 cm²
Brachioradialis	1.5 cm²

Triceps brachii	
Medial head	6.1 cm²
Lateral head	6.0 cm²
Short head	6.7 cm²

The capacity of the muscle to produce force is related to the cross-sectional area of the muscle by a constant of about 30 N•cm⁻². This constant is referred to as **specific tension** and varies from 16 to 30 N•cm⁻² in careful measurements (McDonagh & Davies, 1984). In other words, muscle can generate 30 N of force for each square centimeter of tissue. *Specific tension, therefore, is a measure of the capability of muscle to exert force that is independent of the amount of muscle.* The relation for estimating muscle force (F_m) is given as

$$F_m = \text{specific tension} \times \text{cross-sectional area} \qquad (2.7)$$

From the value above, biceps brachii with a cross-sectional area of 4.6 cm² can develop about 138 N of force. The total muscular cross-section of the human body (i.e., the sum of the cross-sections of all muscles) has been measured at about 0.56 m². If all the muscles were to contract simultaneously and in the same direction, the resulting force would be about 168 kN.

What accounts for the spread in the specific-tension constant that relates force capability to area (i.e., 16-30 N•cm⁻²)? Is it influenced by any single factor such as training, muscle-fiber type, muscle function, or the gender of the individual? Some evidence suggests that force production capability of muscle does depend on the percentage of fast-twitch fibers (e.g., Schantz, Fox, Norgren, & Tydén, 1981), but the specific tension of fast-twitch muscle fibers (25.4 N•cm⁻²) has not been found to be different from that of slow-twitch fibers (23.8 N•cm⁻²; Lucas, Ruff, & Binder, 1987). In addition, not everyone agrees that specific tension is constant for all muscle fibers (Bodine, Roy, Eldred, & Edgerton, 1985; McDonagh, Binder, Reinking, & Stuart, 1980). If the specific tension of type-identified fibers is the same, the differences observed by Schantz et al. (1981) and others may be due to variation in muscle mass and differences in the activation provided by the nervous system. Antigravity muscles—those involved with the maintenance of an upright posture (e.g., knee extensors)—are twice as strong as their counterparts (e.g., knee flexors), but this is supposedly due to a difference in size rather than variation in specific tension. Similarly, males are generally stronger than females (when strength is defined as the capacity to produce force in an isometric contraction), but this is due to differences in muscle mass (Figure 2.19). The cause for these differences is hormonal: Testosterone (male) is better than estrogen (female) at stimulating the protein synthesis that results in muscle growth. For the population depicted in Figure 2.19, Ikai and Fukunaga (1968) determined a mean constant of 61.1 N•cm^{-2} for the elbow flexors. That is,

on the average, an individual is capable of generating 61 N of force for each square centimeter of muscle tissue. (The specific-tension value of 61.1 N•cm^{-2} is larger than usual because Ikai and Fukunaga did not correct for the internal architecture of muscle.) In summary, apart from the effects of the nervous system and the mechanical arrangement of the muscle, the force a muscle can exert depends on its size (as indicated by its cross-sectional area) and not its function, its fiber-type composition, or the gender of the individual.

Torque

All human motion involves the rotation of body segments about their joint axes. These actions are produced by the interaction of forces associated with external loads and muscle activity. In particular, *human movement is the consequence of an imbalance between the components of these forces that produce rotation*. The capability of a force to produce rotation is referred to as **torque** or **moment of force**. Torque represents the rotational effect of a force with respect to an axis—the tendency of a force to produce rotation.

Suppose an individual was exercising on a device such as a Cybex. A number of different exercises can be performed on the Cybex, such as extension and flexion about the knee joint. Figure 2.20A illustrates the position of the subject for a knee-extension task. The knee joint is positioned in line with an axis about which a lever rotates. The subject pushes the lever and causes it to rotate. One of the features of the Cybex is that it can measure the pushing effort of the subject; however, there is often confusion as to what the Cybex actually measures. To measure force, it would be necessary for the transducer to

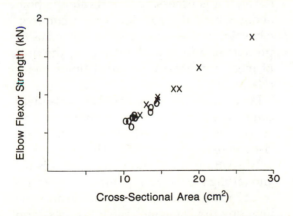

Figure 2.19. Relationship between elbow-flexor strength and the cross-sectional area of the flexors for 129 male (x) and 126 female (o) subjects, grouped according to age. (Adapted from Ikai & Fukunaga, 1968.)

be located along the line of action of the force vector. According to Figure 2.20B, the transducer is located at a distance from the line of action of the force exerted by the subject on the lever, and thus the *Cybex measures torque and not force*.

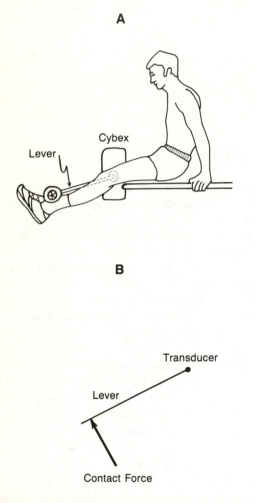

A

B

Figure 2.20. The measurement capability of a Cybex. (A) The subject performs a knee-extension exercise and pushes against the lever to cause it to rotate. (B) The line of action of the pushing force (contact force) that the subject exerts on the lever acts at a distance from the transducer. For this reason the Cybex measures torque and not force.

Torque is a vector that is equal to the magnitude of the force times the perpendicular distance from the line of action of the force to the axis of rotation. This distance is known as the **moment arm**. Algebraically,

$$\mathbf{T} = \mathbf{F} \times \text{moment arm} \qquad (2.8)$$

where $\mathbf{T}$ = torque and $\mathbf{F}$ = force. Since the moment arm is a perpendicular distance, it is the shortest distance from the line of action of the force to the axis of rotation. Both $\mathbf{F}$ and the moment arm indicated in Equation 2.8 are vector quantities; therefore, the direction of the torque vector is perpendicular to the plane in which the force and the moment arm exist. In other words, it is at right angles to the plane of this page. For graphic convenience torque is often represented as a curved arrow in the same plane as the force and moment arm (e.g., Figure 2.21C). Torque or moment of force is always determined with respect to a specific axis and therefore must be expressed with reference to the same axis. For example, to discuss the rotary effect of activating a muscle group (e.g., elbow flexors), it is necessary to indicate the point about which the rotation will occur (e.g., elbow joint). Since torque is calculated as the product of a force and a distance, the units of measurement are newtons times meters (N•m).

Let us consider an example of these ideas. Suppose a person was recovering from knee surgery by doing seated knee-extension exercises with a weight boot. The exercise involves sitting at the end of a trainer's bench and raising the leg from a vertical (knee angle = 1.57 rad) to a horizontal position and then lowering the leg again. What torques about the knee joint would be involved in this exercise? Figure 2.21A depicts the appropriate system, from the knee joint down to the toes, and the four forces (joint reaction force, resultant muscle force, limb weight, and boot weight) that represent the interaction of this system with its surroundings. The first step in determining the torques is to draw in the moment arms. This involves extending the line of action for each force and then drawing a perpendicular line from the line of action to the axis of rotation (Figure 2.21B). As the line of action of the joint reaction force passes through the axis of rotation, its moment arm, and therefore the moment of the joint reaction force about the knee joint, is equal to zero. Thus, for the system indicated in Figure 2.21, there are three forces that produce a torque about the knee joint. These effects can be represented as in Figure 2.21C, the direction of the curved torque arrow being the same as the rotation that the torque causes.

The calculation of the moment of force (or torque) is a straightforward procedure that often involves the use of trigonometric functions. Suppose the person illustrated in Figure 2.21A had a body weight of 700 N, a magnitude and direction of the resultant muscle force vector of 1,000 N and 0.25 rad, respectively, a leg length of 0.36 m, and a distance of 0.05 m from the knee joint to the point of application of the resultant muscle force vector, and was using an 80-N weight boot. What are the magnitudes of the three torques? First, if we focus on the moment produced by the resultant muscle force, the appropriate part of the free-body diagram appears as follows:

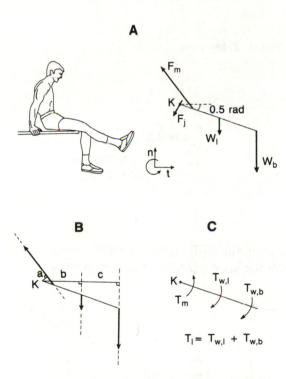

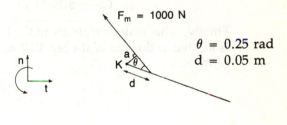

$F_m = 1000$ N

$\theta = 0.25$ rad

$d = 0.05$ m

Figure 2.21. Free-body diagrams of the leg of a person performing leg-extension exercises. (A) Four forces acting on the system. (B) The moment arms (a, b, c) for the three forces (F_m, W_l, W_b) that produce a moment about the knee joint. (C) Graphic representation of the three torques (T_m, $T_{w,l}$, $T_{w,b}$). F_j = joint reaction force; K = knee joint; T_l = resultant load torque; F_m = resultant muscle force; T_m = resultant muscle torque; $T_{w,b}$ = torque due to W_b; $T_{w,l}$ = torque due to W_l; W_b = boot weight; W_l = limb weight.

$$T_m = F_m \times a$$
$$= 1{,}000 \times a$$

$$\sin 0.25 = \frac{a}{0.05}$$
$$a = 0.05 \sin 0.25$$
$$= 0.0124$$

$$= 1{,}000 \times 0.0124$$
$$T_m = 12.37 \text{ N} \cdot \text{m}$$

The moment due to the weight of the limb can be determined in a similar manner. The weight of the leg (shank) and foot can be estimated from the combined leg and foot regression equations in Table 2.1, with the center of gravity (i.e., point of application for the weight vector) for the leg plus foot located at a distance of 43.4% of leg length measured from the knee joint. Hence,

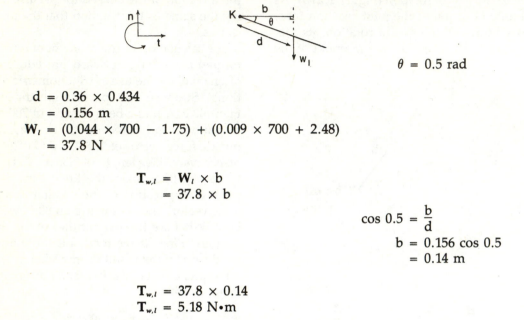

$\theta = 0.5$ rad

$d = 0.36 \times 0.434$
$\quad = 0.156$ m
$W_l = (0.044 \times 700 - 1.75) + (0.009 \times 700 + 2.48)$
$\quad = 37.8$ N

$$\mathbf{T}_{w,l} = \mathbf{W}_l \times b$$
$$= 37.8 \times b$$

$$\cos 0.5 = \frac{b}{d}$$
$$b = 0.156 \cos 0.5$$
$$= 0.14 \text{ m}$$

$$\mathbf{T}_{w,l} = 37.8 \times 0.14$$
$$\mathbf{T}_{w,l} = 5.18 \text{ N} \cdot \text{m}$$

Finally, what is the torque about the knee joint due to the weight boot? The boot is located at the end of the leg, 0.36 m from the knee joint, and has a magnitude of 80 N.

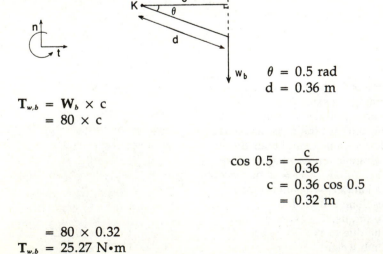

$\theta = 0.5$ rad
$d = 0.36$ m

$$\mathbf{T}_{w,b} = \mathbf{W}_b \times c$$
$$= 80 \times c$$

$$\cos 0.5 = \frac{c}{0.36}$$
$$c = 0.36 \cos 0.5$$
$$= 0.32 \text{ m}$$

$$= 80 \times 0.32$$
$$\mathbf{T}_{w,b} = 25.27 \text{ N} \cdot \text{m}$$

Note that the direction of the weight vector is always vertically downward, and, because a moment arm is perpendicular to the line of action of a vector, *the moment arm of a weight vector is always horizontal.*

The net moment of force about the knee in this example can be determined by summing the magnitudes and taking into account the direction of each torque (i.e., counterclockwise indicated as positive). The direction of each torque vector can be determined with the **right-hand-thumb rule**. The effect of each force on the system is considered separately by taking the right hand, curling the fingers into a loose fist, and extending the thumb. The right hand is positioned so that the curled fingers indicate the direction in which the force will cause the system to rotate. The extended thumb then indicates the direction of the torque vector that produces such a rotation. Recall that *a torque can be represented by a vector that is directed perpendicular to the plane of this page.* If such a vector extends toward you, it will cause the system to rotate in a counterclockwise direction. Throughout this text, torques producing counterclockwise rotation are indicated as positive. In the present example, the forces W_l and W_b produce clockwise rotation and thus are identified as negative torques.

To determine the net effect of these forces on the system, we sum (Σ) the moments of force about the knee joint (M_K):

$$\sum M_K = (F_m \times a) - (W_l \times b) - (W_b \times c)$$
$$= 12.37 - 5.18 - 25.27$$
$$\sum M_K = -18.08 \ N \cdot m$$

The net moment of force, therefore, has a magnitude of 18.08 N•m and acts in a clockwise direction. However, the fact that the torque acts in a clockwise direction says nothing about the direction of the limb displacement. For example, recall the elbow flexion-extension problem we considered in the "Acceleration and Muscle Activity" section. As indicated in Figure 1.5, displacement and force (torque) are often offset so that the direction of one does not necessarily tell us about the direction of the other. We need to have position, velocity, and acceleration (torque) information to get a complete description of the motion.

Since the torque is equal to the product of force and moment arm, the rotary effect of a force can be altered by either factor, singly or in combination. There are many examples of anatomical structures (e.g., calcaneus, patella, olecranon process, vertical spines of vertebrae), the mechanical effect of which is to alter (usually increase) the moment arm of associated muscles (Németh & Ohlsén, 1985). For example, consider the attachment of the patellar tendon to the tibia (Figure 2.22). If two individuals could generate the same amount of muscle force in the quadriceps femoris muscle group, the person with the greater perpendicular distance (due to a difference in the patella) from the line of action of the muscle-force vector to the axis of rotation would be able to generate the greater plantarflexor torque about the ankle joint. Since strength is a measure of the capacity to develop torque, it includes not simply a measure of muscle force but also the influence of the moment arm.

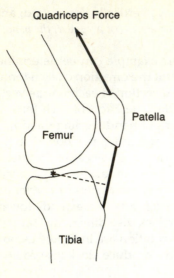

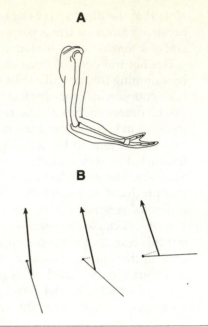

Figure 2.22. The effect of the patella on the length of the moment arm of the quadriceps femoris muscle group relative to the center of the knee joint. *Note.* From ''Patellar Forces During Knee Extension'' by R. Nisell and J. Ekholm, 1985, *Scandinavian Journal of Rehabilitation Medicine*, **17**, p. 64. Copyright 1985 by Almquist & Wiksell International. Adapted by permission.

Figure 2.23. Change in the moment arm for the resultant elbow flexor force over a 1.3-rad range of motion. (A) Schematic of the upper extremity. (B) Associated stick figures of the upper extremity, indicating moment arm length (dotted line) for three selected positions.

Table 2.3 Moment Arms (cm) Associated With the Elbow Flexor and Extensor Muscles for Fully Extended and 1.75 rad of Flexion and for the Hand in Two Positions (Neutral and Supinated)

| | Elbow extended | | Elbow flexed | |
Muscle	Neutral	Supinated	Neutral	Supinated
Flexor				
Biceps brachii	1.47	1.96	3.43	3.20
Brachialis	0.59	0.87	2.05	1.98
Brachioradialis	2.47	2.57	4.16	5.19
Extensor				
Triceps brachii	2.81	2.56	2.04	1.87

Note. Data from An et al. (1981).

In general, muscles have a shallow angle of pull and, consequently, anatomical moment arms are short. However, *moment arms change throughout the range of motion* (Figure 2.23). Data from An et al. (1981), for example, indicate that the moment arms for the major elbow flexors double as the elbow goes from a fully extended position to 1.75 rad (100 degrees) of flexion whereas the moment arm for triceps brachii (elbow extensor) decreases by about one-third over the same range of motion (Table 2.3). Similar observations have been made about the hip extensor (gluteus maximus, hamstrings, adductor magnus) muscles (Németh & Ohlsén, 1985).

Let us take a moment to see if the numbers in Table 2.3 make any sense. Consider an individual who performs push-ups to exhaustion. The prime mover for push-ups is the elbow extensor muscle, triceps brachii. Suppose this muscle was maximally active as the individual approached exhaustion and, based on the cross-sectional data presented previously, was exerting a force of 550 N. According to the data in Table 2.3, the moment arm for the triceps brachii is about 2.81 cm with the elbow extended (Figure 2.24A) and about 2.04 cm with the elbow flexed to 1.75 rad (Figure 2.24B). You can think of this variation in moment-arm length as a change in length of d in Figure 2.24C. Because of this variation in the moment arm, the maximum torque would be approximately 14.05 and 10.2 N•m for the extended and flexed position, respectively. That is, in the flexed position the torque due to the triceps-brachii force, the prime mover for the exercise, is less than in the extended position.

Consequently, failure to perform any more push-ups is more likely to occur in the flexed position, where there is a minimal amount of torque. (In this case, failure is the inability to raise body weight, a constant load, up and down.) A similar rationale applies to the point of failure during pull-ups to exhaustion. The moment arms for the elbow-flexor muscles are minimal with complete elbow extension, and, assuming the muscle force is reasonably constant throughout the range of motion, that is the point at which failure occurs.

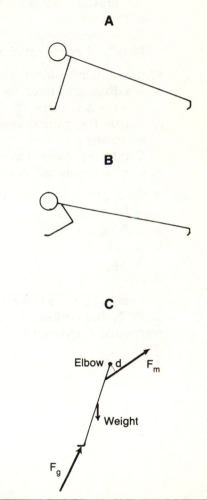

Figure 2.24. A person performing a push-up. (A) Straight-arm position. (B) Bent-arm position. (C) A free-body diagram that isolates the resultant muscle force (F_m) about the elbow joint. The net torque about the elbow joint is equal to the product of F_m and the moment arm (**d**).

Problems

2.1.   Which statement(s) represent assumptions that are necessary in the analysis of human movement?
   a. Weight is a distributed force.
   b. The deformation of soft tissue and the movement of fluids within a body segment have a negligible effect during movement.
   c. In a gravitational environment, movement occurs due to an imbalance of forces.
   d. Forces can be represented as vectors.
   e. Muscles have point attachments.

2.2.   Which statement about weight is incorrect?
   a. Is a distributed force due to the attraction between the Earth and a body.
   b. Always acts vertically downward.
   c. Equals the ground reaction force when the object (e.g., person) is stationary.
   d. Can be represented to act through a fixed point, the center of gravity.
   e. Can be calculated as mass times velocity.

2.3.   A 550-N person standing stationary on one leg, on a weight scale, would record a weight of
   a. 22.5 kg
   b. 225 N
   c. 55 kg
   d. 550 N

2.4.   The medial (M) and lateral (L) heads of gastrocnemius both exert a force of 350 N that is directed 0.25 rad to the left and right of a vertical midline, respectively. Determine the magnitude and direction of the resultant.

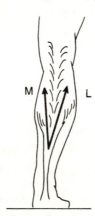

2.5.   The three muscles primarily involved in producing elbow flexion are biceps brachii, brachialis, and brachioradialis. Suppose that the elbow joint is flexed to 1.57 rad and that these muscles are generating 290, 440, and 95 N of force, respectively, and pulling at angles of 0.7, 0.2, and 0.3 rad, respectively. For simplicity, assume the three muscles share a common point of attachment on the radius. What is the direction and magnitude of the resultant muscle force?

2.6. The amount of fluid resistance experienced by an object depends upon the extent to which the fluid is disturbed by the object. From the fluid resistance equation, which two variables have a substantial effect on this disturbance?

2.7. During knee extension the patella moves in the groove between the medial and lateral condyles of the femur. An imbalance between the four muscles that pull on the patella can result in the patella's not tracking correctly. This can occur, for example, if the knee has been immobilized in a cast for a period of time and the vastus medials and lateralis muscles have not atrophied at the same rate. Given the following magnitudes and direction for the four muscle force vectors, determine the resultant vector:

Rectus femoris—130 N, 0.25 rad to the left of vertical

Vastus lateralis—180 N, 0.50 rad to the left of vertical

Vastus intermedius—165 N, 0.15 rad to the left of vertical

Vastus medialis—210 N, 0.62 rad to the right of vertical

2.8. A person performing sit-ups is generating a 480-N force with the hip flexor muscles in the position indicated. What are the magnitudes of the normal and tangential components? Complete the free-body diagram for this situation.

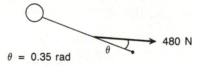

$\theta = 0.35$ rad   480 N

2.9. Which statement about muscle torque is incorrect?

a. Is synonymous with moment of force.
b. Equals muscle force times moment arm.
c. Represents the rotational effect of a muscle force.
d. Cannot vary during a movement.
e. Is independent of the stabilizing component.

2.10. Consider a movement in which the elbow joint goes from complete extension to a right angle (1.57 rad).

a. Does the moment arm of the resultant elbow-flexor force to the elbow joint increase, stay the same, or decrease as the joint flexes?
b. If the muscle force remains constant, does the resultant muscle torque increase, stay the same, or decrease as the joint flexes?
c. If the muscle torque remains constant, does the resultant muscle force increase, stay the same, or decrease as the joint flexes?

2.11. A manufacturer has designed and built a machine to strengthen the elbow-flexor muscles. Draw the appropriate free-body diagram to analyze the effect of the machine on the force developed by these muscles.

2.12. An individual weighs 523 N. Based on the regression equations in Table 2.1 (Chandler et al., 1975), how much does this person's trunk weigh and what percentage is this of total-body weight?

2.13. A 1.72-m person has thigh and lower leg (shank) lengths of 36 cm each and upper arm and forearm lengths of 25 cm each. For which of these limb segments is the CG furthest, and for which is the CG closest, to the proximal joint?

2.14. The specific tension of muscle is about 30 N•cm^{-2}.

    a. The cross-sectional areas of the prime movers for elbow flexion and extension have been measured as

        biceps brachii   4.6 cm^2
        brachialis   7.0 cm^2
        brachioradialis   1.5 cm^2
        triceps brachii   18.8 cm^2

    Determine the maximum force that the elbow flexors (as a group of muscles) can exert.

    b. For an individual whose triceps brachii had a cross-sectional area of 9.4 cm^2, what would be the value of the specific tension?

    c. As the elbow joint is flexed from an extended position to an angle of 1.75 rad, the moment arm for the elbow flexors doubles in size. If the specific tension was 30 N•cm^{-2} in the extended position, what would it be in the flexed position?

2.15. The kicking coach of a football team would like to know what force the knee extensors of his punter produce during a punt. How would you define your system to address this question? Draw your free-body diagram.

2.16. For each of the four positions shown below draw in the moment arms for the two weight vectors relative to the knee joint.

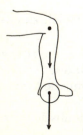 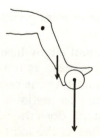 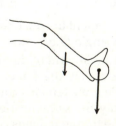 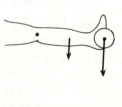

2.17. In most activities involving throwing or hitting an object, coaches emphasize the follow-through. Justify this advice in terms of the force-mass-acceleration relationship.

2.18. In each case below, determine the moment produced by the force about Point B. The beam is pivoted at Point B and is thus free to rotate.

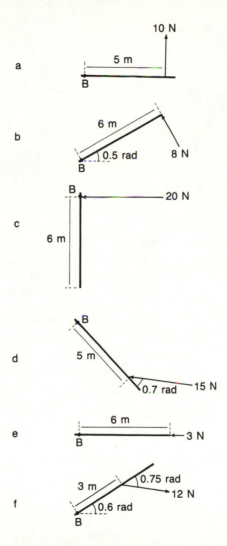

2.19. Imagine doing pull-ups to failure. Draw a free-body diagram (e.g., Figure 2.24) to help explain the point at which you would expect the failure to occur during the exercise. Use the cross-sectional data (An et al., 1981) from page 58 and the moment-arm data (Table 2.3) for the elbow flexors to estimate the torque exerted by the elbow flexors at the extremes of the movement (i.e., extended vs. flexed).

3

Types of Movement Analysis

The motion of an object, which is described in terms of position, velocity, and acceleration, is characterized as the consequence of the interaction between the object and its surroundings. This interaction is commonly represented as a force. The nature of the relationship between force and motion is outlined in Newton's laws of motion, a set of three laws which form the basis of the Newtonian approach to the analysis of motion. The particular algebraic relationship between force and motion that is used in an analysis depends upon the objective of the analysis (e.g., Miller, 1981). In general, the alternatives are to focus on (a) the *instantaneous* value of force (force-mass-acceleration), (b) the effect of a force applied over an *interval of time* (impulse-momentum), or (c) the application of a force that causes an object to move through *some distance* (work-energy).

Force-Mass-Acceleration

When the force-mass-acceleration approach ($F = ma$) is used, a system may exist in one of the two states; that is, a may be either zero (static) or nonzero (dynamic).

Static Analysis

When the focus of an analysis is on the value of force at one instant in time, the appropriate procedure is to use the force-mass acceleration approach, so-named because it is based upon Newton's law of acceleration,

$$\sum F = ma$$

Recall that the left-hand side of this relationship ($\Sigma\mathbf{F}$) represents the interactions between a system and its surroundings whereas the right side indicates the kinematic effects of the interactions on the system. A force-mass-acceleration analysis can be further categorized depending upon the magnitude of acceleration (**a**), that is, whether it is zero or nonzero. **Statics** is a special case of Newton's law of acceleration in which acceleration is zero because the object is either stationary or moving at a constant velocity. *In a static analysis the system is in equilibrium and the sum of the forces in any given direction is zero ($\Sigma\mathbf{F} = 0$).* That is, the interactions are balanced, and therefore the system will not experience an acceleration. Similarly, the sum of the moments of force (i.e., torque) about any designated point or axis is equal to zero ($\Sigma\mathbf{M}_o = 0$). At most, three independent equations are available to solve **coplanar** (i.e., forces confined to the same plane) statics problems:

$$\sum\mathbf{F}_x = 0 \qquad (3.1)$$

$$\sum\mathbf{F}_y = 0 \qquad (3.2)$$

$$\sum\mathbf{M}_o = 0 \qquad (3.3)$$

Equations 3.1 and 3.2 refer to the sum (Σ) of the forces in any two directions in a plane, the directions being perpendicular to one another. These directions are commonly horizontal-vertical or normal-tangential.

In what follows, we shall examine four examples of static analyses: determination of the magnitude and direction of an unknown force, calculation of a resultant muscle torque, resolution of the magnitude and direction of a resultant muscle force and a joint reaction force, and location of the total-body CG using a segmental analysis. For the first example, consider the following system in Figure 3.1A, which is in equilibrium and upon which are acting three known and one unknown forces. What is the magnitude of the unknown force?

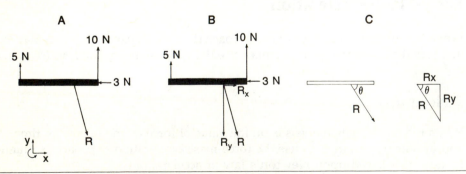

Figure 3.1.   Distribution of forces acting on an object.

The first step is to identify the two directions, at right angles to one another, that will be used and the sense of each that will be denoted as positive. This includes specification of the positive angular direction. These have been indicated to the left of the system: The selected directions are horizontal (x) and vertical (y) and the positive senses are to the right and upward, respectively. Thus any horizontal force directed to the right will be regarded as positive and any to the left will be indicated as negative. The declaration of the horizontal-vertical directions is also an indication that only forces in these directions can be handled in the analysis and thus any force (e.g., **R**) not in either direction must be resolved into such directions (e.g., Figure 2.2).

The next step in the analysis, therefore, is to resolve **R** graphically into horizontal ($\mathbf{R}_x$) and vertical ($\mathbf{R}_y$) components (Figure 3.1B). Once all forces are resolved into the x and y directions, the forces in each direction can be summed to determine the magnitude of the unknowns. Thus

$$\sum \mathbf{F}_x = 0 \qquad\qquad \sum \mathbf{F}_y = 0$$
$$\mathbf{R}_x - 3 = 0 \qquad\qquad 5 + 10 - \mathbf{R}_y = 0$$
$$\mathbf{R}_x = 3 \text{ N} \qquad\qquad \mathbf{R}_y = 15 \text{ N}$$

In determining the magnitudes of $\mathbf{R}_x$ and $\mathbf{R}_y$ note that each calculation began with specification of one of the three independent equations (3.1, 3.2, or 3.3). It is of little consequence whether an inappropriate equation is chosen, for if the calculation proceeds logically, it will soon become evident that such was the case. For example, suppose $\sum \mathbf{M}_o = 0$ has been selected to determine $\mathbf{R}_x$ or $\mathbf{R}_y$. It is not possible to sum the moments in this problem because no distances are given with which to determine the torques. Thus one of the other two equations must be chosen.

With the calculated values of $\mathbf{R}_x$ and $\mathbf{R}_y$, the resultant (**R**) can be obtained by the Pythagorean relationship:

$$\mathbf{R} = \sqrt{\mathbf{R}_x{}^2 + \mathbf{R}_y{}^2}$$
$$= \sqrt{3^2 + 15^2}$$
$$\mathbf{R} = 15.3 \text{ N}$$

This result, however, specifies only the magnitude of the resultant and not its direction. We can actually indicate the direction of **R** relative to several references; for example, we could determine the angle relative to a horizontal ($\mathbf{R}_x$) or a vertical ($\mathbf{R}_y$) reference. Let us calculate and determine the angle of **R** relative to the system (Figure 3.1C). By the parallelogram rule, **R** is the diagonal of the rectangle, which has $\mathbf{R}_x$ and $\mathbf{R}_y$ as its sides. Thus $\mathbf{R}_x$, $\mathbf{R}_y$, and **R** represent the sides of a triangle and we can determine θ as:

$$\cos \theta = \frac{\mathbf{R}_x}{\mathbf{R}} \qquad\qquad \sin \theta = \frac{\mathbf{R}_y}{\mathbf{R}} \qquad\qquad \tan \theta = \frac{\mathbf{R}_y}{\mathbf{R}_x}$$

Accordingly,

$$\cos \theta = \frac{R_x}{R}$$

$$\theta = \cos^{-1} \frac{R_x}{R}$$

$$= \cos^{-1} \frac{3}{15.3}$$

$$= \cos^{-1} 0.1961$$

$$\theta = 1.37 \text{ rad}$$

Another example of a static force-mass-acceleration analysis was indicated in Figure 2.21 (see Figure 3.2). In that instance, the object of the analysis was to determine the magnitude and direction of the resultant muscle torque about the knee joint given a specific value for the resultant muscle force. However, suppose the individual had to hold the limb at an angle of 0.5 rad below the horizontal: What resultant muscle torque must the person generate to accomplish this task? First, reconstruct the free-body diagram. Next, select the appropriate equation (3.1, 3.2, or 3.3) and proceed to sum the forces or moments of force. If you choose Equation 3.3 and sum the moments of force about the knee joint, then you can ignore the joint reaction force. Also, since the purpose of the analysis is to determine the resultant muscle torque, it would seem appropriate to use Equation 3.3. Consequently,

$$\sum M_K = 0$$

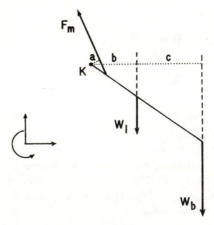

Figure 3.2. Free-body diagram of the leg and foot of an individual performing a knee extension exercise (Figure 2.21). **a, b, c** = moment arms = 0.0124, 0.110, 0.320 m, respectively; F_m = resultant muscle force; W_l = leg weight = 40.6 N; W_b = weight boot = 80.0 N.

Because there are three forces that will produce a rotation of the system about point K (the axis of rotation), these need to be indicated. The calculation, therefore, proceeds as follows:

$$\sum M_K = 0$$
$$(\mathbf{F}_m \times \mathbf{a}) - (\mathbf{W}_l \times \mathbf{b}) - (\mathbf{W}_b \times \mathbf{c}) = 0$$
$$(\mathbf{F}_m \times \mathbf{a}) = (\mathbf{W}_l \times \mathbf{b}) + (\mathbf{W}_b \times \mathbf{c})$$
$$= (40.6 \times 0.11) + (80.0 \times 0.32)$$
$$= 4.63 + 25.27$$
$$(\mathbf{F}_m \times \mathbf{a}) = 29.90 \text{ N} \cdot \text{m}$$

The product of the resultant muscle force ($\mathbf{F}_m$) and its moment arm equals the resultant muscle torque; therefore, the individual must exert a torque of 29.90 N•m to maintain the limb in the indicated position. What resultant muscle torque was the person exerting when the example (Figure 2.21) was solved previously? What is the magnitude of $\mathbf{F}_m$? Which muscle group would have to be dominant to obtain this direction?

As the third, more involved example of a static analysis, consider a student who sits at the end of a trainer's bench and uses a rope-pulley apparatus to strengthen her quadriceps femoris muscle group with isometric exercises. Her leg weighs 30 N, and a force of 100 N is applied to the rope pulley. The quadriceps group is attached 7 cm from the knee joint, the center of gravity for the limb is 20 cm from the knee joint, and the distance between the knee joint and rope-pulley apparatus is 45 cm. The rope-pulley apparatus involves an ankle strap with a rope connecting the strap to a weight stack at the back of the bench. The weight stack can be set so that it does not move, and hence the individual performs an isometric contraction. The free-body diagram of the system, from the knee (K) joint down to the toes, is shown in Figure 3.3. Find

1. the magnitude of the net quadriceps femoris force ($\mathbf{F}_{m,q}$) necessary to maintain the illustrated position,
2. the magnitude of the normal ($\mathbf{F}_{j,n}$) and tangential ($\mathbf{F}_{j,t}$) components of the joint reaction force, and
3. the magnitude and direction of the resultant joint reaction force ($\mathbf{F}_j$).

The initial step is to identify the two independent directions in which the forces are to be summed and the positive senses for these linear and the angular directions. Since this problem concerns the application of forces and torques to a body segment, it is most appropriate to choose the normal and tangential directions. These are indicated to the right of the system.

To determine the magnitude of $\mathbf{F}_{m,q}$ the same three equations (3.1 through 3.3) are available. Since there are three unknown forces acting on the system ($\mathbf{F}_{j,n}$, $\mathbf{F}_{j,t}$, $\mathbf{F}_{m,q}$), it would seem sensible to sum the moments about point K. Alternatively, especially since $\mathbf{F}_{j,n}$ and $\mathbf{F}_{j,t}$ must be addressed subsequently, each force could be resolved into its normal and tangential components and then the appropriate products summed. If the weight of the limb is designated as $\mathbf{W}$, and

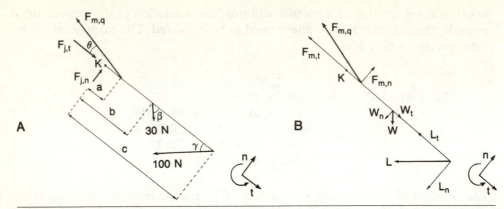

Figure 3.3. Free-body diagram of the forces acting on the leg of an individual as she performs an isometric exercise to strengthen her quadriceps muscle group. $\theta = 0.25$ rad, $\beta = 0.87$ rad, $\gamma = 0.70$ rad.

the force applied to the rope pulley as **L**, these components will appear as shown in Figure 3.3B.

Combining the information in the two diagrams, we can determine the magnitude of the various components trigonometrically as

$$\mathbf{F}_{m,n} = \mathbf{F}_{m,q} \sin 0.25 \qquad \mathbf{F}_{m,t} = \mathbf{F}_{m,q} \cos 0.25$$
$$\mathbf{W}_n = \mathbf{W} \sin 0.87 \qquad \mathbf{W}_t = \mathbf{W} \cos 0.87$$
$$\mathbf{L}_n = \mathbf{L} \sin 0.70 \qquad \mathbf{L}_t = \mathbf{L} \cos 0.70$$

Since the line of action of each tangential (t) component is directed through point K, these components ($\mathbf{F}_{m,t}$, $\mathbf{W}_t$, $\mathbf{L}_t$) produce no moment of force with respect to K. Therefore, the summation of moments about point K reduces to

$$\sum \mathbf{M}_K = 0$$
$$(\mathbf{F}_{m,n} \times 7) - (\mathbf{W}_n \times 20) - (\mathbf{L}_n \times 45) = 0$$
$$7\,\mathbf{F}_{m,n} = 20\,\mathbf{W}_n + 45\,\mathbf{L}_n$$
$$7\,(\mathbf{F}_{m,q} \sin 0.25) = 20\,(\mathbf{W} \sin 0.87) + 45\,(\mathbf{L} \sin 0.7)$$
$$\mathbf{F}_{m,q} = \frac{20\,(\mathbf{W} \sin 0.87) + 45\,(\mathbf{L} \sin 0.7)}{7 \sin 0.25}$$
$$= \frac{20\,(30 \times 0.7643) + 45\,(100 \times 0.6442)}{7 \times 0.2474}$$
$$= \frac{458.60 + 2898.90}{1.73}$$
$$\mathbf{F}_{m,q} = 1{,}941 \text{ N}$$

To determine the magnitude of $\mathbf{F}_{j,t}$ and $\mathbf{F}_{j,n}$ we simply have to sum the forces in each direction, a task that is not too involved since each force has already been resolved into its normal and tangential components.

$$\sum F_t = 0$$

$$F_{j,t} - F_{m,t} + W_t - L_t = 0$$

$$F_{j,t} = F_{m,t} - W_t + L_t$$

$$F_{j,t} = F_{m,q} \cos 0.25 - W \cos 0.87 + L \cos 0.7$$

$$= 1,941 \cos 0.25 - 30 \cos 0.87 + 100 \cos 0.7$$

$$= (1,941 \times 0.9689) - (30 \times 0.6448) + (100 \times 0.7648)$$

$$= 1,880.7 - 19.3 + 76.5$$

$$F_{j,t} = 1,938 \text{ N}$$

The magnitude of the normal component can be found in a similar manner:

$$\sum F_n = 0$$

$$F_{j,n} + F_{m,n} - W_n - L_n = 0$$

$$F_{j,n} = -F_{m,n} + W_n + L_n$$

$$= -(1,941 \sin 0.25) + (30 \sin 0.87) + (100 \sin 0.7)$$

$$= -480.2 + 22.9 + 64.4$$

$$F_{j,n} = -393 \text{ N}$$

The magnitude of $F_{j,n}$ is determined as a negative 393 N. How can a force be negative? Surely the sign must refer to the direction of the force. But reference to the free-body diagram will indicate that $F_{j,n}$ is acting in the positive direction. Actually, if a force is calculated as negative, this means that the direction of the force is opposite to that which is indicated in the free-body diagram. Thus $F_{j,t}$ and $F_{j,n}$ and the associated resultant (F_j) act on point K in the manner illustrated in Figure 3.4. Now that we know the magnitude of $F_{j,t}$ and $F_{j,n}$ we can determine the magnitude of the resultant joint reaction force (F_j) with the Pythagorean relationship:

$$F_j = \sqrt{F_{j,t}^2 + F_{j,n}^2}$$

$$= \sqrt{1,938^2 + 393^2}$$

$$F_j = 1,977 \text{ N}$$

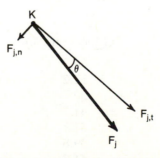

Figure 3.4. Determination of the resultant knee-joint reaction force for the free-body diagram outlined in Figure 3.3.

And we can calculate its direction with respect to the axis of the leg as

$$\tan \theta = \frac{F_{j,n}}{F_{j,t}}$$

$$\theta = \tan^{-1} \frac{F_{j,n}}{F_{j,t}}$$

$$= \tan^{-1} \frac{393}{1,941}$$

$$\theta = 0.2 \text{ rad}$$

In the final example, the principles of statics are used to determine the location of the total-body CG. This approach is known as a segmental analysis. Previously the center of gravity (CG) of an object was defined as a balance point. As a consequence, *the location of the total-body CG for multisegmented objects, such as the human body, can be determined using the static version of Newton's law of acceleration* ($\Sigma F = 0$). This is accomplished by finding the point about which the body segments are balanced. In other words, the CG can be located by requiring that the system be in equilibrium and then finding the point (the CG) about which this is true. Since the body is actually in equilibrium (i.e., balanced) with respect to the CG, the sum of moments about the CG is equal to zero. That is, the CG is the point about which the moments of force due to segmental weights is balanced.

As an example of this technique, let us determine the location of the total-body CG of a gymnast about to perform a backward handspring (Figure 3.5). The necessary steps include the following:

1. Identify the appropriate body segments. The human body is typically divided into 14 segments: head, trunk, upper arms, forearms, hands, thighs, legs, and feet. These segments are identified in Figure 3.5A by indicating the joint centers that represent the proximal and distal markers for each segment (Chandler et al., 1975; Appendix D).
2. Join the joint-center markers to construct a stick diagram (Figure 3.5B).
3. From Table 2.1, determine the location of the CG for each segment as a percentage of segment length. These lengths are measured from the proximal end of each segment (Figure 3.5B).

Segment	CG location (%)	Proximal end
Head	66.3	Top of the head
Trunk	52.2	Top of the neck
Upper arm	50.7	Shoulder
Forearm	41.7	Elbow
Hand	51.5	Wrist
Thigh	39.8	Hip
Leg	41.3	Knee
Foot	40.0	Ankle

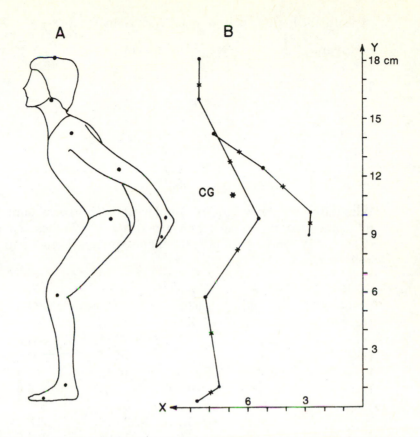

Figure 3.5. Location of whole-body center of gravity (CG) as a function of the position of the body segments. (A) Joint centers (dot) mark the limits of the respective body segments. (B) Location of the segmental CGs (x) as a percentage of segment length.

4. Estimate segmental weights as a function of body weight (BW) with the Chandler et al. (1975) regression equations (Table 2.1). Suppose the gymnast weighed 450 N.

Segment	Equation	Weight (N)
Head	0.032 × BW + 18.70 =	33.10
Trunk	0.532 × BW − 6.93 =	232.47
Upper arm	0.022 × BW + 4.76 =	14.66
Forearm	0.013 × BW + 2.41 =	8.26
Hand	0.005 × BW + 0.75 =	3.00
Thigh	0.127 × BW − 14.82 =	42.33
Leg	0.044 × BW − 1.75 =	18.05
Foot	0.009 × BW + 2.48 =	6.53

5. Measure the location of segmental CGs relative to an x-y axis (Figure 3.5B).

Segment	X-coordinate (cm)	Y-coordinate (cm)
Head	8.6	16.8
Trunk	6.9	12.8
Upper arm	6.5	13.3
Forearm	4.2	11.5
Hand	2.8	9.6
Thigh	6.6	8.2
Leg	8.0	3.9
Foot	8.0	0.8

6. With the segmental weight (SW) and location (x, y) data, sum the segmental moments of force about the y-axis (ΣM_y = SW times x) and the x-axis (ΣM_x = SW times y). Double the limb segmental weights to account for both limbs.

Segment	x (cm)	y (cm)	SW (N)	ΣM_y (N•cm)	ΣM_x (N•cm)
Head	8.6	16.8	33.10	284.7	556.1
Trunk	6.9	12.8	232.47	1,604.4	2,975.6
Upper arm	6.5	13.3	29.32	190.6	390.0
Forearm	4.2	11.5	16.52	69.4	190.0
Hand	2.8	9.6	6.00	16.8	57.6
Thigh	6.6	8.2	84.66	558.8	694.2
Leg	8.0	3.9	36.10	288.8	140.8
Foot	8.0	0.8	13.06	104.5	10.5
				3,018.0	5,014.7

7. Find the location of the point that would produce the same moment as that due to the sum of the segmental effects. *The net moment of force due to segmental weights about the x- and y-axes (3,018.0 N•cm and 5,014.7 N•cm, respectively) is the same as the net moment due to total body weight.* Thus

$$\text{body weight} \times \text{moment arm} = \sum (\text{segmental weight} \times \text{moment arm})$$

$$\text{moment arm} = \frac{\sum (\text{segmental weight} \times \text{moment arm})}{\text{body weight}}$$

To find the x- and y-coordinates for the total-body CG,

$$x = \frac{3,018.0 \text{ N•cm}}{450 \text{ N}} \qquad y = \frac{5,014.7 \text{ N•cm}}{450 \text{ N}}$$
$$= 6.71 \text{ cm} \qquad\qquad = 11.14 \text{ cm}$$

With these coordinates, the location of the total-body CG is indicated in Figure 3.5B.

Dynamic Analysis

A static analysis is the most elementary approach to the kinetic analysis of human movement. In contrast, when the system experiences an acceleration, the right-hand side of Equation 2.3 (Newton's law of acceleration) is nonzero and the analysis becomes correspondingly more difficult. Use of the force-mass-acceleration approach in situations where acceleration is nonzero is referred to as a **dynamic** analysis. The general form of the three independent equations (3.1, 3.2, 3.3) used in the static approach also applies to the dynamic problem, with the exception that the right-hand side of the equations is now equal to the product of mass and acceleration. Hence,

$$\sum \mathbf{F}_x = m\mathbf{a}_x \qquad (3.4)$$

$$\sum \mathbf{F}_y = m\mathbf{a}_y \qquad (3.5)$$

$$\sum \mathbf{M}_g = I_g \alpha \qquad (3.6)$$

As in the static case, these equations are independent and represent two perpendicular linear directions (x and y) and one angular direction. They can be applied to movements that occur in a single plane, each providing a solution for its respective direction. In expanded form, Equation 3.4 states that the sum (Σ) of the forces (**F**) in the x direction is equal to the product of the mass (m) of the system and the acceleration of the system's center of gravity in the x direction ($\mathbf{a}_x$). The product of mass and acceleration is often referred to as an **inertia force**. Equations 3.5 and 3.6 similarly address forces and accelerations in the y (perpendicular to x) and angular directions, respectively. The angular equivalent of the inertia force is the **inertia torque** ($I_g \alpha$), which is determined as the product of the moment of inertia about the center of gravity (I_g) and angular acceleration (α). Inertia was previously defined as the resistance of an object to a linear change in its state of motion. Likewise, the **moment of inertia** (I) is a quantity that indicates the resistance of an object to an angular change in its state of motion. *It is a measure of the distribution of the mass of the object with respect to the axis or point about which it is rotating*. The greater the distribution of mass of the object, the greater the moment of inertia. Thus the moment of inertia is not a fixed quantity but may be altered by shifting the mass within the object. For example, a springboard diver performing somersaults rotates about an axis that passes from side to side through the center of gravity. This axis of rotation is known as the somersault axis. In the pike position (straight legs) the body segments are spread further from this axis than in the tuck position, and, accordingly, the moment of inertia of the diver about the somersault axis is greater in the pike position. Similarly, the axis that passes front to back through the center of gravity is known as the cartwheel axis, and the axis that passes from head to toe through the center of gravity is referred to as the twist axis. In general, the moment of inertia of the human body is least about the twist axis and greatest about the cartwheel axis. The moment of inertia about the somersault axis, however, can be made to vary over a substantial range by going from a tuck to a layout position.

Since the right-hand side of Equations 3.4 and 3.6 is nonzero, the free-body diagram of the system can be equated to a **mass-acceleration diagram**. That is, by Newton's law of acceleration ($\mathbf{F} = \mathbf{ma}$), force (free-body diagram) equals mass times acceleration (mass-acceleration diagram). In this context the free-body diagram (FBD) represents the left-hand side of the equation and the mass-acceleration diagram (MAD) the right-hand side. In other words, the free-body diagram defines the system and how it interacts (forces shown as arrows) with its surroundings. The mass-acceleration diagram shows the effects of these interactions on the system—that is, how the interactions alter the motion of the system. For example, consider a weight lifter as he raises a barbell to his chest. An analysis is performed to determine the torque developed by the back and hip extensor muscles when the barbell is about knee-height. An appropriate system (as identified previously) would include the upper body from the lumbosacral (LS) joint to the head (Figure 3.6).

We can identify five forces that act on this system: the resultant muscle force ($\mathbf{F}_m$) about the LS joint, the joint reaction force ($\mathbf{F}_j$), the weight of the barbell ($\mathbf{W}_b$), the weight of the body ($\mathbf{W}_u$) above LS, and a force ($\mathbf{F}_i$) generated by the pressure within the abdominal cavity (intraabdominal pressure). The object of the analysis is to determine the magnitude of $\mathbf{F}_m$. As with the static situations, the most obvious approach is to sum the moments about the LS joint, therefore eliminating $\mathbf{F}_j$ from consideration. To sum the moments of force about the LS joint we have to add a transfer term (md^2) to the inertia torque about the center of gravity

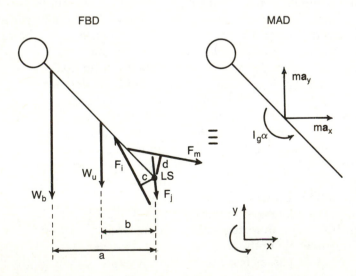

Figure 3.6. A dynamic analysis (free-body diagram [FBD] = mass-acceleration diagram [MAD]) of a weight lifter performing a clean. $\mathbf{W}_b = 1{,}003$ N, $\mathbf{W}_u = 525$ N, $\mathbf{F}_i = 1{,}250$ N, $\mathbf{a} = 38$ cm, b = 24 cm, c = 9 cm, $I_g + md^2 = 7.43$ kg•m², $\alpha = 12.59$ rad/s/s.

$(I_g\alpha)$; in this transfer term, m = segment mass, and d = the distance from the center of gravity to the joint. The analysis would proceed as follows:

$$\sum M_{LS} = (I_g + md^2)\alpha$$

$$(\mathbf{W}_b \times \mathbf{a}) + (\mathbf{W}_u \times \mathbf{b}) - (\mathbf{F}_i \times \mathbf{c}) - (\mathbf{F}_m \times \mathbf{d}) = (I_g + md^2)\alpha$$

$$(\mathbf{F}_m \times \mathbf{d}) = (\mathbf{W}_b \times \mathbf{a}) + (\mathbf{W}_u \times \mathbf{b}) - (\mathbf{F}_i \times \mathbf{c})$$
$$- (I_g + md^2)\alpha$$
$$= (1{,}003 \times 0.38) + (525 \times 0.24)$$
$$- (1{,}250 \times 0.09) - (7.43 \times 12.59)$$
$$= 381.14 + 126.00 - 112.50 - 93.56$$
$$(\mathbf{F}_m \times \mathbf{d}) = 301.08 \ \text{N} \cdot \text{m}$$

The main difference between the static and dynamic analyses, therefore, is the latter's inclusion of values for the moment of inertia and angular acceleration (i.e., consideration of the inertia forces and torques). Although these appear to have been obtained with minimal effort in this weight-lifting example, both measurements, particularly the angular acceleration, usually are the consequence of substantial data processing. In fact, a dynamic analysis is more difficult than a static analysis not because of gross differences associated with the theoretical construct but largely because of the general effort required to obtain the necessary data. In this example, the moment of inertia value was obtained from measurements made on cadavers whereas the angular acceleration value was derived from position-time data that were obtained from a film of a weight lifter performing the movement.

Impulse-Momentum

It is possible to conceive of human movement as the consequence of an interaction between the force developed by muscle and that provided by the surroundings, but these forces do not occur only at an instant in time. Rather, *motion is the result of forces applied over intervals of time*, a concept referred to as **impulse**. Figure 3.7, which illustrates the vertical component of the ground reaction force ($\mathbf{R}_z$) during running, provides an example of an application of a force over a period of time. An impulse is determined graphically as the area under a force-time curve (Figure 3.7), or numerically as the product of the mean force (N) and time (s). If the mean force ($\mathbf{R}_z$) in Figure 3.7 were 1.3 kN and the time of application 0.29 s, the impulse would be 377 N•s. It should be apparent that the magnitude of the impulse could be altered by varying, singly or in combination, either mean force or time of application.

If Newton's law of acceleration is interpreted to focus on epochs rather than instants of time, the law indicates that *the application of an impulse will result in a change in momentum of the system*. This is precisely the premise upon which the impulse-momentum approach to the analysis of motion is based. Momentum was previously used to describe the quantity of motion possessed by a system; it is

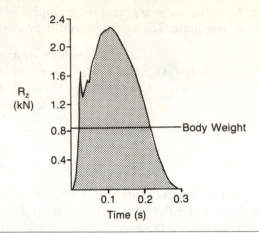

Figure 3.7. Graphic representation of an impulse as an area (shaded) under a force-time curve.

defined as mass times velocity (Equation 2.2) or, in angular terms, as the product of moment of inertia and angular velocity. If $\overline{\mathbf{F}}$ is the average force over a time interval (t), then the impulse-momentum relationship can be stated as

$$\overline{\mathbf{F}} \cdot t = \Delta m v \qquad (3.7)$$

The equation suggests that if the magnitude of the impulse is known, then its effect upon the momentum of the system can be calculated. Conversely, if the change in momentum can be measured, it is possible to determine the applied impulse.

For example, by filming a person spiking a volleyball and measuring the mass (m) of the ball, we can determine the impulse applied to the ball. From the film it would be necessary to measure both the velocity of the ball before (v_b) and after (v_a) contact and the total time the hand is in contact with the ball (t_c). Given these measurements,

$$v_b = 3.6 \text{ m} \cdot \text{s}^{-1}$$
$$v_a = 25.2 \text{ m} \cdot \text{s}^{-1}$$
$$m = 0.27 \text{ kg}$$
$$t_c = 18 \text{ ms}$$

And applying Equation 3.7,

$$\overline{\mathbf{F}} \cdot t = \Delta m v$$
$$= m \Delta v$$
$$= m(v_a - v_b)$$
$$= 0.27 (25.2 - 3.6)$$
$$\overline{\mathbf{F}} \cdot t = 5.83 \text{ N} \cdot \text{s}$$

Since we know the contact time (t_c), we can determine the average force (**F**) exerted by the spiker during the contact:

$$\overline{F} \cdot t = 5.83$$
$$\overline{F} = 5.83/t_c$$
$$= 5.83/0.018$$
$$\overline{F} = 324 \text{ N}$$

Thus, although the impulse appeared to be insignificant (5.83 N•s), the brief duration of the force application resulted in forces that were quite substantial ($\overline{F} = 324$ N). Incidentally, the time of contact with the volleyball in this example is quite similar to those (10-16 ms) recorded during the kicking of a ball (Asami & Nolte, 1983).

In most contact events, such as spiking a volleyball, the momentum of an object is altered by applying relatively high forces for brief periods of time. There are instances, however, in which the change in momentum is accomplished by applying smaller forces for longer periods. A good example (Brancazio, 1984) of this is the distinction between the consequences of a person jumping off a 15-m building onto the pavement and the consequences of another person diving off a 15-m cliff into the ocean. In both instances the individual will have a speed of about 17.3 m•s^{-1} just prior to contact. Eventually, however, the speed (and thus momentum) of each person will reach zero. The jumper will experience large forces (probably fatal) for a brief interval whereas the diver will encounter smaller forces over a longer period of time, but the change in momentum for each individual will be the same.

The running data included in Figure 2.12 provide yet another example of the impulse-momentum relationship. Consider the forward-backward component (R_y) of the ground reaction force during the support phase. The graph illustrates that the runner experiences two horizontal impulses during support; initially R_y is directed backward creating a retarding or braking impulse, and then R_y changes direction eliciting a propulsive impulse. Since these impulses act in opposite directions, the change in momentum that the runner (the system) experiences in the R_y direction depends on the difference between the braking and propulsion impulses. When the individual is running at a constant speed (no change in momentum), the two impulses will be equal. For a runner to increase speed, however, the propulsive impulse must exceed the braking impulse; to decrease speed, the converse is true.

Recall that statics presents a special case to the force-mass-acceleration approach in situations where one of the quantities of the equation is zero; the same is true for equations in the impulse-momentum context. Specifically, if there is no impulse applied to a system, then the left-hand side of Equation 3.7 is zero, a state in which momentum is said to be conserved. That is, *if there is no change in momentum then the momentum of the system must remain constant*; this can occur in linear and angular motion, the occurrence representing the principle of the **conservation of momentum**. However, conservation in both the linear and angular directions does not always occur at the same time. This is particularly evident in

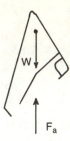

Figure 3.8. Forces experienced by a diver during free-fall. $\mathbf{F}_a$ = air resistance, $\mathbf{W}$ = weight.

free-fall, including such activities as gymnastics (e.g., Dainis, 1981; Nissinen, Preiss, & Brüggemann, 1985) and diving (e.g., Bartee & Dowell, 1982; Frohlich, 1980; Stroup & Bushnell, 1970; Wilson, 1977), and is classically demonstrated by the cat, which always lands on its feet when it is dropped (Kane & Scher, 1969; Magnus, 1922; Marey, 1894).

$$\text{impulse} = \Delta \text{ momentum}$$

Linear	Angular
$\bar{\mathbf{F}} \cdot t = \Delta mv$	$(\bar{\mathbf{F}} \times d) \cdot t = \Delta I_g \omega.$
Because	Because
$\bar{\mathbf{F}} = \mathbf{W} + \mathbf{F}_a$	$(\bar{\mathbf{F}} \times d) = 0$
then	then
$0 \neq \Delta mv.$	$0 = \Delta I_g \omega.$

Thus mv changes during free-fall. Thus $I_g \omega$ remains constant during free-fall.

Consider again the springboard diver mentioned earlier. Once the diver has left the board, there is no change in the angular momentum (quantity of angular motion) until contact is made with the water, but the linear momentum does change throughout the event. That is, the forces (weight and air resistance) acting on the diver exert a linear but not an angular (because they act through the CG and d = 0) effect (Figure 3.8). Since angular momentum remains constant and is equal to the product of moment of inertia and angular velocity, any change in one parameter (i.e., moment of inertia or angular velocity) will be accompanied by a complementary change in the other parameter. For example, suppose the diver was performing a multisomersault event in the pike position. If, during the dive, it became apparent that the diver would not make the appropriate number of revolutions, then one alternative (because angular momentum [**L**] remains constant) would be to assume a tuck position, which would be accompanied by an increase in the speed of rotation. The moment of inertia (I_g) of the diver about a horizontal axis that passes through the center of gravity is about 7.5 kg•m² in the pike position, as opposed to 4.5 kg•m² in the tuck. If, in the pike position, the person had an angular velocity (ω) of 6 rad•s⁻¹, then on changing to a tuck the speed would increase to 10 rad•s⁻¹ such that the product of the two parameters would remain constant (45 kg•m²•s⁻¹). Specifically,

$$L = I_g\omega$$

Pike	Tuck
L = 7.5 kg•m² × 6 rad/s	L = 4.5 kg•m² × 10 rad/s
L = 45 kg•m²•s⁻¹	L = 45 kg•m²•s⁻¹

and thus angular momentum (**L**) remains constant. If the diver wishes to slow the speed of rotation, then this is accomplished by increasing the moment of inertia, in this case, assuming a greater layout position (e.g., Miller, 1981).

The concept of momentum conservation is also applicable to linear motion, as exemplified by events that occur during collisions. Many sports activities are based on collisions, such as those between players (e.g., rugby, boxing), between a participant and an inanimate object (e.g., handball, soccer), and between inanimate objects (e.g., badminton, golf). *A collision does not create or destroy momentum; rather, the sum of the momentum of the colliding objects remains constant*. Consider, for example, the effects of two football players involved in a head-on tackle:

	Running back	Defensive back
mass:	100 kg	85 kg
velocity:	7.2 m•s⁻¹ (to the right)	−5.9 m•s⁻¹ (to the left)

$$
\begin{aligned}
\text{momentum after tackle} &= \text{momentum before tackle} \\
&= (100 \times 7.2) + (85 \times -5.9) \\
&= 720.0 - 501.5 \\
&= 218 \text{ kg•m•s}^{-1}
\end{aligned}
$$

Since momentum is a vector with the same direction as that of velocity, after the head-on tackle the running back will continue to move to the right albeit with a lesser momentum. At what speed will the two players, now joined in a tackle, move? In addition, the change in velocity experienced by each player will be inversely proportional to his mass—hence the advantage of size (mass) in contact sports.

Work-Energy

In contrast to the consideration of force at instants and epochs of time, the third type of analysis addresses *the ability of force to move objects*. If an object or system is moved some distance as the result of a force, it is described as having had **work** performed on it, where work is defined as the product of force and the distance the object has moved in the direction of the force. If a muscle force is applied

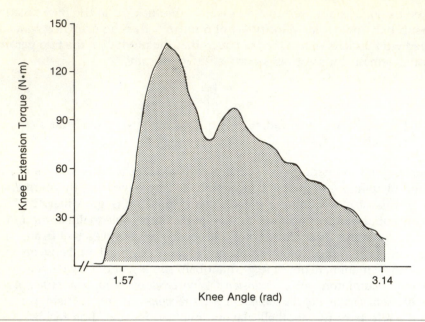

Figure 3.9. Idealized knee extensor torque-displacement curve for a single knee extension contraction, as measured with a Cybex II isokinetic dynamometer.

to an immovable object, then no work has been done on the object. Of course, energy had to be provided for the muscle contraction and thus metabolic work was performed, but since the object did not move, no (mechanical) work was done.

Work can be represented graphically as the area under the force-displacement (distance or length) curve. For example, a person rehabilitating from knee surgery uses a machine that can measure the resultant muscle torque (e.g., Cybex). Figure 3.9 depicts the torque exerted by the knee extensor muscles against the machine over a 1.57-rad range of motion. The work ($\overline{\mathbf{F}} \cdot d$) performed by these muscles on the machine can be calculated by measuring the area under the torque-displacement curve. If the average torque for the contraction illustrated in Figure 3.9 is 50 N•m, then work can be determined as follows:

$$\text{work} = \text{torque} \times \text{displacement}$$
$$\overline{\mathbf{F}} \cdot d = 50 \text{ N•m} \times 1.57 \text{ rad}$$
$$= 78.5 \text{ J}$$

where the quantity of work is measured in joules (J; 1 J = 1 N•m).

In the impulse-momentum approach the relationship between the two variables was such that the application of an impulse resulted in a change in the momentum of the system. Work and energy have a parallel relationship in that *the perfor-*

mance of work requires an expenditure of energy. **Energy** can be described as the capacity to do work; thus it can be regarded as a measure of the fuel available to the system for the performance of work. In fact, almost every process or change that occurs in nature can be considered in terms of the transformation of energy from one form to another. In this context, however, the word *fuel* refers to mechanical rather than metabolic parameters. Energy can exist in many forms, including several that are generally classified as mechanical—potential and kinetic energy represent two such forms. An object acquires potential energy when a force does work on it against another maintained force. An object acquires kinetic energy when a force does work against its inertia.

When work is done on an object to counteract the effect of another force, the object is described as possessing **potential energy**. In other words, once the force maintaining the object in the new position is removed, the object will tend to return to its original position and, in the process, will perform work. Thus the energy that an object has due to its position is referred to as potential energy (i.e., the object has the potential to do work). In the analysis of human movement, we commonly encounter two types of potential energy: (a) gravitational—potential energy due to the location of an object or system in a gravitational field above some baseline (e.g., the height of an object above the ground), and (b) elastic or strain—potential energy due to the stretch of an object (e.g., tennis racket) or tissue (e.g., muscle) beyond its resting length.

The magnitude of the gravitational potential energy (PE) can be determined by

$$PE = mgh \qquad (3.8)$$

where m represents mass, g indicates the acceleration due to gravity ($9.8 \text{ m} \cdot \text{s}^{-2}$), and h is the height of the system above the baseline (e.g., ground). For example, a 60-kg (mass) acrobat about to leap off a 10-m tower has a potential energy of 5.88 kJ. The instant the acrobat leaves the tower, there will be no supporting surface to provide a ground reaction force, and, because of gravity, the acrobat will fall. Mechanically, this observation can be explained as a conversion of energy from one form to another. **Kinetic energy** is defined as *the capacity of an object to perform work because of its motion*; therefore, the fall can be described as a change of the acrobat's energy from potential to kinetic. Because the acceleration due to gravity is constant, the speed of falling increases with the distance covered in the fall. This correlates with an increasing conversion from potential to kinetic energy.

Consider the system energy after the acrobat has fallen 4 m. At this position, the potential energy of the acrobat is 3.53 kJ, a decrease of 2.35 kJ. The kinetic energy (KE) of the system is determined by

$$KE = 1/2 \ mv^2 \qquad (3.9)$$

To calculate the kinetic energy of the acrobat after falling 4 m, it is necessary to determine the acrobat's velocity (**v**) at that point. Velocity can be calculated by using Equation 1.4 to determine the time (0.9045 s) it took the acrobat to fall 4 m and then using the definition of acceleration:

$$\mathbf{a} = \frac{\Delta \mathbf{v}}{\Delta t}$$

$$\mathbf{a} = \frac{\mathbf{v}_f - \mathbf{v}_i}{t}$$

$$9.81 = \frac{\mathbf{v}_f - 0}{0.904}$$

$$\mathbf{v}_f = 8.86 \text{ m} \cdot \text{s}^{-1}$$

where $\mathbf{v}_i$ and $\mathbf{v}_f$ refer to the initial (at the beginning of the fall) and the final (at 4 m) velocities, respectively. The final-velocity value (8.86 m·s⁻¹) can then be used in Equation 3.9 to determine the acrobat's kinetic energy at 4 m.

Alternatively, because KE = 1/2 mv² and because we know how much PE has been reduced (2.35 kJ) due to the law of conservation of mechanical energy ($PE_f + KE_f = PE_i + KE_i$), then we can determine $\mathbf{v}$ by rearranging this relation:

$$KE = 1/2 \, m\mathbf{v}^2$$

$$\mathbf{v} = \sqrt{\frac{2 \times KE}{m}}$$

$$= \sqrt{\frac{2 \times 2{,}350}{60}} \left(\frac{J}{kg} = \frac{N \cdot m}{kg} = \frac{kg \cdot m \cdot m}{kg \cdot s^2} \right)$$

$$= \sqrt{78.33 \quad m^2/s^2}$$

$$= 8.85 \text{ m/s}$$

Either way, we get a final velocity of about 8.85 m/s.

Thus the kinetic energy changed from zero as the acrobat began to fall to a value of 2.35 kJ after 4 m, an increase that matched the decrease in potential energy. This simple example, however, has assumed that the acrobat experienced no angular motion; but, in general, the kinetic energy of a system comprises both linear (1/2 mv²) and angular (1/2 Iω²) contributions, and hence,

$$KE = 1/2 \, m\mathbf{v}^2 + 1/2 \, I\omega^2 \tag{3.10}$$

Suppose the acrobat were to land on a trampoline. Upon contact the trampoline bed would begin to be stretched or strained, where **strain** refers to the change in length of an object per unit of the original length. The stretching of the trampoline bed can be described as the conversion of kinetic to potential (elastic or strain) energy. Elastic energy is a type of potential energy in that it represents the energy that an object possesses because of its tendency to return to its pre-stretched position. *Elastic energy, therefore, represents a restorative capability*. In human movement performance there are several instances in which consideration of the elastic energy capability of an object is essential to an analysis (e.g., diving board, archery bow, tennis racket). An equally important consideration is the elastic energy properties of biological tissue. Given the appropriate forces, biological tissue can be subjected to strains. Whether or not the tissue recovers its prestrain form depends upon the magnitude of the strain. If the magnitude is small and the tissue can recover, the strain exists within the **elastic** capabilities of the tissue. The ability of activated muscle to use energy in this form will be examined later in the text. However, if the amount of the strain exceeds the elastic capability of the material and the tissue cannot recover its prestrain length, the strain will induce **plastic** changes in the tissue. When people use stretching techniques to increase muscle length, they are actually attempting to cause plastic changes in the connective tissue (Sapega, Quedenfeld, Moyer, & Butler, 1981).

In terms of the work-energy relationship, work is equivalent to the change (Δ) in energy of the system:

$$\text{work} = \Delta \text{ energy}$$
$$\text{work} = \Delta PE + \Delta KE$$

An analysis based on this perspective involves determining the difference in system energy between two positions, the result of which represents the work done on or by the system. If the energy is transferred from the system to the surroundings, the work is done by the system. If the energy transfer proceeds in the opposite direction, work is done by the surroundings on the system. For example, when a person lifts a barbell by using the elbow flexors, the muscles shorten (concentric contraction) and perform work on the barbell, a situation that physiologists refer to as **positive work**. When the person lowers the barbell, however, the activated elbow flexors are lengthened (eccentric contraction) and the barbell does work on the muscles, an energy transfer known as **negative work**.

If we assume that the universe is a closed system, then we can use the idea that energy is not created or destroyed but rather conserved. As a consequence, when energy is used to perform work, it is not lost but changed into kinetic or potential energy of a system. However, the work-energy relationship is not a one-for-one exchange in that not all the energy made available is used to perform work; some of the energy is converted to heat. The proportion of the available energy (input) that provides fuel for the work (output) varies and depends on the efficiency of the conversion process. Muscle is often described as having an efficiency of about 25%, which means that 25% of the energy is used to perform work while the remaining 75% is converted into heat or used in recovery processes. This energy balance is derived from the first law of thermodynamics and can be represented as

$$\Delta C = \Delta H + W \tag{3.11}$$

where C = chemical energy, H = heat or thermal energy, and W = work.

These transformations can be quite difficult to follow during such complex events as human movement. Ward-Smith (1984), among others, has attempted to analyze various events in these terms. Figure 3.10 represents one such effort by a flow-diagram representation of sprinting. In this scheme, ATP (chemical energy) is provided by a variety of metabolic processes to the muscles for the performance of work. As mentioned, some of the ATP is converted into heat (H1). Although

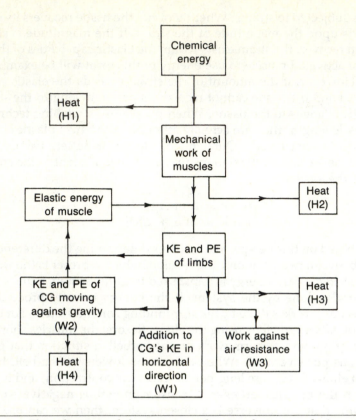

Figure 3.10. Flow-diagram of the energy exchanges that occur during running. *Note.* From ''Air Resistance and Its Influence on the Biomechanics and Energetics of Sprinting at Sea Level and at Altitude'' by A.J. Ward-Smith, 1984, *Journal of Biomechanics,* **17**, p. 340. Copyright 1984 by Pergamon Journals, Ltd. Adapted by permission.

the net result of these interactions is the performance of work by the runner on the environment, this is accomplished by the angular motion of the body segments. Accordingly, the work (positive and negative) done by the muscles provides kinetic (both translational and rotational) and potential energy to the limbs. In the process, however, some of the mechanical energy is degraded to heat (H2) due to frictional effects within joints and muscles. The mechanical energy (kinetic and potential) acquired by the limbs is transferred into kinetic and potential energy of the runner's CG and into work against air resistance (W3). Functionally, the mechanical energy of the CG can be partitioned into two effects: (a) W1—the addition of kinetic energy to its horizontal component; and (b) W2—an addition to the vertical component, which amounts to doing work against gravity. The kinetic and potential energy of the limbs and of the CG moving against gravity (W2) results in the storage of elastic energy in the muscles (including tendons) that can be recycled—this phenomenon is referred to as the storage and utilization of elastic energy. Over a number of strides, the net vertical displacement of the runner's CG is zero, and thus no work is done against gravity. Consequently, the ATP supplied to the muscles is ultimately converted into heat (H1 + H2 + H3 + H4) or used to do work (W1 + W3). The process of running, therefore, can be described as a repetitive sequence of the $\Delta C = \Delta H + W$ relationship.

In many short-duration events (e.g., 100-m sprint, Olympic weight lifting, arm wrestling), the rate at which muscles can produce work is often cited as the variable limiting performance. This ability is known as **power** and is measured as the amount of work done per unit of time. Thus power can be determined as work (**F** • d) divided by an amount of time (Δt), or as the product of force (**F**) and velocity (**v**). Since distance is synonymous with displacement ($\Delta \mathbf{r}$) in this context, the two expressions can be demonstrated as equivalent by the following:

$$\mathbf{F} \cdot d \cdot \Delta t^{-1} = \mathbf{F} \cdot \mathbf{v}$$
$$\mathbf{F} \cdot \Delta \mathbf{r} \cdot \Delta t^{-1} = \mathbf{F} \cdot \mathbf{v}$$
$$\mathbf{F} \cdot \frac{\Delta \mathbf{r}}{\Delta t} = \mathbf{F} \cdot \frac{\Delta \mathbf{r}}{\Delta t}$$

As a measure of the rate of work performance, power is measured in watts (W). Because work represents a change in the energy of the system, power can also be envisaged as the rate of energy utilization. Unlike the variables of position, velocity, acceleration, force, impulse, and momentum, which are vector quantities, the variables of work, energy, and power are scalar quantities (Appendix B).

Recall the elbow extension-flexion example (Figure 1.5) considered previously. Since power can be determined as the product of force and velocity and due to the proportionality between acceleration and force, the power-time profile associated with the movement would be obtained by multiplying the velocity and acceleration curves. When velocity and acceleration have the same sign (positive or negative), *power is positive and represents an energy flow from the muscles to the arm.* Conversely when *power is negative* (i.e., velocity and acceleration have opposite signs), *energy flows from the arm to the muscles.* These conditions are known as power **production** and **absorption**, respectively, indicating energy flow from and to the muscles. With regard to the elbow flexion-extension movement, positive velocity (above zero) indicates elbow extension, positive acceleration represents an extension-directed force, and positive power (production) represents energy flowing from the appropriate muscles to the system (forearm-hand). The power-time curve is determined by multiplying the velocity and acceleration (force) graphs. Whenever the velocity or acceleration graph crosses zero (i.e., changes sign) so does the power curve. The resulting power-time graph for the elbow flexion movement is depicted as a four-epoch event (Figure 3.11). The first two epochs, power production and absorption, respectively, occur during elbow extension (see velocity-time graph) and represent periods of positive and negative work. During positive work, the muscles do work on the system, and during negative work the system (due to its inertia) does work on the muscles. A

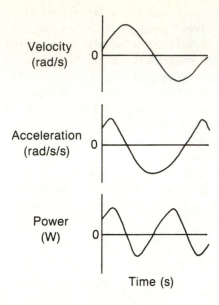

Figure 3.11. Power-time profile associated with the muscles across the elbow joint during the event depicted in Figure 1.5. Positive velocity represents an extension movement; positive acceleration indicates an acceleration in the direction of extension; positive power (production) refers to the power produced by the system. The four phases of the power-time graph (production, absorption, production, absorption) correspond to the four bursts of muscle activity (concentric extensor, eccentric flexor, concentric flexor, eccentric extensor) associated with this movement.

similar sequence (power production then absorption) occurs during the flexion phase of the movement.

This example emphasizes the correlation between the concepts of positive and negative work, power production and absorption, and concentric and eccentric muscle activity. As shown in the lower panel of Figure 3.11, the elbow extension-flexion movement is associated with a four-phase power-time profile. The epochs of power production correspond to periods of positive work and, therefore, concentric muscle activity. Recall that in chapter 1 we determined that this movement involved a sequence of activity: concentric extensor, eccentric flexor, concentric flexor, and eccentric extensor activity. According to this scheme, therefore, power absorption is related to negative work and eccentric muscle activity (Figure 3.11).

Such an analysis, however, is only a first approximation, because in reality not all the power observed during the production phase (especially the second production phase) is produced by the muscle. Some is probably due to the elastic stretch applied to the muscles and tendons. We will consider this possibility in more detail in Part III.

Problems

3.1. The following systems are in equilibrium, acceleration is equal to zero, and thus

$$\sum F_x = 0$$
$$\sum F_y = 0$$
$$\sum M_o = 0$$

Determine the magnitude of the unknown forces.

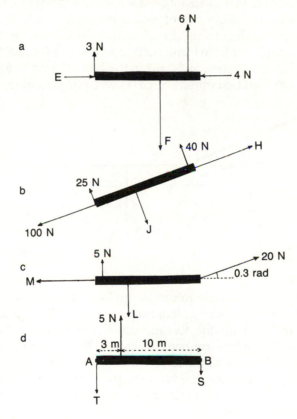

3.2. The following are x- and y-coordinates for the lower limb:

Hip   0.47, 0.74

Knee 0.71, 0.47

Ankle 0.63, 0.09

Toes   0.73, 0.00

Plot these points on graph paper and join them to form a stick figure of the lower limb. Use the regression equations listed in Table 2.1 to find the location of the CG for the lower limb.

3.3. The product of mass and acceleration is referred to as
  a. inertia torque
  b. moment of inertia
  c. inertia force
  d. impulse
  e. contact force

3.4. Find the resultant elbow flexor force (F) that is required to keep the forearm and hand in a horizontal position. The forearm and hand together weigh 30 N, and the center of gravity for the system is located 12 cm from the axis of the elbow joint (E). The resultant muscle force is applied 5 cm along the segment from E and pulls at an angle of 0.4 rad. If a 100-N weight is added to the system and held in the hand (25 cm from the elbow joint axis), what resultant muscle force (F) is required to maintain equilibrium?

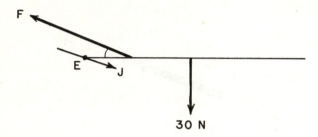

3.5. What resultant muscle force (F), pulling at an angle of 0.6 rad to the forearm-hand and acting 5 cm from the elbow (E) joint axis, would be required to maintain the forearm-hand in a position 0.2 rad above the horizontal? The forearm-hand weighs 45 N, with the point of application of the weight vector located 10 cm from E. Before beginning the calculation, draw an accurate free-body diagram of the system. How much of the resultant muscle force (F) tends to cause rotation, and how much contributes to stabilization?

3.6. In 1680, Borelli observed that a man can support a mass (R) of 20 libra (probably a weight of 67 N) from the tip of his thumb (A in Figure Problem 3.6). What resultant force (F_m) must the muscles (flexor and extensor pollicis longus) across the distal phalangeal (P) joint exert to support this weight? (B) The appropriate free-body diagram is indicated, where W represents the phalanx weight (0.5 N) and F_j the joint reaction force.

A   **B**

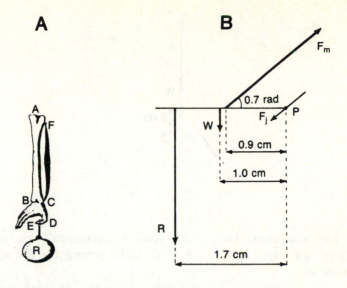

Note. From "Mechanics of Skeleton and Tendons" by R.M. Alexander, 1981, in V.B. Brooks (Ed.), *Handbook of Physiology: Sec. I. The Nervous System: Vol. II. Motor Control. Part I* (p. 28), Bethesda, MD: American Physiological Society. Copyright 1981 by the American Physiological Society. Adapted by permission.

3.7. Consider the following free-body diagram of a forearm-hand system in which the system is oriented vertically: the cross-sectional area of the elbow flexors ($F_{m,e}$) is 14 cm², the weight (**W**) of the system is 40 N, the joint reaction force (F_j) has a magnitude of 850 N, and the $F_{m,e}$ vector is at an angle of 0.3 rad to the forearm-hand.

   a. If muscle has a specific tension of 27 N•cm⁻², determine the maximum torque that $F_{m,e}$ can exert about the elbow joint (E) in the position shown.

   b. Determine the magnitude of the normal and tangential components of the force exerted by $F_{m,e}$.

   c. If the forearm-hand has a length of 43 cm, and the center of gravity (g) is located at 32% of that length from the proximal end of the segment, how far is it from E to g?

   d. Calculate the magnitude of the net muscle torque required to maintain the system in a vertical position.

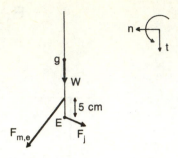

3.8. Which statements (a-e) about types of movement analysis are incorrect? Only one part (i-vi) of a-e needs to be wrong for the statement to be incorrect.

    i. The right-hand side of Newton's law of acceleration is nonzero in a dynamic analysis.
    ii. The mass-acceleration diagram includes all the external forces.
    iii. Impulse is the term that describes the application of a force over a period of time.
    iv. Momentum describes the quality of motion.
    v. Strain energy is a form of potential energy.
    vi. As a muscle performs positive work, it is described as producing power.

    a. iii, v
    b. vi, i
    c. iv, iii
    d. i, v
    e. ii, iv

3.9. Identify the correct statement(s) (a-e) about the work-energy relationship. Both parts (i-v) of a-e have to be correct for the statement(s) to be correct.

    i. Energy can be described as the capacity to do work.
    ii. Work can be determined as the area under a force-time curve.
    iii. Kinetic energy is not affected by the height of the object above the ground.
    iv. Positive work refers to the performance of work by the system.
    v. Power is calculated as the product of force and distance.

    a. v, ii
    b. iii, i
    c. iv, v
    d. ii, iii
    e. i, iv

3.10. A photograph was taken of an athlete rehabilitating from knee surgery. The lower leg-foot (W_l) weighed 120 N and the ankle weight (W_a) was 250 N.

a. What is the magnitude of the load torque in this position?

b. If the leg were being lowered,

    i.   what muscle group would be controlling the movement?

    ii. what is the maximum torque (T_m) that the muscle group may exert and still allow the leg to be lowered?

c. Suppose the moment of inertia of the system about the knee joint (K) had a magnitude of 0.11 kg•m². What magnitude of torque (T_m) would the athlete have to exert to obtain a system acceleration of 9.4 rad/s²? (Hint: Perform a dynamic analysis including the drawing of free-body and mass-acceleration diagrams.)

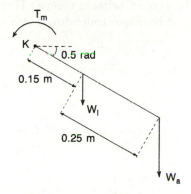

3.11. A golf ball has a mass of 46 g. When a golf ball is hit with a driver its speed will change from 0 to about 60 m•s⁻¹.

a. What is the change in momentum of the ball?

b. If the time of contact of the club with the ball is 0.5 ms, what is the average force on the ball?

c. If the clubhead has a mass of 200 g and a speed of 28 m•s⁻¹ just prior to contacting the ball, what is the speed of the clubhead after hitting the ball?

3.12. A baseball weighs 1.43 N and has a speed of 24.4 m•s⁻¹ just prior to being caught by the catcher. What is the kinetic energy of the ball?

3.13. A skier (weight = 653 N) leaves from the top of a ski jump that is 90 m above the takeoff area of the jump. Neglecting friction and air resistance, what is the jumper's speed at takeoff?

3.14. In walking across a tightrope sideways, a circus performer begins to fall backward. According to the conservation of momentum principle, in which direction (forward or backward) will the performer's arms be circled so that balance is maintained? Explain the reason for your choice—a diagram would be helpful.

3.15. A soccer ball (weight = 4.17 N) was traveling at 7.62 m•s⁻¹ until it was contacted by the head of a soccer player and sent traveling at 12.8 m•s⁻¹ in the opposite direction. If the ball were in contact with the player's head for 22.7 ms, what was the average force applied to the ball?

3.16. According to Stevenson (1985), a diver (58 kg) entering the water from a 10-m tower experiences a change in vertical velocity of 16.8 m/s to 5.2 m/s in 133 ms. What was the average force exerted by the water on the diver to get this change in momentum?

3.17. Vaughan (1980) obtained the following position-, velocity-, and acceleration-time histories for the CG of a person bouncing on a trampoline. Use these data to graph qualitatively the power-time relationship during this event; use the same approach as in Figure 3.11. Once you have drawn the graph, explain what it means. The person is in contact with the trampoline bed between touchdown and takeoff.

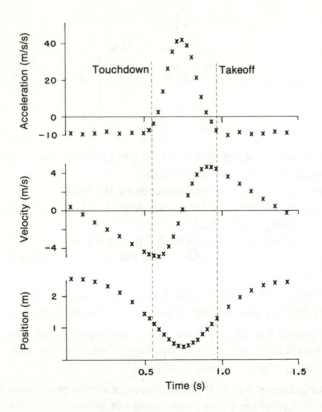

Note. From "A Kinetic Analysis of Basic Trampoline Stunts" by C.L. Vaughan, 1980, *Journal of Human Movement Studies*, **6**, p. 241. Copyright 1980 by Henry Kimpton (Publishers) Ltd. Adapted by permission.

Summary—Part I

In this first part of the text (chapters 1-3), the goal has been to define the mechanical bases of movement. At the beginning of Part I a number of specific objectives were listed. At this point it seems appropriate to list the major concepts with which you should now be familiar:

- Understand the definitions of and relationships (numeric and graphic) between the kinematic variables position, velocity, and acceleration.
- Know how to read a graph carefully and to interpret the relationship (between two or more variables) that is shown.
- Realize that many of the details of projectile motion can be determined from the definitions of position, velocity, and acceleration, without the use of lengthy formulae.
- Consider force as a concept used to describe an interaction the magnitude of which can be determined using Newton's laws, particularly the law of acceleration.
- Use a free-body diagram to define the conditions of an analysis and the free-body and the mass-acceleration diagrams as a graphic version of Newton's law of acceleration.
- Conceive of torque as the rotary effect of a force in which torque is defined as the product of force and moment arm.
- Realize that force acting over time (impulse) causes a change in the momentum (quantity of motion) of a system.
- Understand that the performance of work (force × distance) requires the expenditure of energy and that the work can be done by the system (positive) or on the system (negative).
- Consider power as a measure of the rate of doing work or the rate of using energy.

II

The Simple Joint System

Human movement is a complex phenomenon. To examine the neuromechanical bases of human movement it is necessary to make a variety of simplifying assumptions. For example, in Part I ("The Force-Motion Relationship") we assumed that the force exerted by muscle acts on rigid body segments, and we ignored the complexity of muscle with its great variety of structure and attachment sites in that we described muscle as either a generic flexor or extensor of a joint. Although these simplifications are barely acceptable, they do allow us to address some of the basic concepts associated with the study of movement. Part II continues this focus by describing the human body as a system of rigid links that are rotated by muscles about pinned frictionless joints. The activation of muscle is controlled (neurons) and monitored (sensory receptors) by the nervous system. *These five elements (i.e., rigid link, synovial joint, muscle, neuron, sensory receptor) comprise the basic apparatus for the production of human movement and thus form a biological model that is called the simple joint system* (Figure II.1). It is important to realize that Figure II.1 is just a model. Although the model only includes one neuron, there are generally hundreds of neurons that innervate each muscle and provide both motor commands (motoneurons) and sensory

information (sensory receptors). Similarly, about each joint there are generally groups of muscles, each of which controls movement in one direction (e.g., flexion vs. extension). In Part II we shall first review simplified descriptions of these five elements ("System Components") and then consider several of the interactions between the elements ("System Operation") that are important in the elaboration of movement.

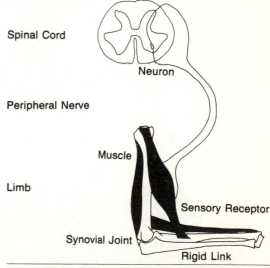

Figure II.1. The five elements of the simple joint system: neuron, muscle, rigid link, synovial joint, and sensory receptor.

Objectives

The goal of this text is to describe movement as the interaction of a biological model (a simplified version of us) with the physical world in which we live. In Part I, we examined the mechanical bases of movement, focusing on the relationship between force and motion. The aim of this second part is to define a biological model and to describe the interactions among its elements. Specific objectives include the following:

- To describe the simple joint system and to explain why it is an adequate model for the study of the basic features of movement.
- To list the details of the structural characteristics of the five elements of the simple joint system.
- To define the basic functional unit of the system.
- To explain the means by which information is transmitted rapidly throughout the system.
- To outline the link between the neural signal and muscle contraction.
- To examine the role of afferent information in the operation of the system.

4

Simple Joint System Components

It is anticipated that you have been exposed to much of the chapter 4 material in a prior anatomy course. The material is repeated here to emphasize a functional focus. Indeed, perhaps the most important task in chapter 4 is to emphasize that *the morphological and mechanical features of the simple joint system elements are determined largely by the functions they serve*. To realize this emphasis, the central focus of each topic is the function of the structure.

Rigid Link

Many different tissues provide a structural framework for the simple joint system. In general these are known as connective tissue and comprise living (cells) and nonliving (intercellular material) substances that are bathed in tissue fluid. The cells (e.g., fibroblasts, macrophages, fat cells, mast cells) perform functions necessary for the maintenance of the tissue. The intercellular material, which forms the matrix in which the cells live and includes the proteins collagen, elastin, and

reticulum, determines the physical characteristics of the tissue. The connecting elements that comprise the rigid link of the simple joint system include bone, tendon, and ligament.

Bone

Bone is a living tissue consisting of a protein matrix upon which calcium salts (especially phosphate) are deposited. Water accounts for 20% of the wet weight of bone; the protein matrix, which is mainly osteocollagenous fibers, represents 35%, and the bone salts account for 45% of the wet weight. The osteocollagenous fibers determine the strength and resilience of bone. The strength of bone (the force necessary to break the bone) depends on the angle and the direction at which the force is being applied. The human femur has a strength of 132 $MN \cdot m^{-2}$ when a tensile force is applied along the length of the bone (tangential) but a strength of only 58 $MN \cdot m^{-2}$ for tensile forces acting perpendicular (normal) to the bone; compressive strength is 187 and 132 $MN \cdot m^{-2}$ for tangential and orthogonal forces, respectively, that are applied to the femur (Cowin, 1983). These numbers underscore the notion that *bone is strongest in the direction that it is most frequently stressed*. Put another way, function has a major effect on the mechanical characteristics of bone. In engineering terms, it appears that bones are designed with safety factors of between two and five; that is, bones are two to five times stronger than the forces they commonly encounter in everyday activities (Alexander, 1984a).

Bone performs several functions essential to movement production, including (a) providing mechanical support as the central structure of each body segment, (b) producing red blood cells, and (c) serving as an active ion reservoir for calcium and phosphorous. As a living tissue, the status of bone is related to the stress that is imposed upon it. **Wolff's law** characterizes this relationship by stating that all changes in the function of bone are attended by alterations in its internal structure. For example, an increase in weight bearing results in an increase in the thickness and density of bone. Living bone is continually undergoing processes of growth, reinforcement, and resorption, which are collectively termed **remodeling** (Lanyon & Rubin, 1984). The time required for one complete cycle of remodeling (replacement of all the structures) seems to be about 10-20 years for limb bones of the adult human (Alexander, 1984a). These processes generally occur over months or years. For example, Shumskii, Merten, and Dzenis (1978) found a greater deposition and density of bone in the tibia of athletes compared to control subjects. Similarly, Dalén and Olsson (1974) found that bone mineral content for cross-country runners (25 years experience) was 20% greater in appendicular sites (distal radius, ulna, calcaneus) but less than 10% greater in axial sites (lumbar vertebrae and head of the femur) compared to a control group of subjects. At the other end of the

spectrum, it appears that one of the major problems that will be faced by people who spend several months on the space station will be loss of bone tissue. It has been quite well documented that the zero-gravity conditions of space flight cause bone **demineralization**, the excessive loss of salts from the skeleton (Anderson & Cohn, 1985). These results strongly suggest that *cyclic loading* plays a major role in modulating bone mass.

Tendon and Ligament

As connecting elements, tendon links muscle to bone and ligament connects bone to bone. The structural organization of these two elements differs to accommodate their respective functions. Since the function of tendon is to transmit muscle force to bone or cartilage, the structure of tendon is such that it is least susceptible to deformation from **tensile** forces (i.e., the pulling force exerted by muscle). Tendon can withstand **stress** (force per unit area) of up to 80 MN•m⁻² before the tissue is damaged. The greater the cross-sectional area of tendon the greater the force it can transmit. In contrast, only small longitudinal-pushing (**compressive**) and side-to-side (**shear**) forces are required to deform tendon. In contrast, the primary function of ligament is joint stabilization. Since a joint can be subjected to tensile, compressive, and shear forces, the structure of ligament has evolved to provide multidirectional stability.

The collagen **fibril** (Figure 4.1) is the basic load-bearing unit of both tendon and ligament. The structure of the fibril from the alpha chains of the triple helix to the packing of the collagen molecules in the microfibril is the same for tendon and ligament. The major distinction between the two connecting elements concerns *the way in which the fibrils are arranged*. In tendon, the fibrils are arranged

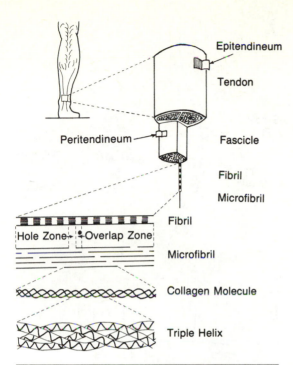

Figure 4.1. The hierarchical organization of tendon to the level of the triple helix of collagen.

longitudinally in parallel to maximize the resistance to tensile forces. In ligament, the fibrils are aligned in parallel, oblique, or spiral arrangements to accommodate forces in different directions.

The **triple-helix** structure of collagen indicates that the molecule consists of three intertwined polypeptide chains. Each polypeptide chain consists of a sequence of about 1,000 amino acids (e.g., proline, hydroxyproline, glycine) and is known as an **alpha chain**. The three-stranded collagen molecules are then arranged end to end (in series), and five such rows are stacked in parallel (side to side) to form the **microfibril**. The collagen fibril, which is the basic load-bearing unit of ten-

don and ligament, consists of bundles of microfibrils held together by cross-linkages. Since these cross-links bind the microfibrils together, *the number and state of the cross-links are thought to have a substantial effect on the strength of the connective tissue* (Bailey, Robins, & Balian, 1974). Thus the functional focus of tendon and ligament is the fibril, a collection of units (microfibrils) bound together by cross-links. The strength of the fibril depends on these cross-links. The number and state of the cross-links are thought to be determined by function.

The connective tissue proteins (collagen, elastin, reticulum) are not merely inert structural proteins; they are known to play active roles in developmental and regenerative processes, cell attachment, chemotaxis, and the binding of antigen-antibody complexes. One radical example that challenges traditional thought on connective tissue suggests that the primary function of ligaments is not structural but neurosensory; that is, ligaments provide the nervous system with information about the state of the joint (Brand, 1986). The distinction between adjacent tissues is not abrupt but rather involves a gradual transition from one to the other. For example, elements of tendon often extend into a muscle, especially pinnate muscles, well beyond the musculotendinous junction. Similarly, the insertion of tendon into bone involves a transition from tendon to fibrocartilage, to mineralized fibrocartilage, to lamellar bone. It is these junctions between bone-ligament and bone-tendon that are the most susceptible to injury (separation). As with other connecting elements, however, these junctions as well as tendon and ligament strength are known to be affected by activity; increased use results in increased strength (Woo et al., 1980; Wunder, Matthes, & Tipton, 1982a, 1982b) and enhances the healing process (Vailas, Tipton, Matthes, & Gart, 1981).

Synovial Joint

There are about 206 bones in the human body, and these form approximately 200 joints or articulations. Joints are generally classified as belonging to one of three groups: the fibrous joint, which is relatively immovable (e.g., sutures of skull, interosseus membrane between radius and ulna or tibia and fibula); the cartilaginous joint, which is slightly movable (e.g., sternocostal, intervertebral discs, pubic symphysis); or the synovial joint, which is freely movable (e.g., hip, elbow, atlanto-axial). Since the synovial joint most closely approximates the frictionless pinned joint of the rigid-link assumption, it is taken as the joint component of the simple joint system.

Figure 4.2 illustrates the characteristics of a **synovial joint**. The surfaces of the bones that form the joint are lined with a viscoelastic gel reinforced with collagen known as **articular cartilage**. The function of articular cartilage is to absorb impacts, to prevent direct wear to the bones, and to modify the shape of the bone to insure better contact with the next bone. Articular cartilage is thicker in more active individuals and increases in thickness when an individual goes from a resting to an active state. The thickness of the articular cartilage is altered by the amount of fluid that is absorbed; the more fluid absorbed, the less compressible the cartilage becomes and therefore the more protection the cartilage provides. The articulating surfaces are enclosed in a **joint capsule**, which attaches to the two bones and thus separates the joint cavity from surrounding tissues. The internal aspect of the capsule and those areas of the articulating bones that are not covered with articular cartilage are lined with **synovial membrane**, a vascular membrane that secretes synovial fluid into the joint cavity. The synovial fluid provides nourishment for the articular cartilage and

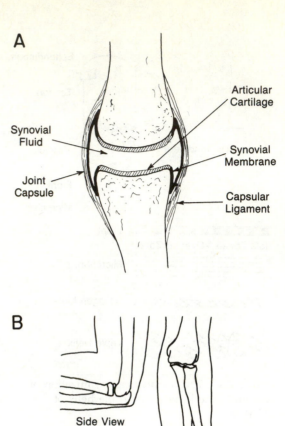

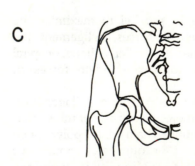

Figure 4.2. Selected features of the synovial joint. (A) Gross morphological elements. (B) A one-degree-of-freedom joint, the elbow. (C) A three-degree-of-freedom joint, the hip. Architectural differences largely determine the range of motion of a joint.

lubricates the joint. The joint capsule is a loose structure that surrounds the entire joint and, in some places, fuses with capsular ligaments, which are typically thought to keep the articulating surfaces in close proximity.

In one sense, the structure of the synovial joint shown in Figure 4.2 is an oversimplification. The structure of the joint (i.e., bone-on-bone architecture, ligaments, capsule) is quite variable and largely determines the *quality* of motion between two adjacent body segments. The joint will permit rotation about one to three axes. These axes could pass through the joint (figuratively) from side to side, from front to back, or up and down. Each axis is referred to as a **degree of freedom**. The only motion possible at the elbow joint is in the flexion-extension plane, which is rotation about an axis that passes side to side through the joint. In contrast, the hip and shoulder joints have three degrees of freedom, which means that rotation is possible about each of the axes due to the joint structure. Motion at these joints can occur in the flexion-extension plane, the abduction-adduction plane, and rotation about a longitudinal axis.

Muscle

Muscles are molecular machines that convert chemical energy, initially derived from food, into force. The properties of muscle include (a) irritability—the ability to respond to a stimulus, (b) conductivity—the ability to propagate a wave of excitation, (c) contractility—the ability to modify its length, and (d) a limited growth and regenerative capacity. In histology, there are three types of vertebrate muscle: cardiac, smooth, and skeletal. Only skeletal muscle is considered in the simple-joint-system analysis of human movement. Cardiac muscle, which makes up

most of the heart wall, is composed of a network of individual cells that show obvious striations. Smooth muscle, which is found in the viscera and in the walls of blood vessels, consists of individual cells that are separated by a thin cleft and that lack apparent striations. Skeletal muscle comprises fused cells in which the striations are well defined. With the exception of some facial muscles, skeletal muscles act across joints to produce rotation of body segments. The ensuing comments on muscle refer specifically to skeletal muscle (Figure 4.3). The role of muscle in the simple joint system is to provide a force that interacts with those exerted by the environment on the system. This interaction, in turn, causes the rigid links to rotate about their joint.

Muscle contains a great many identifiable elements. In the process of piecing together these elements, you are encouraged to focus on the function of muscle and the process by which the function is carried out. In particular, you are encouraged to focus on the elements related to *two critical aspects of muscle function: the relationship between the sarcolemma and the sarcoplasmic reticulum and the components of the sarcomere.* As we shall note in chapter 5, these two sets of elements are functionally associated with the connection between the nervous system and muscle (sarcolemma-sarcoplasmic reticulum) and the force that muscle can exert (sarcomere).

Gross Structure

Muscle fibers are linked together by a three-level network of collagenous connective tissue; **endomysium** surrounds individual fibers, **perimysium** collects bundles of fibers into fascicles, and **epimysium** ensheaths the entire muscle. Fibers vary from 1 to 400 mm in length and 10 to 60 μm in diameter. The cell membrane encircling each set of myofilaments that comprises a muscle fiber is

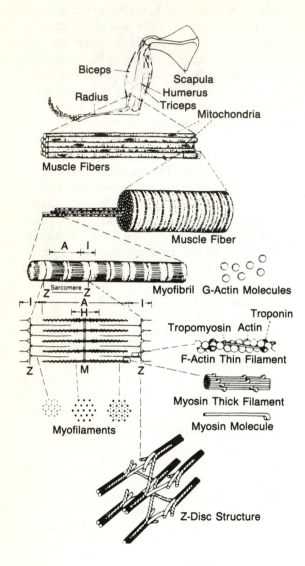

Figure 4.3. Organization of skeletal muscle from the gross to the molecular level. The figure emphasizes the bands and zones that comprise the sarcomere and the molecular components of the thick and thin filaments. *Note.* From T.A. McMahon, *Muscles, Reflexes, and Locomotion*. Copyright © 1984 by Thomas A. McMahon. Published by Princeton University Press. Figure 3.2 reprinted with permission of Princeton University Press.

known as the **sarcolemma**. As a plasma membrane, the sarcolemma provides active and passive selective membrane transport—this is an essential property of excitable membranes. That is, the sarcolemma allows some material to pass through (passive transport) whereas it actually helps other material to pass through (active transport). The sarcolemma is about 7.5-nm thick. The fluid enclosed within the fiber by the sarcolemma is referred to as **sarcoplasm**. Within the sarcoplasm are fuel sources (e.g., lipid droplets, glycogen granules), organelles (e.g., nuclei, mitochondria, lysosomes), enzymes (e.g., myosin ATPase, phosphorylase), and the contractile machinery (bundles of **myofilaments** arranged into **myofibrils**).

In addition, the sarcoplasm contains an extensive, hollow, membranous system that is linked to the surface sarcolemma and assists the muscle in conducting commands from the nervous system. This membranous system includes the sarcoplasmic reticulum, lateral sacs (terminal cisternae), and transverse (T) tubules (Figure 4.4). The **sarco-**

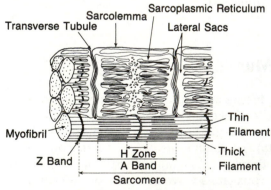

Figure 4.4. Alignment of the transverse tubules and sarcoplasmic reticulum with respect to the myofibrils. *Note.* From *A Textbook of Histology* (9th ed.) (p. 281) by W. Bloom and D.W. Fawcett, 1968, Philadelphia: W.B. Saunders. Copyright 1968 by W.B. Saunders. Adapted by permission.

plasmic reticulum runs longitudinally along the fiber, parallel to and surrounding the myofibrils. At specific locations along the myofibril, the sarcoplasmic reticulum bulges into **lateral sacs**. Perpendicular to the sarcoplasmic reticulum and associated with the lateral sacs are **transverse** tubules, branching invaginations of the sarcolemma. The term **triad** refers to one transverse tubule plus two terminal cisternae of the sarcoplasmic reticulum, one on each side of the T tubule. As we shall see in more detail later, this triad aids in the rapid communication between the sarcolemma and the contractile machinery.

Sarcomere

Skeletal muscle fibers can be regarded as a series of repeating units, each of which comprises the same characteristic banded structure. Histologically, this unit is defined as a **sarcomere** and represents the zone of a myofibril from one **Z band** to another. In other words, a myofibril is a series of sarcomeres added end to end. The sarcomere is the basic contractile unit of muscle and comprises an interdigitating set of thick and thin contractile proteins (Figure 4.3). Because a sarcomere has a length of about 2.5 μm in resting muscle, a 10-mm myofibril represents 4,000 sarcomeres added end to end. Each myofibril is composed of bundles of myofilaments (thick and thin contractile proteins). In many muscles, however, myofibrils are difficult to identify, and hence it is more appropriate to emphasize the myofilaments (Hoyle, 1983).

The obvious striations of skeletal muscle are due to the differential refraction of light as it passes through the contractile proteins. The thick-filament zone, which includes some interdigitating thin filaments, is doubly refractive (i.e., the formation of two refracted rays of light from a single incoming ray) and forms the dark or **A band** (anisotropic). With-

in the A band is a zone that contains only thick filaments. Since this zone is clear of thin filaments, it is known as the **H band** (Hellerscheibe or clear disk). The area between the A bands contains predominantly thin filaments and, as it is singly refractive, is called the **I band** (isotropic).

Each set of filaments (thick and thin) is attached to a central transverse band; the thick filaments attach to the **M band** (Mittelscheibe or middle disk; the band located in the middle of the A band), and the thin filaments connect to the **Z band** (Zwischenscheibe or between disk). A cross-sectional view through the A band illustrates the relationship between the interdigitating filaments. As shown in Figure 4.3, each thick filament (the large dots) is surrounded by six thin filaments (the small dots) whereas a single thin filament can interact with only three thick filaments.

Myofilaments

Both the thick and thin filaments are comprised of several different proteins. The structure of the thin filament is dominated by actin but also includes the regulatory proteins tropomyosin and troponin. Each actin filament is composed of two helical strands of **F** (**fibrous**) **actin** (Figure 4.3). Each F-actin strand is a polymer (i.e., chemical union of two or more molecules) of some 200 **G-** (**globular**) **actin** molecules.

A G-actin molecule is a protein containing about 374 amino acids. Located in each groove of the F-actin helix are two coiled strands of **tropomyosin** (Figure 4.5A). The structure of tropomyosin is referred to as a two-chain coiled-coil; each of these chains contains approximately 284 amino acids. The **troponin** (TN) complex has a globular structure (Figure 4.5A) that includes three subunits (Figure 4.5B); the **TN-T** unit binds

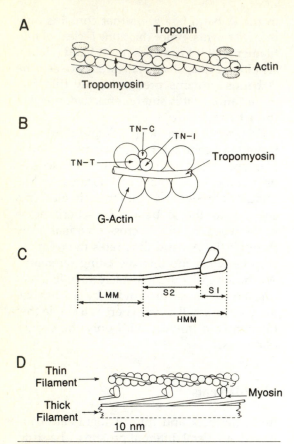

Figure 4.5. Organization of the myofilaments. (A) The thin filament. (B) Troponin (TN) elements. (C) Fragments of the myosin molecule. (D) Alignment of the thick and thin filaments.

same way during a muscle contraction; *tropomyosin and troponin impose their influence on the activity of actin*.

A set of thin filaments that projects longitudinally into one sarcomere connects in the Z-band region to another set, which projects in the opposite direction into an adjacent sarcomere. At this connection, each thin filament appears to be linked to its four closest opposing neighbors. A region of considerable flexibility, the Z band changes its shape under different conditions. Z-band width can vary from one muscle fiber to another (e.g., different muscle-fiber types), and it probably also varies as a consequence of training (Sjöström et al., 1982; Sjöström, Kidman, Larsén, & Ängquist, 1982).

Of the thick filament proteins, most is known about the **myosin** molecule. It is a long, two-chain, helical tail that terminates in two large globular heads (Figure 4.5C). The myosin molecule can be decomposed into **light meromyosin (LMM)** and **heavy meromyosin (HMM)** fragments, the latter of which is further subdivided into **subfragments 1** and **2 (S1** and **S2)**. The globular heads, one of which contains an ATP- and the other an actin-binding site, are known as S1. The remaining portion of HMM is called S2.

Since LMM binds strongly to itself under physiological conditions, approximately 400 myosin molecules aggregate to form the dominant element of the thick filament (Pepe & Drucker, 1979). The union is not random but rather quite structured. The molecules are aligned in pairs, and the S1 element of each molecule is oriented to its partner at 3.14 rad (180 degrees). The next pair is displaced by a translation of about 0.0143 μm and a rotation of 2.1 rad (120 degrees). The result is an ordered alignment of myosin molecules in which the HMM projections encircle the thick filament (Figure 4.3). Each sarcomere actually contains two such sets of myosin molecules; however, because the S1 elements of the two

troponin to tropomyosin, **TN-I** inhibits four to seven G-actin molecules from binding to myosin when tropomyosin is present, and **TN-C** can reversibly bind Ca²⁺ ions as a function of calcium concentration. TN-C has four binding sites, two for Ca^{2+} and two for Ca^{2+} or Mg^{2+}. Thus the thin filament has as its backbone two strands of actin molecules (F actin) upon which are superimposed (wrapped around or attached) two-strand (tropomyosin) and globular (troponin) proteins. These proteins operate in much the sets point in opposite directions, the LMM fragments unite in the M band (Figure 4.3) to form a single thick filament.

The myosin molecules contain two hinge regions (i.e., regions of relatively greater flexibility). These occur at the LMM-HMM and S1-S2 junctions. In the resulting alignment, the HMM fragment can extend from the thick filament to within close proximity of the thin filament (Figure 4.5D). Due to the ability of S1 to interact with actin, *the HMM extension has been called the **crossbridge***. Each thick filament is surrounded by and can interact with six thin filaments (Figure 4.3) since the HMM projections encircle the thick filament.

Neuron

We have thus far described the rigid-link elements, a joint about which they rotate, and an organ known as muscle that is capable of exerting a force on the rigid links. Next we turn our attention to the nervous system and its cellular components, which represent the means by which we activate muscle. The nervous system comprises several functional elements:

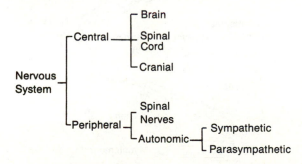

The organization of the central nervous system within the human body is illustrated in Figure 4.6. The spinal cord is described as

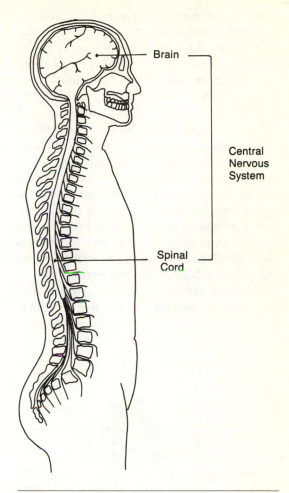

Figure 4.6. The gross organization of the central nervous system.

a process that extends from the brain. Both components are encased in bony protective structures: the brain in the skull and the spinal cord in the vertebral column. Branches (roots) extend from the spinal cord between each pair of vertebrae. These branches contribute to peripheral nerves that innervate various structures, including muscle.

There are only two cell types in the nervous system: **neurons** and **neuroglia**. The neuron is characterized by a distinctive cell shape, an outer membrane (axolemma) capable of generating and conducting an electrical signal, and a unique structure (synapse) for the transfer of information. Less is known about the neuroglia, which are nine times more numerous than neurons. They are primarily thought to provide structural, metabolic, and protective support for the neurons. For example, two prominent functions known to be performed by glial cells are myelination and phagocytosis. Myelination is accomplished by oligodendrocytes in the central nervous system and by Schwann cells in the peripheral nervous system. In this process, the surface membrane of the glial cell (oligodendrocyte or Schwann cell) wraps around the axon, a branch of the neuron that is involved in sending out commands (Figure 4.7). One consequence of this myelination is

that the commands sent by the neuron travel at a much greater speed. With regard to phagocytosis, glial cells are known to proliferate around damaged neurons and to assume the appearance of phagocytes. It is believed, for example, that glial cells are able to disrupt the normal connections between neurons by displacing the contact of intact neurons onto a neuron that has been damaged. These two examples (i.e., myelination and phagocytosis) of neuroglial function probably represent just the tip of the iceberg. This area of research is currently experiencing rapid growth (Abbott, 1985).

Although neurons are a morphologically diverse group of cells, their common function

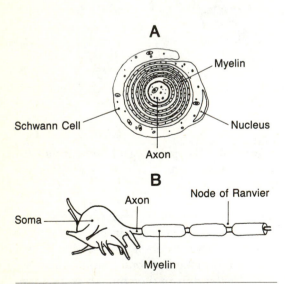

Figure 4.7. Myelination of an axon by a Schwann cell. (A) Cross-sectional view of a Schwann cell ensheathing an axon. (B) An axon is ensheathed by many Schwann cells that provide an interrupted covering of myelin. The gaps in the myelin are known as nodes of Ranvier.

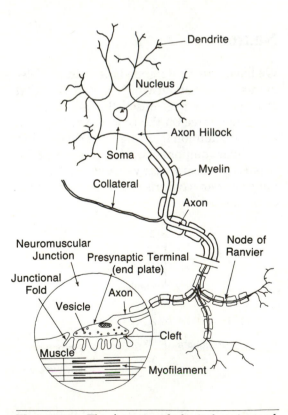

Figure 4.8. The four morphological regions of a typical neuron: dendrites, soma, axon, and presynaptic terminals.

is performed in three distinct phases. These include (a) the reception of information, (b) a computation to determine whether a signal should be transmitted, and (c) the transmission of the electrical signal. A typical neuron has four morphological regions (dendrites, soma, axon, presynaptic terminal; Figure 4.8), which interact to accomplish these tasks. The cell body (**soma**) contains the apparatus (e.g., nucleus, ribosomes, rough endoplasmic reticulum, Golgi apparatus) needed for the synthesis of macromolecules. The **axon** is a tubular process that arises from the soma at the **axon hillock** and functions as a cable for transmitting the electrical signal (action potential). The axon hillock is the most excitable portion of the axon and represents the computing center and site of action potential initiation. The axon usually gives off branches that are referred to as **collaterals**. Large axons are surrounded by a fatty insulating sheath called **myelin**, which, in peripheral nerves, is provided by Schwann cells. The myelin increases the rate at which the action potential is conducted. Gaps between adjacent Schwann cells are referred to as nodes of Ranvier. Near its end, the axon divides into many fine branches that form functional contacts with the receptive surface of cells. These contacts are referred to as **synapses**. The ending of the axon involved in a synapse is identified as the **presynaptic terminal** and includes the means for transferring the signal from the neuron to the target cell. In neuron-to-neuron interactions, the most common receptive site is the **dendrites**, the other processes extending from the soma. Although synapses can occur between any neuronal parts (e.g., axo-dendritic, axo-somatic, axo-axonic, dendro-dendritic, dendro-somatic), dendrites provide about 80% of the sites for the reception of information.

In the simple joint system, the neural elements of greatest interest are the neurons

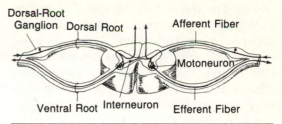

Figure 4.9. Segmental organization of the spinal cord.

that innervate the skeletal muscles; they are known as **motoneurons**. The somas of these neurons are located in the gray matter of the spinal cord, and their axons exit the cord and are bundled together into peripheral nerves that course to the target muscles (Figure 4.9). The spinal cord is often described as a segmented structure in which the segments correspond to the vertebrae. Between each pair of vertebrae, a set of axons exits and another set enters on each side (left and right) of the cord. The **Bell-Magendie** law states that the axons exiting in the **ventral** (front or belly-side) roots serve an **efferent** (motor) function whereas those entering in the **dorsal** (back) roots are **afferent** (sensory).

A nerve-muscle connection is known as a **motor end plate**, or a **neuromuscular junction**. The presynaptic membrane (axon) is separated from the postsynaptic membrane (muscle) by a 1- to 2-μm cleft. The transfer of the signal across the cleft is an electrochemical process in which the electrical energy embodied in the nerve action potential is converted to chemical energy in the form of a neurotransmitter. The electrical change (or excitement) of the presynaptic terminal elicits a release of a chemical neurotransmitter into the cleft. The neurotransmitter, in turn, causes a change in the permeability and, subsequently, the electrical status of the postsynaptic membrane. At the neuromuscular junction the neurotransmitter is **acetylcholine**

(**ACh**). The transfer of the signal is accomplished by an interaction between the presynaptic membrane and ACh-containing organelles known as **vesicles**. On the muscle side of the junction, the neurotransmitter (chemical energy) is converted back to electrical energy; the final product is a muscle action potential (Figure 4.8).

Sensory Receptors

Now we turn our attention to the fifth and final element of the simple joint system. The reason for including the first four elements in this biological model is intuitively obvious, but why include sensory receptors? The basic function of sensory receptors is to provide information to the system on both its state and its environment. This type of information flow, from the sensory receptors to the central nervous system, is known as **feedback**. *It appears as a general principle, both in engineering design and in biological systems, that the more maneuverable a system the more feedback it requires to maintain its stability* (Hasan & Stuart, in press). As biological systems, we are highly maneuverable in that we can perform all sorts of movements, which require a great deal of feedback to control.

The function of sensory receptors is to convert energy from one form to another. This process is known as **transduction**. Energy can exist in a variety of forms, such as light, pressure, temperature, and sound, but the common output of sensory receptors is electrochemical energy manifested as a sequence of action potentials. The information embodied in the action potentials is transmitted centrally and is used by the central nervous system to monitor the status of the musculoskeletal system. The human body contains many different types of sensory receptors, which can be distinguished on the basis of their location (exteroceptors, proprioceptors, interoceptors), function (mechano-

receptors, thermoreceptors, photoreceptors, chemoreceptors, nocioceptors), and morphology (free nerve endings, encapsulated endings). From the perspective of the simple joint system, we are most interested in receptors that appear to be involved in the moment-to-moment control of movement. The two most likely candidates are the muscle spindle and the tendon organ (Stuart,

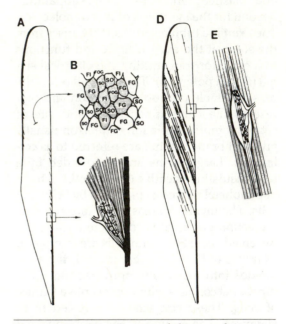

Figure 4.10. Distribution of the muscle spindle and tendon organ in the medial gastrocnemius muscle of the cat. (A) Tendon organs associated with the aponeurosis. (B) Mixture of muscle-fiber types throughout the muscle. (C) Enlarged view of a single tendon organ in series with the skeletomotor fibers. (D) Muscle spindle distribution throughout the belly of the muscle. (E) Muscle spindle in parallel with the skeletomotor fibers. *Note.* From ''Functional Anatomy of the Association Between Motor Units and Muscle Receptors'' by B.R. Botterman, M.D. Binder, and D.G. Stuart, 1978, *American Zoologist*, **18**, p. 136. Copyright 1978 by the American Society of Zoologists. Reprinted by permission.

1987b). Both of these receptors respond to mechanical stimuli and hence are mechano-receptors. Similarly, both receptors are located in muscle and its associated connective tissue (Figure 4.10) and, because they respond to muscle activity, are known as proprioceptors.

Muscle Spindle

Provided a muscle operates across a joint and is subject to unexpected loads, it will contain a variable number of spindles (6-1,300) that are distributed throughout the muscle. The spindles are fusiform-shaped and lie in parallel with the skeletal muscle fibers (Figure 4.10). Although the spindle is a morphologically and functionally complex sensory receptor, it is essentially a collection of (2-12) miniature skeletal muscle fibers that are partially enclosed by a connective tissue capsule (Figure 4.11). These smaller muscle fibers are referred to as **fusimotor** fibers in contrast to those outside the spindle, the **skeletomotor** fibers. Because of the greater myofilament content of a skeletomotor fiber, it can generate approximately 36 times more force than a fusimotor fiber. There are two types of fusimotor fibers, which differ as to the arrangement of their nuclei. In particular, the nuclei of the **chain** fiber are arranged

end to end as the links in a chain whereas those of the **bag** fiber cluster in a group. Both types of fiber, however, are devoid of myofilaments in their central or **equatorial** region. The bag fiber is the longer of the two, extending at both ends beyond the capsule.

As a sense organ, the muscle spindle has an afferent supply over which the action potentials are centrally transmitted. In general, afferent fibers are classified into four groups, primarily due to differences in axonal diameter. Group I fibers have the greatest diameters and Group IV the smallest; the larger the axon diameter, the faster the action potentials can be conducted. We tend to think that receptors that possess a Group I axon must carry an urgent signal because they can be conducted so rapidly. Each spindle has a variable number (8-25) of Group I and II afferent fibers. The larger of the two, the **Group Ia** afferent, has an ending that spirals around the equatorial regions of both the chain and bag fibers. The **Group II** (spII) afferent has a nonspiral ending that connects principally to the chain fibers. Not all spindles have an spII afferent but all include an Ia afferent. The somas of the Ia and spII afferents are located in the spinal ganglia just outside the spinal cord (Figure 4.9).

One of the abbreviations that has evolved in the neuroscience literature is the term *afferent* or *efferent* fiber. Also, we may talk about a particular group of afferents or efferents. In all cases we are referring to the *axons* of an afferent or efferent neuron. The word axon is usually not stated but implied. For example, a Group Ia afferent signifies the axon identified as a Group Ia afferent.

In addition to an afferent system, the fusimotor fibers of the muscle spindle receive efferent input. In general, skeletal muscle fibers are innervated by three groups of motoneurons, which can be distinguished by size and by the fibers that they innervate. The

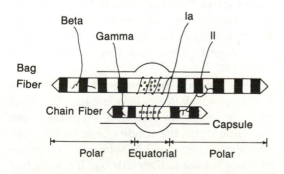

Figure 4.11. A schematized muscle spindle.

alpha motoneurons are the largest and serve skeletomotor fibers; **gamma** motoneurons are the smallest and connect exclusively to fusimotor fibers; and **beta** motoneurons, which connect to both types of skeletal fibers, serve a skeletofusimotor function. The beta and gamma motoneurons contact the fusimotor fibers in their myofilament-rich **polar** regions. When an action potential is initiated at the axon hillock and transmitted over a beta or gamma axon, the net effect is a contraction (shortening) of the fusimotor fibers in their polar regions and a stretch of the equatorial region and the afferent (Ia and spII) endings. *The stretching of the fusimotor fibers within the vicinity of the afferent connections results in excitation of the Ia and spII endings.* This can be accomplished by either stretching the entire muscle (passive activation) or activating the fusimotor fibers through the gamma or beta motoneurons (active activation).

Tendon Organ

In contrast to the muscle spindle, the tendon organ is a relatively simple sensory receptor in that it includes a single afferent and no efferent connections. Few tendon organs are located in the tendon proper. Rather, most are arranged around a few skeletomotor muscle fibers as they connect with an aponeurosis of attachment. An aponeurosis refers to the tendinous sheaths that usually extend along and deep into the belly of the muscle (Stuart, 1987b). Due to this location the tendon organ is described as being in series with the skeletomotor fibers. The ending of the afferent, a **Group Ib** fiber, is contained within a capsule and branches out to encircle several strands of collagen that comprise the aponeurosis (Figure 4.12). It is estimated that there are about 10 skeletomotor fibers included in a typical tendon organ capsule and that each skeletomotor fiber is inner-

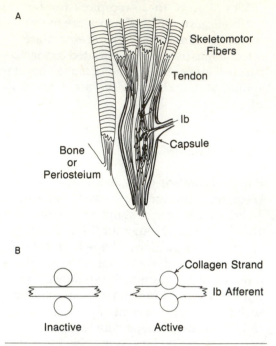

Figure 4.12. The tendon organ. (A) The encapsulated Ib afferent encircles the tendons of several skeletomotor fibers. (B) Contraction of the skeletomotor fibers causes the collagen strands (tendon) to squeeze and thus activate the Ib afferent.

vated by a different motoneuron. When a muscle-connective tissue system is stretched, by either pulling the muscle (passive force) or activating the skeletomotor fibers through their motoneurons (active force), the strands of collagen pinch and thus excite the Ib afferent.

As a consequence, *the tendon organ is described as a monitor of muscle force*. The level of force necessary to excite a tendon organ depends upon the mode of excitation; passive stretch requires 2 N, whereas the activity of a single muscle fiber (30-90 μN) is sufficient in active-force conditions.

Joint Receptors

Among the functions of mechanoreceptors are those of position- and movement-sense (Clark, Burgess, Chapin, & Lipscomb, 1985). In addition to the muscle spindle and tendon organ, the joint receptor is a significant contributor to these senses. In contrast to the muscle spindle and tendon organ, however, the joint receptor is not a single, well-defined entity. Joint receptors vary in their location (e.g., joint capsule, ligament, loose connective tissue surrounding the joint), type (e.g., Ruffini, Golgi, Pacinian corpuscle, free nerve endings), and presumably function. These receptors are served by Group II, III, and IV afferents.

The activation of joint receptors is related to joint angle and, in some cases, angular velocity. With passive joint rotation, the receptors usually respond vigorously to one or both extremes of the range of motion. However, activation of muscles that insert on a joint capsule can result in a discharge in the absence of movement. Consequently, joint receptors can generally be described as responding to both joint angle and muscle force.

Problems

4.1. Consider the biological model we call the simple joint system.
  a. Why is it necessary to use such a model?
  b. What are the five elements of the model?
  c. Why does the model not include such elements as the lungs and heart?

4.2. Bone has a strength of 58 MN•m^{-2} for tensile forces applied to the long axis of the bone.
  a. What mechanical variable (Appendix A) do the SI units MN•m^{-2} represent?
  b. Since human bone does not have the dimensions of m², convert 58 MN•m^{-2} into cm² values.

4.3. Bone is stronger in the direction of compression than in the direction of tension (132 vs. 187 MN•m^{-2}). What does this suggest about the cellular organization of bone?

4.4. Which of the following is not a function of bone?
  a. Provides mechanical support.
  b. Secretes synovial fluid into the joint cavity.
  c. Produces red blood cells.
  d. Serves as an active ion (Ca^{++}, Mg^{++}) reservoir.

4.5. Given what we know about the maintenance of bone mass (i.e., cyclic loading), what types of exercise might be best for astronauts to prevent bone demineralization during space flight?

4.6. Tendon can withstand stress (force per unit area) of up to 80 MN•m^{-2}. What area measurement is this? (Hint: Think about the function of tendon).

4.7.   Why is the fibril referred to as the basic load-bearing unit of tendon and ligament?

4.8.   Although the fibril is the basic load-bearing unit of tendon and ligament, the strength of the connective tissue depends on the state of the cross-links. What are cross-links, and why does connective-tissue strength depend on them?

4.9.   Which of the following is not an element of the simple joint system?
a. Neuroglia
b. Sensory receptor
c. Rigid link
d. Muscle
e. Synovial joint

4.10.   Where does the fluid in the synovial joint come from?

4.11.   Why does articular cartilage increase in thickness when an individual goes from a resting to an active state?

4.12.   Fluid in a joint cavity helps minimize impact forces and is retained there by the joint capsule and the articular cartilage. Why does the joint need the articular cartilage rather than just the capsule to keep the fluid within the cavity?

4.13.   What is a degree of freedom?

4.14.   Which of the following are not properties of muscle?
a. Limited growth and regenerative capacity
b. Conductivity
c. Transduction
d. Irritability
e. Contractility
f. Demineralization

4.15.   What is the difference between the endomysium and the sarcolemma?

4.16.   The regulatory proteins in muscle are
a. actin and myosin.
b. troponin and tropomyosin.
c. Ca^{++}.
d. light and heavy meromyosin.
e. subfragments 1 and 2.

4.17.   The term *muscle cell* refers to what level of hierarchy of muscle?
a. Fascicle
b. Sarcomere
c. Fiber
d. Myofibril
e. Contractile proteins

4.18. How many sarcomeres (average width = 2.5 μm) are there in a 7.2-mm muscle fiber?

4.19. Which statement (a-e) is correct about the contractile proteins? Both parts (i-v) of each statement have to be correct.

    i.   Subfragment 1 is part of the light meromyosin unit.

    ii. The hinge areas of crossbridges are part of the tropomyosin molecule.

    iii. Troponin is associated with the actin filament.

    iv. Troponin is attached to the heavy meromyosin unit adjacent to sub-fragment 2.

    v. Troponin covers the myosin-binding site.

  a. iii, v

  b. i, iii

  c. v, ii

  d. i, v, iii

  e. iv, ii

4.20. Which band refers to the zone where two sets of thick filaments of opposite polarity (pointing in opposite directions) are joined together?

  a. M

  b. H

  c. I

  d. Z

  e. A

4.21. How many strands of F actin are there in each thin filament?

4.22. How many tropomyosin strands per thin filament?

4.23. Which statement(s) about muscle is (are) correct?

  a. The sarcolemma is the connective-tissue sheath surrounding each muscle fiber.

  b. The sarcomere does not include the thick filaments.

  c. Tropomyosin covers the thin filament binding site.

  d. The HMM extension is known as the crossbridge.

  e. The thick filament contains mainly myosin.

4.24. Identify the incorrect statement(s) about the thick filament.

  a. There is more than one myosin molecule per filament.

  b. The actin-binding site is on S1.

  c. The crossbridge refers to the LMM fragment.

  d. Each sarcomere contains two sets of thick filaments joined at the Z band.

  e. Each thick filament is surrounded by six thin filaments.

4.25. Which one of the following is not part of a neuron?

  a. Sarcoplasmic reticulum

  b. Axon hillock

    c. Soma

    d. Dendrites

    e. Collateral

    f. Nucleus

4.26. Neurons can be described as cells capable of receiving, computing, and transmitting information. Identify neuronal structures associated with each of these functions.

4.27. The Bell-Magendie law refers to

    a. the myelination of large axons.

    b. the location of motoneurons within the spinal cord and sensory neurons in dorsal root ganglia.

    c. axons that give off branches known as collaterals.

    d. axons that exit the spinal cord via the ventral root and serve an efferent function.

    e. input to the neuron that arrives through the dendrites and output that is sent along the axon.

4.28. Why does the simple joint system need a sensory receptor as one of its elements?

4.29. Muscle spindles and tendon organs are both mechanoreceptors and proprioceptors. What aspects of sensory receptors do these terms describe?

4.30. Muscle spindles possess both afferent and efferent innervation.

    a. What axons provide the efferent innervation?

    b. What axons provide the afferent innervation?

    c. Muscle spindle afferents can be excited by active or passive means. What is this distinction?

4.31. Why do fusimotor fibers not contribute any significant force to whole-muscle force?

4.32. The presence of gamma-motoneuron innervation of fusimotor fibers is like having a variable-gain control.

    a. What is gain?

    b. What does variable-gain control mean?

    c. Why would such a control mechanism be useful in the control of movement?

    d. Does the tendon organ have a peripheral variable-gain control?

4.33. Which statement (a-e) is correct about muscle spindles? Both parts (i-v) need to be correct for the statement to be correct.

    i.   Muscle spindles lie in parallel with skeletomotor fibers.

    ii. Ia and Group II axons carry sensory information via the ventral horn to the spinal cord.

    iii. Muscle spindles monitor changes in length.

    iv. Nuclear chain fibers cannot contract.

    v. Muscle spindles receive efferent input via the beta and gamma systems.

  a. i, ii

  b. v, i

  c. ii, iii, iv

  d. iv, ii

  e. v, iii

4.34. Although a force of 2 N delivered by passive stretch is required to activate a tendon organ, an activated muscle fiber that exerts a force of 50 μN can activate a tendon organ.

  a. How many times smaller is the 50 μN compared to 2 N?

  b. What mechanical reason can you think of to explain this difference?

  c. What advantage is there for the simple joint system to have these two different thresholds?

4.35. Select one of the elements of the simple joint system and describe how its structure is affected by its function.

CHAPTER
5

Simple Joint System Operation

Given the morphological characteristics of the five elements (rigid link, synovial joint, muscle, neuron, sensory receptor) of the simple joint system, it is now appropriate to consider how these elements interact to produce movement. In the study of human movement, particularly elite performance, it is easy to become entranced with the accomplishments and to forget that each movement is the consequence of a multitude of minute interactions between nerve and muscle cells. When these are taken into consideration, movement becomes all the more awesome. In this chapter we shall consider four key features of the operation of the simple joint system: (a) the basic functional unit (the motor unit), (b) the means by which information is transmitted rapidly throughout the system (excitable membranes), (c) the link between the neural signal and muscle contraction (excitation-contraction coupling), and (d) the role of afferent information in the operation of the system (proprioceptive feedback).

Motor Unit

In Part I ("The Force-Motion Relationship") we discussed the concept that activated muscle exerts a force on a rigid link and that, depending on the relationship between the load on the link and the force exerted by the muscle, the link either rotates or remains stationary. In this scheme, we characterized the muscle as being able to exert a force that could vary in magnitude, a variation that is profoundly influenced by the nervous system. In a functional sense, therefore, the analysis of movement as the consequence of muscle activation must include consideration of the associated neural factors. The concept of a motor unit represents such a perspective. Specifically, a **motor unit** is defined as *the cell body and dendrites of a motoneuron, the multiple branches of its axon, and the muscle fibers that it innervates*. Each muscle fiber is innervated by a single motoneuron, but each motoneuron will innervate more than one muscle fiber (Figure 5.1). The number of muscle fibers innervated by a single motoneuron is referred to as the **innervation ratio** and may vary from about 1:1,900 (e.g., gastrocnemius, tibialis anterior) to 1:15 (e.g., extraocular muscles). That is, one motoneuron may innervate from 15 to 1,900 muscle fibers. Each time a moto-neuron is activated in the central nervous system, it sends an action potential(s) to all of its muscle fibers (except perhaps under fa-tigue conditions); hence, the lower the inner-vation ratio, the finer the control of muscle force in terms of motor unit activation. The innervation ratio is also indicative of the number of times an axon must branch out to contact all of its muscle fibers (cf. Figure 4.7).

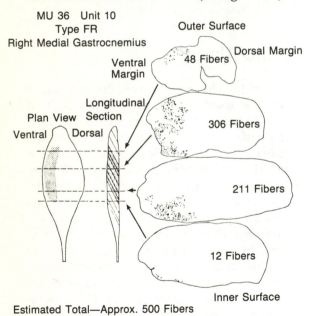

MU 36   Unit 10
Type FR
Right Medial Gastrocnemius

Outer Surface

Dorsal Margin

Ventral Margin

48 Fibers

Longitudinal Section

Plan View

Ventral   Dorsal

306 Fibers

211 Fibers

12 Fibers

Inner Surface

Estimated Total—Approx. 500 Fibers

Figure 5.1. Distribution of the muscle fibers belonging to a single Type FR motor unit in the medial gastrocnemius muscle of a cat. The motor unit appeared to include 500 muscle fibers. The distribution of these fibers is shown in the cross-sectional views to the right. *Note.* From ''Anatomy and Innervation Ratios in Mo-tor Units of Cat Gastrocnemius'' by R.E. Burke and P. Tsairis, 1973, *Journal of Physiology*, **234**, p. 755. Copyright 1973 by Cambridge Univer-sity Press. Reprinted by permission.

Physiologically, motor units can be com-pared to one another based upon a number of properties; these include the characteris-tics of discharge, the speed of contraction, the magnitude of the force exerted, and the resistance to fatigue. Over the years two methodologies have emerged for evaluating these parameters, one direct and the other in-direct. The direct evaluation refers to the physiological measurement of the motor-unit properties. Such an assessment can be made by an evaluation of the discharge characteris-tics of motor units (Gydikov & Kosarov, 1974) or the mechanical response of motor units to different inputs (Burke, Levine, Tsairis, & Zajac, 1973). We shall consider the former ap-proach in chapter 6. For now, we will con-fine our attention to the effect of two types of input on motor-unit output (Figure 5.2); the first, a single action potential, generates a **twitch**, and the second, a series of action potentials, produces a **tetanus**. The terms *twitch* and *tetanus* refer to the force-time pro-file of muscle in response to qualitatively different types of input. A twitch represents a unit response of muscle to a single input and can be characterized by three measure-ments: the time from force onset to peak force (**contraction time**), the magnitude of the peak force, and the time from the peak force to the time at which the force has declined to one-half of its peak value (**one-half relax-ation time**; Figure 5.2A). *Contraction time is used as a measure of the speed of the contractile machinery.* If contraction time is long the mo-tor unit is described as **slow twitch**; the term **fast twitch** refers to a twitch response that in-volves a brief contraction time (Figure 5.2B). For example, contraction times for slow- and fast-twitch motor units of the human biceps brachii muscle are 90 and 36 ms, respectively (Saltin & Gollnick, 1983). The peak force exerted in a twitch response appears to in-crease with training (Duchateau & Hainaut, 1981).

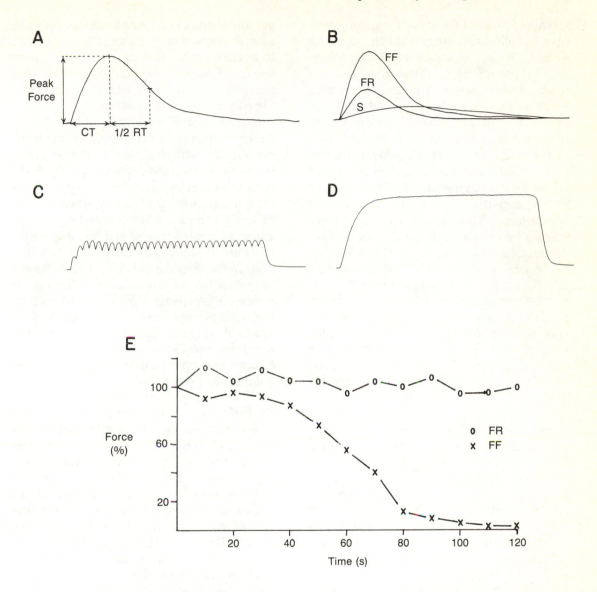

Figure 5.2. The response of motor units to single (twitch) and multiple (tetanus) neural inputs. (A) Type FF motor unit: contraction time (CT) = 24 ms, 1/2 relaxation time (1/2 RT) = 21 ms, peak force = 0.03 N. (B) Twitch responses for Type FF, FR, and S motor units. Note the difference in CT and peak force for the three motor units. (C) An unfused tetanus (stimulated at 28 Hz) for the FF unit: peak force = 0.42 N. (D) A fused tetanus (stimulated at 200 Hz) for the motor unit in C: peak force = 1.30 N. The fused tetanus produces a greater force than the unfused tetanus. (E) Fatigue test for the Type FF and FR motor units in B. The FF motor unit is described as fast-to-fatigue and the FR unit is fatigue resistant. These characteristics are indicated by the force at 120 s relative to the initial force. The axes for all records (A-E) are force and time.

When a series of stimuli are given, each stimulus elicits a single twitch response so that we get a series of twitch responses. As the stimuli occur closer together, the twitches begin to sum and the force profile becomes known as a tetanus. As the time between the stimuli decreases further, the tetanus changes from a sawtooth (**unfused**; Figure 5.2C) to a smooth plateau (**fused**; Figure 5.2D). *The capability of the motor unit to exert force* is not measured from the twitch but rather *assessed from the peak force of a single fused tetanus*. That is, the maximum force exerted by a motor unit (and a muscle) occurs during a fused tetanus. The difference in the peak twitch force and the maximum force in a fused tetanus is referred to as the twitch-tetanus ratio and generally varies from 1:1.5 to 1:10 (i.e., in a fused tetanus the force may be 1.5-10 times greater than the twitch force). In general, the force produced in a single tetanus will decline over time if the motor unit is required to produce a series of tetani. *The ability of a motor unit to prevent such a decline is taken as a measure of its resistance to fatigue*. A standard fatigue test involves eliciting tetani for 2-6 min at a rate of 1 Hz—each tetanus lasts 330 ms and includes 13 stimuli. (*Note.* This protocol was originally designed to elicit muscle fatigue while avoiding neuromuscular-junction fatigue.) The ratio of the peak force exerted after 2 min of this stimulus protocol to that exerted in the initial tetanus is referred to as the fatigue index (Figure 5.2E).

On the basis of two of these parameters, contraction speed and fatigue resistance, motor units can be classified into three groups (Burke, 1981): slow-contracting, fatigue resistant (**Type S**); fast-contracting, fatigue resistant (**Type FR**); and fast-contracting, fast-to-fatigue (**Type FF**). The Type S motor units produce the least force and the Type FF the greatest. This difference

in force is due to variations in the number of muscle fibers within a motor unit (i.e., the innervation ratio) and the size of individual muscle fibers (i.e., the quantity of contractile proteins per muscle fiber). In general, Type FF motor units have the greatest innervation ratios and the largest muscle fibers, although data from the human vastus lateralis muscle, particularly among females, does not support this trend (Stuart & Enoka, 1983).

As indicated by their names, Type S motor units are slow contracting whereas both FF and FR units are fast contracting. Differences in contraction speed among motor units are thought to be due largely to variations in the enzyme myosin ATPase (bound to one of the S1 heads) and to the rate at which Ca^{++} is released from and taken up by the sarcoplasmic reticulum (Kugelberg & Thornell, 1983). As we shall see shortly, the significance of Ca^{++} is that it affects the ability of actin and myosin to interact and, consequently, to exert a force.

The two fatigue-resistant unit types (S and FR) have a fatigue index greater than or equal to 0.75 whereas that for the FF motor units is usually less than 0.25. An index of 0.25 indicates that, after 2 min of the fatigue test (e.g., Figure 5.2E), the force exerted by the unit will be only 25% of that measured at the beginning of the test. These data suggest that activation of the S and FR motor units is more appropriate for sustained contractions because they are more resistant to fatigue.

Motor units can also be classified indirectly based on histochemical and biochemical measurements. Both techniques involve the determination of the enzyme content of the muscle fibers, one qualitative (histochemistry) and the other quantitative (biochemistry). Since enzymes are the catalysts for chemical reactions, measurement of the amount of enzyme provides an index of the speed of the reaction. Thus *the histochemical and biochemical techniques attempt to measure mechanisms responsible for the various physiological properties* (contraction speed, magnitude of force, and fatigue resistance). Once a correlation can be determined between a chemical reaction and a physiological response, the quantity of enzyme can be interpreted as a correlate of the physiological response. Typically, three types of enzymes are measured; one type indicates the contractile speed (myosin ATPase—although the volume of sarcoplasmic reticulum may be more important than myosin ATPase), whereas the other two represent the metabolic basis (aerobic vs. anaerobic) by which the muscle fiber produces its energy for contraction. Commonly assayed enzymes for aerobic metabolism are succinic dehydrogenase (SDH) and nicotinamide adenine dinucleotide-tetrazolium reductase (NADH-TR), and for anaerobic capabilities are phosphorylase and alpha-glycerophosphate dehydrogenase (alpha GPD).

Based upon these enzyme assays of the muscle fibers (note that histochemical and biochemical schemes refer only to the muscular element and ignore the neural component), it is possible to classify the fibers with a tripartite scheme. Two such schemes are commonly encountered in the literature. One scheme classifies fibers solely on the basis of myosin ATPase, of which the nomenclature is Types **I**, **IIa**, and **IIb**. The distinction between Types I and II is based on the amount of ATPase activity remaining after preincubation in a bath with a pH of 9.4. Type I represents the slow-twitch and Type II the fast-twitch muscle fibers. Type II muscle fibers can be further separated into two groups (IIa and IIb) after preincubation in baths with pHs of 4.3 (IIa) and 4.6 (IIb; Brooke & Kaiser, 1974). The other scheme, which uses enzymes for contraction speed (myosin ATPase), aerobic capacity (SDH or NADH-TR), and anaerobic capacity (phos-

phorylase and alpha GPD), employs the terms slow-twitch, oxidative (**SO**), fast-twitch, oxidative-glycolytic (**FOG**), and fast-twitch, glycolytic (**FG**). Although Type I fibers are the same as SO, and Type II are equivalent to FG and FOG, there is sometimes no further equivalency between the two schemes. In particular, the Type IIa fiber is usually the same as an FOG, but a IIb can be either FOG or FG (Nemeth & Pette, 1981). Actually the IIb-FOG/FG correspondence appears to be species-dependent in that IIb and FG are equivalent in the cat but not so in the rat. The SO-FOG-FG nomenclature is preferable because it is based upon a greater number of properties and because the physiological significance of myosin ATPase remains unresolved. The SO muscle fibers belong to a Type S motor unit, FOG to a Type FR, and FG to a Type FF. Because the muscle fibers in a motor unit are all the same type, these fibers all possess the same properties and are therefore described as **homogeneous** (Edström & Kugelberg, 1968; Nemeth, Solanki, Gordon, & Hamm, 1986). For example, a Type S motor unit has only Type SO muscle fibers, and these fibers are homogeneous (i.e., have the same physiological and biochemical characteristics). The same relationship applies to the other two motor-unit types and their muscle fibers. Each human muscle contains a mixture of all three motor-unit types.

Figure 5.3 provides a reasonable view of some of the physiological and histochemical differences among the FF, FR, and S motor units. Each motor unit is shown as a soma, which gives rise to an axon that descends vertically and branches out to innervate four muscle fibers. The differences in size (e.g., soma, axon diameter, muscle-fiber cross-sectional area) indicate general morphologic differences between the unit types. Beneath the motor units are shown the respective force-time (twitch) and fatigability profiles. Accordingly, the Type FF motor unit exerts the greatest twitch force, has the fastest (shortest) contraction time, and is the most fatigable. Figure 5.3 also illustrates the variable effect of the Ia input from the muscle spindle; Type FF units receive fewer Ia afferents and hence produce a lesser response (Ia

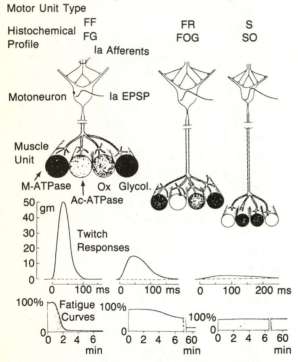

EPSP; excitatory postsynaptic potential) to Ia input.

In addition to the physiological features, Figure 5.3 indicates the histochemical profile for the muscle fibers of the different motor units. Each fiber attached to a motor unit illustrates the histochemical staining pattern for a different enzyme. The four enzyme systems tested were myosin ATPase (M-ATPase), myofibrillar ATPase after acid preincubation (Ac-ATPase—this is used to differentiate between Type IIa and IIb fibers), oxidative (Ox), and glycolytic (glycol.). The staining patterns are dark (indicating a high amount of enzyme), intermediate, and clear. It is possible that myosin ATPase is related to contraction speed; therefore, the muscle fibers that stain dark for myosin ATPase suggest that the motor unit is fast contracting. The first of the four muscle fibers for each motor unit shows the myosin ATPase stain. The histochemical data reveal that the Type FF and FR motor units, which have Type FG and FOG muscle fibers, respectively, are fast contracting. In a similar manner, Type SO and FOG muscle fibers stain dark for oxidative enzymes, and Type FG and FOG fibers show a high glycolytic capability.

Figure 5.3. Physiological and histochemical features of motor units in the medial gastrocnemius muscle of the cat. The diagram is scaled to emphasize differences between the motor units in number of Ia afferents, size of motoneuron soma and axon, diameter of muscle fiber, histochemical staining intensity (dark represents a lot of enzyme), contractile speed, magnitude of force, and fatigue resistance. *Note.* From "Motor Unit Properties and Selective Involvement in Movement" by R.E. Burke and V.R. Edgerton, 1975, in J.H. Wilmore and J.F. Keogh (Eds.), *Exercise and Sport Sciences Reviews*, Vol. 3 (p. 36), New York: Academic Press. Copyright 1975 by Academic Press. Reprinted by permission.

Excitable Membranes

Given that the motor unit represents the basic functional unit of movement control, how does the motoneuron command its muscle fibers into activity? In other words, what is the mechanism by which the two elements communicate? Interaction between the motoneuron and its muscle fibers occurs at a rapid, electrical level and a slower, chemical level. The latter is often neglected in movement analyses, yet it may represent a significant mechanism by which the properties of a motor unit are specified. This possibility is embodied in the concept of **neurotrophism**, which refers to the sustaining influence that one biological element (e.g., neuron) exerts directly on another (e.g., muscle fibers). Although an axon is typically represented as a simple cylinder (cf. Figure 4.7), the internal structure of the axon is complex and comprises systems for transporting materials from the soma to the end plate (**orthograde** transport) and in the reverse direction (**retrograde** transport; Schwartz, 1981). For example, an important step in the electrochemical transfer of information from the neuron to the muscle is the release of the neurotransmitter by the vesicle into the synaptic cleft. After a while the vesicle membrane requires repair, and it is transported back to the soma where the membrane repair occurs; the vesicle is subsequently sent back to the end plate. In a similar manner, the soma manufactures and exports materials that influence the muscle fibers, and, conversely, the muscle fibers appear to send back materials that affect some properties of the soma.

Of the two levels of nerve-muscle interaction, most is known about the rapid electrical form. This type of interaction is possible due to the excitable nature of the axolemma and sarcolemma. These membranes comprise a lipid bilayer on or in which proteins are located, and are semipermeable in that some lipid-soluble substances and smaller molecules can move through them. The membrane proteins, which account for about 50%-70% of the membrane structure and serve structural, enzymatic, receptor, channel, and pump functions, are critical to the membrane's capability to store, transmit, and release energy. The membrane is surrounded by intracellular (e.g., sarcoplasm, axoplasm) and extracellular fluids (Figure 5.4), which contain variable concentrations of certain ions, notably sodium (Na^+), potassium (K^+), and chloride (Cl^-). The concentration ratio

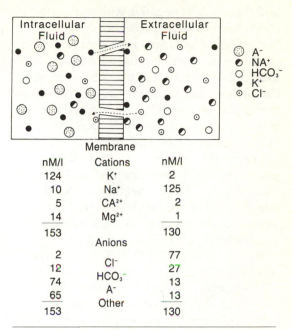

nM/l	Cations	nM/l
124	K^+	2
10	Na^+	125
5	CA^{2+}	2
14	Mg^{2+}	1
153		130
	Anions	
2	Cl^-	77
12	HCO_3^-	27
74	A^-	13
65	Other	13
153		130

Figure 5.4. Distribution of ions about a mammalian excitable membrane. The membrane has pores through which K^+ and Cl^- can move easily, Na^+ with difficulty, and A^- not at all.

(outside the cell with respect to the inside) differs for each of these ions (e.g., muscle cell of a warm-blooded animal: Na^+ = 12.08, K^+ = 0.03, Cl^- = 30.00) such that the net effect is a charge distribution (voltage or **electrical potential**) across the membrane. *The particular distribution of an ion represents an equilibrium between two forces, the electrical and concentration gradients*; electrically unlike charges attract and like charges repel. The effect of differences in concentration is to cause ions to move from an area of high concentration to one that is lower.

When a membrane is at rest or in a steady-state condition (i.e., not conducting a signal), the electrical potential across the membrane remains relatively constant and is called the **resting membrane potential**. The resting potential is usually in the order of 60-90 mV, and the inside is negative with respect to the outside. The ions involved in establishing this electrical potential represent just a few of those included in the intracellular and extracellular fluids (Figure 5.5). The ionic distribution across the membrane represents a balance of the electrical forces between the positive and negative ions and the concentration-associated force experienced by each ion. In the resting state, Na^+ is prevented from entering the cell by the pumping activity of a membrane-bound protein (known as the **Na^+-K^+ pump**) that transports Na^+ from the intracellular to the extracellular fluid. K^+ is held internally by both the activity of the Na^+-K^+ pump and an electrical attraction to various organic anions (A^-; negatively charged ions such as amino acids and proteins) that are too large to cross the membrane. Thus Na-K^+ pump activity keeps Na^+ in the extracellular fluid and K^+ in the intracellular fluid. The charges provided by Na^+ (attraction) and A^- (repulsion) cause Cl^- to be concentrated in the extracellular

fluid. *The distribution of these ions (Na^+ and Cl^- externally, K^+ and A^- internally) largely determines the electrical potential that exists across an excitable membrane.*

The forces acting on these ions (Na^+, K^+, and Cl^-), and their flux across the membrane in a steady-state condition, are schematized in Figure 5.6. The forces driving the ions across the membrane (driving force) are due to chemical and electrical effects. Chemically, each ion experiences a force that is directed from high to low concentration; in each case the magnitude of this effect is illustrated by the length of the arrow. For example, Na^+ has a greater external (Out) concentration, as in-

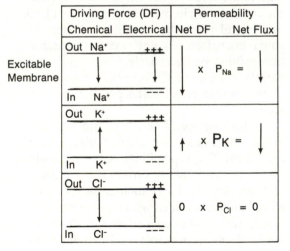

Figure 5.6. The net driving force and flux for Na^+, K^+, and Cl^- ions across a membrane with a steady-state membrane potential of -60 mV. The net flux of an ion across a membrane depends on the net driving force it experiences and the permeability (P) of the membrane to that ion. *Note.* Reprinted by permission of the publisher from "Resting Membrane Potential and Action Potential" by J. Koester, 1984, in E.R. Kandel and J.H. Schwartz (Eds.), *Principles of Neural Science* (2nd ed.), p. 55. Copyright 1985 by Elsevier Science Publishing Co., Inc.

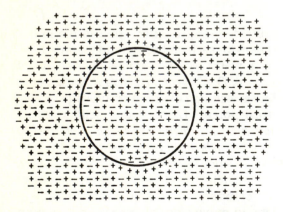

Figure 5.5. Conceptual view of the ionic charge distribution inside and outside a cell. *Note.* Reprinted by permission of the publisher from "Resting Membrane Potential and Action Potential," by J. Koester, 1984, in E.R. Kandel and J.H. Schwartz (Eds.), *Principles of Neural Science* (2nd ed.), pp. 49-57. Copyright 1985 by Elsevier Science Publishing Co., Inc.

dicated by the larger Na+ symbol on the outside of the membrane, and hence chemically it experiences a force that tends to drive it inward. The membrane is electrically negative inside (In) with respect to the outside (Out). Positive ions (Na+ and K+) are electrically attracted inward, and negative ions (Cl−) experience a force that drives them out. The net driving force (Net DF) experienced by each ion can then be determined by summing the chemical and electrical effects. For example, Na+ is subject to inward chemical and electrical effects, which result in a large, inward Net DF. By similar reasoning, K+ experiences a small, outward Net DF, whereas the chemical and electrical components for Cl− cancel, resulting in a zero Net DF. The Net DF for each ion combines with its permeability (P) to determine the net magnitude and direction of the ion's flux at a steady-state membrane potential. The ease with which an ion crosses a membrane (i.e., the permeability of the membrane to an ion) is indicated by the size of the symbol; excitable membranes are most permeable to K+ (P_K) and least to Na+ (P_{Na}). Due to these differences in permeability, the amount of an ion that crosses a membrane (net flux) depends upon the combination of the net driving force experienced by an ion and its permeability. The result (Figure 5.6, net flux column) indicates that, *in steady-state conditions, approximately equal quantities of Na+ and K+ cross the membrane, whereas Cl− remains internally.* However, once Na+ and K+ cross the membrane, they are quickly returned to their original sides of the membrane by the Na+-K+ pump such that the ionic distribution, and hence the electrical potential, remains relatively constant under steady-state conditions.

Disruption of this ionic distribution, however, is possible and results in changes in the membrane potential. For example, the movement of negative ions across the membrane to the outside or vice versa (positive ions to the inside) will produce a decrease in the membrane potential, a change referred to as **depolarization**—that is, the membrane potential becomes less polarized or closer to zero. In contrast, the movement of negative ions internally or the deposition of additional positive ions externally causes the membrane to become **hyperpolarized** (more polarized).

The shift of ions across the membrane is due to changes that occur within the membrane. These changes can be induced chemically (e.g., by a neurotransmitter) or electrically (e.g., by variations in membrane potential) and are described as gated changes in membrane permeability. For example, although Na+ crosses the membrane in the resting state with considerable difficulty, the membrane is able to alter its permeability to Na+ by about 500-fold, which makes this crossing much easier. This change is referred to as an increase in Na+ **conductance** or permeability. Once Na+ can cross the membrane it does so, moving down its concentration gradient (Figure 5.6) from the extracellular to the intracellular fluid. As the positive ions move inside the cell, the membrane becomes depolarized, which causes an additional increase in sodium conductance leading to a further depolarization, and so on. *Such changes in Na+ conductance are voltage-gated*, since changes in the electrical potential (voltage) lead to changes in conductance, which, in turn, lead to further changes in the electrical potential and so on. A hypothetical model of a voltage-gated channel is shown in Figure 5.7 (Koester, 1981). In this model, a gating molecule blocks the passage of Na+ through a channel (pore). The orientation of the gating molecule depends on the potential across the surrounding membrane. In the resting state (Figure 5.7A) the molecule is positioned so that it blocks the channel. As the potential across the membrane reverses (Figure 5.7B), the molecule shifts its position, thus opening the channel (Figure 5.7C).

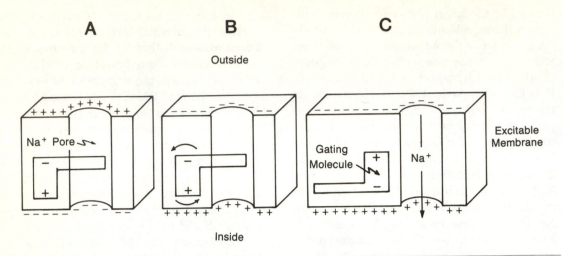

Figure 5.7. Model of a voltage-gated Na⁺ channel. A gating molecule (A) blocks the channel in the steady-state condition but (C) moves its position when (B) the potential across the membrane reverses. *Note.* Reprinted by permission of the publisher from ''Active Conductances Underlying the Action Potential'' by J. Koester, 1981, in E.R. Kandel and J.H. Schwartz (Eds.), *Principles of Neural Science* (2nd ed.), p. 61. Copyright 1981 by Elsevier Science Publishing Co., Inc.

Communication within the neuromuscular system is accomplished by such gated changes in membrane potential. In general, these alterations are of two types: **local-graded potentials** and **action potentials**. Both involve the same mechanism, an ionic shift across the membrane, but the local-graded potential decreases in amplitude as it is conducted along the membrane whereas the action potential involves a self-regenerative process that minimizes changes in amplitude. As an example of this distinction, both local-graded and action potentials are forms of communication in which the local-graded potential is like a suggestion that one individual might make to another whereas the action potential is like a command issued by someone in authority. Furthermore, the differences between these two potentials extend to the ways in which they are transmitted; the action potential is **propagated** rather than conducted. To distinguish between propagated and conducted, consider the ripples in a pond after a stone has been thrown into the pond. From the place that the stone contacts the water, ripples are set up in concentric circles, and these ripples move across the surface of the water away from the point of contact. Focus for a moment on a single ripple. As it travels across the surface it decreases in height, a phenomenon that is comparable to conduction of a potential. If, however, the ripple were able to maintain the same height (a characteristic that would require the addition of energy to the ripple—therefore an active process), then we would say that the ripple was being propagated.

The action potential, which is about 10-100 times larger than a local-graded potential and is generally much briefer in duration, *represents the all-or-none command given by the neuron* (Figure 5.8). In contrast, the local-graded potential is an input to the neuron that is used by the computing center to decide if an

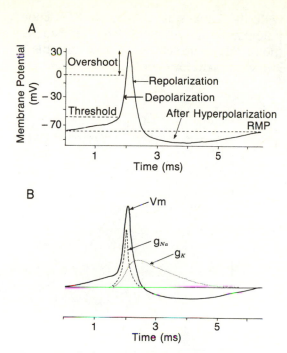

A

B

Figure 5.8. A schematic diagram of the action potential indicating its (A) various phases and (B) conductance changes. The symbols g_K and g_{Na} represent potassium and sodium conductance, respectively; RMP refers to resting membrane potential; and Vm indicates the voltage across the membrane.

action potential should be generated. These local-graded inputs can be **excitatory** or **inhibitory**; the latter is due to an increased conductance to smaller ions, such as K^+ and Cl^-. In reality, much of the communication within the nervous system occurs not by exciting neurons but rather by removing inhibitory input. A neuron can receive up to 10,000 synapses from other neurons; these synapses are distributed over the soma and the dendritic tree. When activated, each input will be in the form of a local-graded potential that will be conducted over the neuron, decreasing in amplitude as it travels along the membrane.

Thus, for a local-graded potential of given amplitude, the further the synapse is located from the computing center, the smaller will be its effect on the decision (made at the axon hillock) to generate an action potential. The neuron does not generate an action potential each time it receives an input; rather, the decision is based on the sum of the local-graded potentials at the axon hillock. When this sum reaches threshold, an action potential is generated. In general, the initiation of an action potential involves voltage-gated mechanisms, whereas local-graded potentials depend upon chemically gated changes.

An ionic shift across the low-threshold region of the axolemma (i.e., axon hillock) or sarcolemma that produces a depolarization of 10-15 mV will reach **threshold** and result in the generation of an action potential (Figure 5.8A). That is, the potential across a membrane will fluctuate as excitatory and inhibitory local-graded potentials are initiated by impinging neuronal contacts. If the net effect of these inputs is large enough (+10 to +15 mV) to reach the trigger level (threshold), then an action potential will be generated. An action potential is characterized by a rapid depolarization from the resting level to a complete reversal of potential (overshoot: the inside becomes positive with respect to the outside), followed by a **repolarization** (return to a polarized state) beyond the resting potential to a hyperpolarized state, and then a slow return to the resting membrane potential. These changes in membrane potential are the consequence of *alterations in Na^+ and K^+ conductances that are temporally offset* (Figure 5.8B). Since Na^+ and K^+ are both positive ions, their simultaneous movement across the membrane would not affect the membrane potential. However, because the net Na^+ **influx** occurs before the K^+ **efflux** and because the increased Na^+ conductance lasts for only a short time, the membrane experiences first a depolarization and then a repolarization. At any instant in time, therefore, the membrane potential (Figure 5.8B) represents the imbalance in the Na⁺ and K⁺ conductances. The number of ions of one species (e.g., Na⁺, K⁺) that cross the membrane depends on the driving force and the permeability experienced by the ion (i.e., Na⁺, K⁺, Cl⁻). At the conclusion of the action potential, for example, sodium conductance has returned to resting levels and potassium conductance has remained greater than normal, the net effect being a hyperpolarization (the **afterhyperpolarization**) of the membrane. The Na⁺-K⁺ pumps gradually reverse the ionic distribution, returning Na⁺ to the extracellular fluid and K⁺ internally; this causes the membrane potential to return to steady-state levels.

Once a neuronal action potential has been initiated, it is propagated along the axon at speeds of up to 120 m•s⁻¹. Since an action potential represents the reversal of the ionic distribution across the membrane (Area 2 in Figure 5.9B), an action potential and its propagation can be depicted as in Figure 5.9, where (A) the electrical potential is shown relative to (B) the ionic distribution. Area 1 (Figure 5.9B) represents the membrane ahead of the action potential (inactive region), and Area 2 represents the active region of the membrane. The depolarization spreads (positive charges on the inside = current flow) from Area 2 to Area 1 in the direction of the action potential propagation. Although the depolarization also spreads from Area 2 to Area 3, the change in K⁺ conductance in the membrane behind the action potential offsets any accumulation of positive charges on the inside.

The speeds at which action potentials are propagated vary with the diameter of the axon, mainly because much of the surface area of the large axons is insulated with myelin and thus prevented from involvement with the ionic shifts. Instead, the action potential jumps from one node of Ranvier (noninsulated axolemma) to another—this is known as **saltatory** conduction.

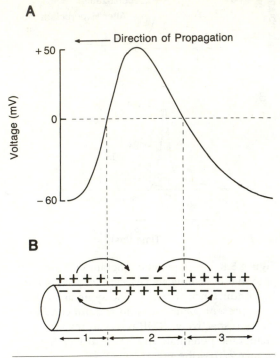

Figure 5.9. Propagation of an action potential and the associated ionic distribution. (A) The voltage across the membrane varies with distance along the membrane. (B) This spatial variation in transmembrane potential depends on the distribution of ions across the membrane. The processes associated with ionic distribution form the basis of action-potential propagation. Depolarization spreads from the active region (B, Area 2) along the membrane ahead of (Area 1) and behind (Area 3) the action potential. *Note.* Reprinted by permission of the publisher from ''Functional Consequences of Passive Membrane Properties of the Neuron,'' by J. Koester, 1985, in E.R. Kandel and J.H. Schwartz (Eds.), *Principles of Neural Science* (2nd ed.), p. 72. Copyright 1985 by Elsevier Science Publishing Co., Inc.

Upon arrival at the end plate, the action potential accelerates the release of neurotransmitter by promoting fusion of the vesicles with the terminal membrane (inside the axon). The action potential causes an increase in Ca^{++} conductance in the axolemma of the synaptic enlargement. The increase in intraaxonal Ca^{++} enhances the release of neurotransmitter by facilitating the vesicle fusion. This process of vesicular fusion and release of neurotransmitter is an example of a general process known as **exocytosis**. The steps involved in this process are depicted in Figure 5.10:

1. The vesicle approaches the active zone (triangular structure).
2. The vesicle attaches to the active zone—the presence of Ca^{++} facilitates this step.

3. By an unknown process the vesicle fuses with the presynaptic membrane.
4. Opening (fission) of the vesicle up into the synaptic cleft.
5. The vesicle membrane collapses.
6. Some vesicle membrane is retrieved for subsequent reuse.
7. The remaining vesicle membrane is returned to the cell body by retrograde transport.
8. The vesicle is replenished with neurotransmitter and moves back to the region around the active zone.

Once released, the neurotransmitter interacts with the postsynaptic membrane (the target cell) to induce further events such as action potentials and local-graded potentials.

Electromyogram

Experimentalists have devised a technique with which to monitor the activity of excitable membranes. The application of this technique to muscle is known as **electromyography** (EMG; *myo* = muscle). Essentially, an EMG represents an extracellular view of changes in membrane potential that are associated with the propagation of action potentials (Denny-Brown, 1949; Hof, 1984; Loeb & Gans, 1986; Perry & Bekey, 1981; Person, 1963). An action potential is actually a mobile reversal of the ion distribution across an excitable membrane (Figure 5.9). This shift in the ion distribution is largely accomplished by the movement of Na^+ and K^+ across the membrane. One result of these ion shifts is that on each side of the membrane (intra- and extracellular) there are adjacent patches of positive and negative membrane (Figure 5.9B). Imagine that each patch of membrane is represented by a single charge, like a center of gravity. The combination of the positive

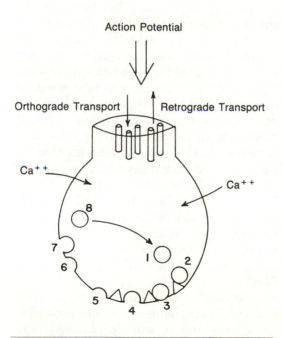

Figure 5.10. Steps involved in the release of neurotransmitter from vesicles.

charge (**cathode**) and the negative charge (**anode**) separated by a distance represents a **dipole**; the dipole can be thought of as a generator potential in that it generates the movement of ions that represent current flow. Because physiological fluids are conductive, this current flow is actually distributed in a field, much like magnetic fields at the end of a magnet (Loeb & Gans, 1986). In this sense, we talk of tissue (e.g., muscle) as being a **volume conductor**. The conductivity of these voltage fields in muscle is greater in the axial (length) direction than in the radial (width) direction by a 10:1 ratio.

These voltage fields are measured with probes known as electrodes. Depending largely on size and location, electrodes can be used to measure the current flow induced by dipole generators in single muscle fibers, single motor units, or whole muscle (Person, 1963). Typically, an electrode is placed in a stationary position over the target (e.g., single fiber, whole muscle) and senses the voltage field generated by the dipole as it approaches, reaches, and moves away from the electrode. For example, consider an electrode located on the left edge of the fiber in Figure 5.9B. As the action potential (the dipole generator) passes by the electrode, it senses the current flow indicated by the arrows (Figure 5.9B): Area 1 (outside positive) represents a current source, Area 2 (outside negative) is a current sink, and Area 3 (outside positive) is another current source. The electrode, therefore, senses a triphasic waveform of positive, negative, and positive phases. However, the actual shape of the waveform is variable and depends on the electrode configuration.

The electrode serves as an antenna (Loeb & Gans, 1986) and can be configured in either a monopolar or a bipolar mode. Although electrodes sense the voltage fields generated by dipoles in a volume conductor, a voltage is the difference in potential between two points. With a monopolar electrode, one electrode is placed over the signal source (e.g., muscle), and the signal that it senses is compared to that at a distant location (ground). In contrast, a bipolar arrangement has two electrodes over the signal source, and the output is the difference between what the two electrodes sense. Consequently, a monopolar arrangement is necessary to determine the magnitude of the signal whereas a bipolar configuration allows us to record selectively from a localized signal source.

When an action potential in an axon exits the spinal cord through the ventral roots, it invades all of its branches (15-600, depending upon the innervation ratio) and initiates a muscle action potential in each of the muscle fibers to which it connects. The action potential in each muscle fiber has the general form shown in Figure 5.11A. This waveform can be quantified easily by measuring its amplitude, duration, and area (voltage-time integral). For the measurement of the EMG of a single motor unit, however, the recorded waveform (Figure 5.11A) represents an average of all the constituent muscle fibers. If these muscle fibers are activated synchronously, then the waveforms sum without much cancellation due to offset positive and negative phases. For the measurement of single-fiber EMG, it is necessary to insert the electrodes into the muscle (e.g., as needle or fine wire electrodes). The EMG of single motor units can be measured with intramuscular, subcutaneous, or surface electrodes. The distance between the active fibers and the electrode will affect the size of the EMG.

In contrast, whole-muscle EMG involves the complicated summation of single-fiber waveforms and is usually obtained noninvasively by placing either one or two electrodes (monopolar or bipolar) on the skin

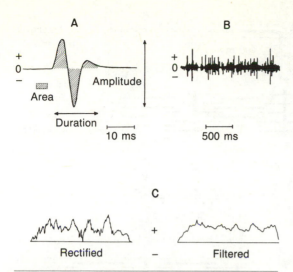

A

B

C

Rectified   +   Filtered
−

Figure 5.11. The EMG as an extracellular voltage-time measure of voltage fields generated by dipoles. (A) Triphasic single muscle-fiber and single motor-unit EMG. The phases are positive, negative, and positive. The EMG can be quantified by measures of amplitude, duration, and area. (B) Whole-muscle EMG, which involves the complicated summation of waveforms shown in A. This EMG is sometimes called an interference pattern. (C) Quantification of the whole-muscle EMG, which is achieved by rectification and filtering (3-300 Hz).

over the main body of the test muscle. Most human muscles contain thousands of fibers so that whole-muscle activation involves the addition and cancellation (positive and negative phases) of temporally offset single-fiber EMGs. For this reason, records of whole-muscle EMG are often referred to as interference patterns (Figure 5.11B). One common way to quantify whole-muscle EMG is to **rectify** (flip the negative phases over so they appear positive) and filter (smooth) the signal (Figure 5.11C).

Excitation-Contraction Coupling

The motor unit represents the operational unit by which the simple joint system modulates muscle force. How is the command (action potential) that is issued by the motoneuron converted by the muscle fibers into a force? This process involves two steps. In the first step, the neural action potential must become a muscle action potential before the excitation embodied in the electrical event (action potential) can effect an interaction of the contractile proteins. In the second step, a muscle action potential is transformed into muscle force—this is referred to as excitation-contraction coupling.

At the neuromuscular junction, the neurotransmitter acetylcholine (ACh) takes less than 100 μs to diffuse across the synaptic cleft and interact with receptors on the postsynaptic membrane. The outcome of the interaction between ACh and the membrane-bound receptors is an alteration in the Na^+ and K^+ conductances of the sarcolemma. As with the neural action potential, *the ions cross the membrane (sarcolemma) down their concentration gradients and produce a depolarization*. In this instance the depolarization is referred to as an end-plate potential, and, since the postsynpatic membrane contains no voltage-gated channels, the end-plate potential is a local-graded potential. It is conducted to the adjacent sarcolemma where, if it is of sufficient magnitude, it will initiate a muscle action potential. Under most circumstances, an end-plate potential that is elicited by a nerve action potential is of sufficient magnitude to generate a muscle action potential.

Ca⁺⁺ Disinhibition

The muscle action potential is propagated along the sarcolemma at speeds of up to

$6 \text{ m} \cdot \text{s}^{-1}$. Interestingly, the conduction velocity (i.e., propagation speed) may vary with training; it has been shown that body builders have a higher conduction velocity for the biceps brachii muscle than control subjects (5.5 vs. $2.8 \text{ m} \cdot \text{s}^{-1}$; Kereshi, Manzano, & McComas, 1983). The action potential also travels down the T tubule (Figure 5.12A), which is an invagination of the sarcolemma. By some unknown mechanism, the presence of the action potential in the T tubules triggers an increase in the calcium (Ca++) conductance of the terminal cisternae. Most of the intramuscular Ca++ is stored within the terminal cisternae (lateral sacs); an increase in Ca++ conductance allows Ca++ to move down its concentration gradient into the fluid surrounding the myofilaments (Figure 5.12B). Once the Ca++ concentration in this fluid is above a threshold level (10^{-7} M), Ca++ binds to the TN-C element of the regulatory protein troponin. Recall that, in the unstimulated muscle, actin and myosin are prevented from interacting and forming an actomyosin complex by the presence of the regulatory proteins troponin and tropomyosin. The binding of Ca++ to troponin is thought to cause a structural change in the thin filament such that the myosin-binding site on actin is uncovered and the two proteins (actin and myosin) are then able to interact (Figure 5.13). Thus, in this process of **disinhibition**, *Ca++ inhibits the inhibitory effect of troponin and tropomyosin.*

Crossbridge Cycle

The interaction of actin and myosin to produce the phenomenon referred to as a muscle contraction can be described by the *three-phase crossbridge cycle of attach-rotate-detach* (Figure 5.14). Once the binding sites on actin have been made available (Figure 5.12C), the S1 (globular heads) of myosin rapidly attaches to actin-forming crossbridges between

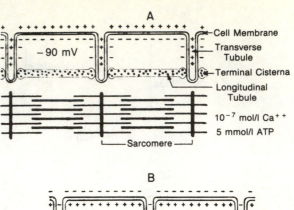

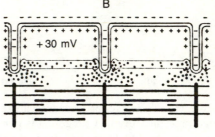

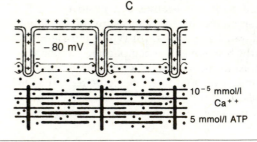

Figure 5.12. Role of Ca++ in excitation-contraction coupling. (A) In the resting state, the potential across the sarcolemma is negative inside with respect to the outside, and most of the Ca++ is stored in the terminal cisternae. (B) Upon arrival of the action potential, as indicated by a reversal of the ionic distribution, Ca++ is released from the terminal cisternae. (C) After the action potential has passed (note ionic distribution), the Ca++ has spread throughout the sarcoplasm and is gradually pumped back into the sarcoplasmic reticulum (longitudinal tubule). *Note.* From ''Muscle'' by J.C. Rüegg, 1983, in R.F. Schmidt and G. Thews (Eds.), *Human Physiology* (p. 37), New York: Springer. Copyright 1983 by Springer-Verlag, Inc. Reprinted by permission.

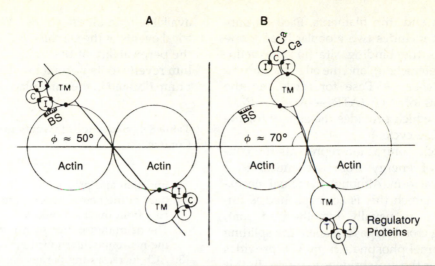

Figure 5.13. Scheme for the uncovering of the binding site (BS) on actin following the attachment of Ca⁺⁺ to the C component of troponin (TN). (A) In the resting state, tropomyosin (TM) is bound to the three components of troponin (T, C, I), and TN-I covers the binding site. (B) Following the attachment of Ca⁺⁺ to TN-C, the TN-I bonds are broken and the complex rotates, uncovering the binding site. *Note.* From "Some Aspects of the Role of the Sarcoplasmic Reticulum and the Tropomyosin-Troponin System in the Control of Muscle Contraction by Calcium Ions" by J. Gergely, 1974, *Circulation Research,* **34** (Suppl. III), p. 79. Copyright 1974 by the American Heart Association, Inc. Adapted by permission of the American Heart Association.

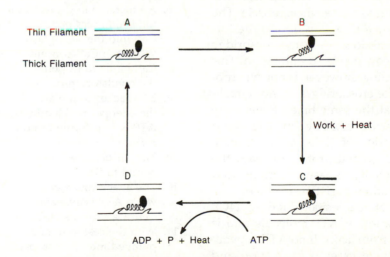

Figure 5.14. The crossbridge cycle. (A) In the resting state, actin and myosin are prevented from interacting. (B) Following Ca⁺⁺ disinhibition, actin and myosin connect, forming the actomyosin complex. (C) The complex uses the energy made available from the hydrolysis of ATP for crossbridge (S1 + S2) rotation, and thus causes sliding of the thick and thin filaments relative to one another. (D) ATP is bound to S1, and myosin detaches from actin.

the thick and thin filaments. Each S1 sub-fragment includes two globular heads; one head has the binding site (for the actin-myosin interaction), and the other has the enzyme myosin ATPase for catalyzing the hydrolysis of ATP (ATP → ADP + Pi + energy), which provides the energy for the crossbridge cycle.

A muscle contraction represents the conversion of energy from a chemical to a mechanical form. Although the actual mechanism by which this is accomplished is unknown, it is usually hypothesized that, following crossbridge formation, the splitting of a terminal phosphate from ATP provides energy for the crossbridges to rotate. In this rotation S1 rotates about S2 toward the LMM fragment (Figure 5.14). Since *the rotation occurs while actin and myosin are bound, the thick and thin filaments slide past one another* (the **sliding-filament theory**) and exert a force at the Z bands. This occurs along the entire myofibril and indeed among all the myofibrils of a muscle fiber, which explains how the force is transmitted to the whole muscle. The force exerted by a muscle is due to the formation and breakdown of many crossbridge connections following Ca^{++} disinhibition. This crossbridge cycling, however, is not synchronous in that the crossbridges do not attach-rotate-detach at the same time. If this were the case, the force exerted by a muscle would comprise a series of jerks rather than a smooth, finely graded profile. Instead, the crossbridge activity is asynchronous and results in a gradual variation in force.

Once in the rotated position (Figure 5.14C), the S1 binds another ATP molecule and is able to detach from actin. If no ATP is available, as in severe cases of starvation and following death, then detachment does not occur and actin and myosin remain bound; this state is known as rigor mortis. Upon detachment, the globular heads return to their prerotated position and search for other available actin-binding sites. When the electrical events of the sarcolemma are finished, the permeability of the sarcoplasmic reticulum reverts to its normal low level, the Ca^{++} pump (located in the sarcoplasmic reticulum)

Table 5.1 Sequence of Events in a Muscle Contraction

1. Initiation and propagation (active conduction) of the neural action potential (AP) occurs from the axon hillock.
2. The neurotransmitter ACh is released at the neuromuscular junction (NMJ).
3. ACh increases the permeability of the postsynaptic membrane (sarcolemma) to Na^+ and K^+, which causes an end-plate potential (EPP).
4. The EPP is conducted away from the NMJ and results in the generation of a muscle AP in the adjacent sarcolemma.
5. Propagation of the muscle AP occurs along the sarcolemma and into the T-tubule system.
6. An increase in g_{Ca} (calcium conductance) of the lateral sacs occurs with a release of Ca^{++} into the sarcoplasm.
7. When the Ca^{++} concentration is adequate, Ca^{++} binds to troponin (TN) and disinhibits the regulatory proteins.
8. S1 attaches to the actin-binding site and the energy provided by the breakdown of ATP is transformed into a crossbridge (XB) rotation.
9. The XB detaches once another ATP has bound to S1.
10. The attach-rotate-detach XB cycles continue while ATP is available and there is sufficient Ca^{++} for disinhibition.
11. With the cessation of muscle APs, Ca^{++} is pumped into the saroplasmic reticulum and returned to the lateral sacs.
12. The removal of Ca^{++} results in the resumption of inhibition by the regulatory proteins (TN and TM); XBs do not attach, and hence the myofilaments relax.

returns Ca^{++} to the sarcoplasmic reticulum, and the inhibitory effect of the troponin-tropomyosin complex is reestablished. Table 5.1 summarizes this entire sequence of events.

It is appropriate at this point to mention that, although the mechanism of muscle contraction may involve the cycling of crossbridges, some muscle physiologists often identify three different types of contractions. Hoyle (1983) refers to these as the major contraction, the basic tonus, and the local contraction. When the sarcolemma is depolarized past the excitation-contraction-coupling threshold, the ensuing crossbridge activity is referred to as a major contraction; until now we have simply called this sequence of events (Table 5.1) a muscle contraction. Accordingly, the term **contraction** is used *to indicate the internal state in which muscle actively exerts a force, whether or not muscle shortens its length*. In addition, however, we have traditionally adopted the view that when the sarcolemma is at a resting potential then the contractile machinery is completely switched off. The notion of **muscle tone** suggests otherwise, claiming that although the sarcolemma is at rest, the contractile machinery is in a state of very low activation (Hník, 1981). This might be accomplished, for example, by small increases in the extracellular K$^+$ concentration. However, muscle tone is generally thought to be due to the mechanical properties of the muscle, connective tissue, and joint (Brooks, 1986). Finally, **local contraction** refers to waves of activation that involve 5-30 sarcomeres and propagate along a fiber at the rate of about 10 μm/s (Hoyle, 1983).

Feedback From Proprioceptors

In the operation of the simple joint system, sensory receptors provide input that origi-

nates from a wide range of stimuli. In this limited discussion we shall draw a distinction between stimuli that arise from outside the system and those that arise from within the system. **Exteroreceptors** detect external stimuli that impinge on the system and include, among others, the eyes and ears, and the skin receptors that respond to temperature, touch, and pain. In contrast, **proprioceptors** detect stimuli generated by the system itself (Sanes & Evarts, 1984), such as those associated with the activation of muscle. One general distinction between these two forms of afferent input is that the exteroreceptors inform the system on the state of its external environment whereas the proprioceptors are more involved in the moment-to-moment control of movement. Both forms of afferent input can affect the motor output, but it appears that the proprioceptive effects are less intense than those generated by the exteroreceptors (Sanes & Evarts, 1984).

Perhaps the best known, but certainly not the only, type of coupling between sensory input and motor output is a class of responses known as reflexes. Traditionally, a **reflex** is defined as a *stereotyped motor response of an organism to a sensory stimulus*. Since the formulation of this concept in 1771, many different types of reflexes have been identified: stretch reflex, tendon jerk, flexor-withdrawal reflex, crossed-extensor reflex, corneal reflex, and so forth. On the basis of experimental evidence obtained in recent years, however, it appears that most reflexes (responses to given inputs) depend very much on the state of the animal—that is, whether the animal is stationary or moving and, if moving, the phase of the movement (e.g., swing vs. stance) (Nashner, 1982; Rossignol, Julien, & Gauthier, 1981). Even the responses associated with pain receptors do not truly satisfy the traditional concept of a reflex as an unmodifiable output in that they can be modulated during locomotion (Crenna & Frigo, 1984). As a consequence of these findings, our understanding of the role of reflexes, particularly during movement, remains rather elementary. The neural connections associated with reflex responses are thought to be as simple as any that exist. Because of our insufficient understanding of the nature and role of reflexes, you can imagine how dangerous it is to extend too far concepts based on neural circuitry. In what follows, the folly associated with carrying these ideas too far is illustrated by a discussion of the use of reflex concepts to develop flexibility protocols.

Reflex Circuitry

Communication within the afferent side of the simple joint system begins with the development of a **generator potential** by the sensing elements of the sensory receptors. For mechanoreceptors (e.g., muscle spindle, tendon organ, joint receptor), the generator potential is created by mechanical deformation of the sensory terminal. As a local-graded potential, the generator potential is conducted along the afferent axon to the trigger zone, and, if the depolarization is greater than threshold, an action potential is initiated. The most excitable portion of the afferent axon (the trigger zone) is located close to the sensing elements, usually within the capsule of the muscle spindle and the tendon organ. The action potential is propagated centrally to the spinal cord where it impinges on various motoneurons and interneurons. In general, neurons located between sensory neurons and motoneurons are referred to as **interneurons** (Figure 4.8).

As proprioceptors, both the muscle spindle and tendon organ are activated by certain stimuli (e.g., changes in length and force) that are experienced by at least some of the fibers in the muscle in which the receptors are located. *One central reflex effect of muscle spindles and tendon organs is to minimize the stimulus that led to their activation.* This is accomplished by the receptors that operate centrally (in the spinal cord) on the alpha motoneurons, which serve the muscle in which the receptors are located (**homonymous** alpha motoneurons; Figure 5.15). Ia input, for example, will generate an excitatory local-graded potential in homonymous alpha motoneurons. If these local-graded potentials are of sufficient magnitude, they will activate the alpha motoneurons and result in contraction of the skeletomotor fibers surrounding the activated spindle. The net effect of the skeletomotor activity is to decrease the change in muscle length that the spindle is detecting. This type of circuit (Figure 5.15A) is an example of **negative feedback**: The Ia input causes activity (contraction of skeletomotor fibers) that tends to reduce the stimulus eliciting the Ia input. It was previously emphasized that a major role of the muscle spindle is to monitor muscle length and that a spindle may be activated passively by stretching the entire muscle or actively by gamma-motoneuron activation of the polar regions of the fusimotor fibers. If a muscle is suddenly stretched, the muscle spindle is excited and it sends a signal along the Ia and spII afferents to the homonymous alpha motoneurons. If the signal is strong enough, the motoneurons generate action potentials, which result in activation of the muscle. This sequence of events is known as the **stretch reflex**. In contrast, Ib input produces, among other effects, an inhibitory local-graded potential in homonymous alpha motoneurons. Such local-graded potentials lower the excitability of the alpha motoneurons and tend to relax the skeletomotor fibers that connect in series with the tendon organ. This response diminishes the muscle-force stimulus that initially activated the tendon organ

(Figure 5.15A)—another negative feedback connection.

The neural connections illustrated in Figure 5.15A oversimplify the central connections made by the Ia and Ib afferents. Each of these afferents branches out many times, making contact with a multitude of motoneurons and interneurons. In addition, many of these branches make connections with neurons that transmit the information up and down the spinal cord, including all the way to the brain. As a consequence, the input

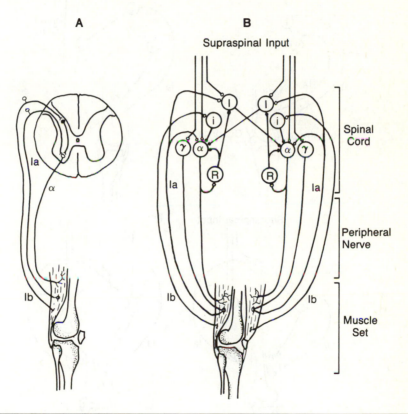

Figure 5.15. Spinal connections between sensory receptors located in muscle and alpha motoneurons. The Ia axon conveys afferent information from the muscle spindle to the central nervous system. The Ib axon represents a similar connection but from the tendon organ. (A) Homonymous relationships—muscle spindles and tendon organs located in a muscle connect with the alpha motoneurons that activate the same muscle. Afferent and efferent axons that service muscles located on the right side of the body enter and exit the spinal cord on the right side, and vice versa. (B) The same connections for an agonist-antagonist muscle set (e.g., the hamstrings and quadriceps for the right leg) but this time emphasizing the complexity of the interneuronal connections. Open synapses circles (○) represent excitatory connections; filled synapses circles (●) indicate inhibitory effects. α = alpha motoneuron, γ = gamma motoneuron, i = interneuron, I = Ia inhibitory interneuron, Ia = muscle-spindle afferent, Ib = tendon-organ afferent, R = Renshaw cell.

from proprioceptors is distributed over much of the nervous system (Binder, Houk, Nichols, Rymer, & Stuart, 1982; Powers & Binder, 1985a, 1985b). For example, in addition to the homonymous effects just de-

scribed, the Ia afferent is known to send a branch to an interneuron that has been labeled the Ia inhibitory interneuron (Figure 5.16B). Activation of this interneuron results in an inhibitory local-graded poten-

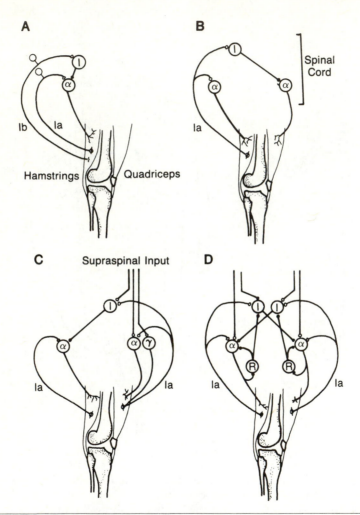

Figure 5.16.   Selected central connections (● = inhibitory, ○ = excitatory) of the muscle spindle (Ia) and tendon organ (Ib) efferents to the schematized quadriceps and hamstrings muscle groups. (A) Effects on homonymous alpha (α) motoneurons. (B) Transmission of the reciprocal-inhibition reflex through the Ia inhibitory interneuron (I). (C) Supraspinal input to the quadriceps muscle group activating the reciprocal-inhibition circuit to the hamstrings. (D) Recurrent inhibition of the alpha motoneuron and the Ia inhibitory interneuron through the Renshaw (R) cell. I = Ia inhibitory interneuron, i = interneuron, R = Renshaw cell, α = alpha motoneuron, γ = gamma motoneuron.

tial in the motoneurons serving antagonist muscles. For example, stretch of the hamstrings may activate muscle spindles located in the hamstrings. The hamstring spindles send input over their Ia afferents to the spinal cord where the afferents connect to, among other neurons, the Ia inhibitory interneuron (I in Figure 5.16B). Once activated, the Ia inhibitory interneuron sends a signal (action potential) to many alpha motoneurons that innervate quadriceps muscle fibers. This interneuron has been so named because its effect is to inhibit these alpha motoneurons (its action potential induces an inhibitory local-graded potential in the motoneurons), thus causing the quadriceps muscle fibers to relax. Thus, as well as activating the homonymous muscle (hamstrings in this example) by the stretch reflex, Ia input may also relax the antagonist muscle (quadriceps in this example) if the appropriate conditions prevail—at least the neural circuitry exists for such an effect. This latter response is referred to as **reciprocal inhibition**. However, reciprocal inhibition appears to be confined to flexor-extensor muscle sets (Jankowska & Odutola, 1980).

In addition to this circuitry, there is another neuron, the Renshaw cell, about which quite a bit is known. We know, for example, that the Renshaw cell is a spinal-cord interneuron that receives some input from collateral branches of alpha-motoneuron axons (Figure 5.16D). Output from the Renshaw cell is distributed among many neurons, including the Ia inhibitory interneuron and alpha motoneurons from which it received the collateral input. The effect of Renshaw-cell input is to generate inhibitory local-graded potentials in both of these neurons. The Renshaw-cell circuit associated with inhibitory effects in alpha motoneurons (Figure 5.16D) is known as **recurrent inhibition**. In addition to these somewhat simple minded interactions, we also know that these neurons send branches

up and down the spinal cord and that many of them receive input from supraspinal structures (Figure 5.16C).

Stretching for Flexibility

One example of the application of these ideas on neural circuitry has been in the area of flexibility training. It has often been claimed that flexibility is one of the indices of fitness, particularly since we tend to lose flexibility as we grow older. Among active athletes, however, it has also been suggested that an individual can be too flexible for a specific event. In both of these contexts, the term *flexibility is used to refer to the range of motion about a joint*. In most instances, flexibility training concerns increasing this range of motion with various stretching exercises. The stretching activities that are employed to enhance flexibility can generally be classified into four groups: ballistic, static, dynamic, and rehabilitation-based. The ballistic and static techniques are the most traditional and can be exemplified by bending forward from an upright position to stretch the hamstrings by touching the toes with a bouncing movement (**ballistic**) versus a slow, prolonged stretch (**static**). Although both techniques appear to be equally effective at enhancing flexibility, static is preferable because it is thought to be less likely to cause injury.

The **dynamic** technique combines a maximum stretch with a concentric activation of the muscle being stretched. The exercise is best done with a partner. A limb is taken to its maximum stretch position and the muscle group being stretched is maximally contracted concentrically for about 8 s as the partner provides an opposing force that is just less than what the muscle group exerts (Figure 5.17). As a consequence, the limb will rotate toward its normal resting position. The limb is then returned to the stretch position, which will be greater than for the previous

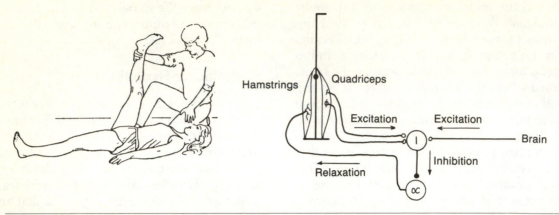

Figure 5.17. Partner-assisted flexibility training. Using the HR-AC technique, the partner stretches the hamstrings maximally while the subject (person lying down) attempts a submaximal concentric activation of the quadriceps muscle group.

repetition, and the exercise is repeated. This is done about four times for each muscle group and direction for which an increased flexibility is sought. This increase in flexibility is probably due to an *increase in muscle-connective tissue core temperature* caused by muscle activation.

A fourth technique, which is based on neural connections (Figure 5.16), has evolved from people's involvement in rehabilitation programs. Essentially, the technique has emerged from Kabat's work on a procedure called *Proprioceptive Neuromuscular Facilitation* (PNF; Knott & Voss, 1968). Among these techniques, Kabat proposed three methods for the relaxation of involuntary muscle spasm. The first was based on the observation that following successive excitations, a motoneuron is inhibited (Kabat, 1950; Thigpen, Moritani, Thiebaud, & Hargis, 1985). In fact, the greater the initial excitation, the greater the subsequent inhibition (decreased excitability). The **hold-relax (HR)** stretch utilizes this response by beginning with an isometric contraction of the muscle to be stretched followed by relaxation and then a stretch of the muscle (Figure 5.17). Since the

muscle is stretched while the alpha motoneurons are least excitable, input from homonymous length detectors (muscle spindles) results in minimal alpha-motoneuron excitation, and there should be less muscle activity (EMG) while the muscle is stretched.

A second PNF-based technique is known as **agonist-contract (AC)**. In this scheme, the muscle to be stretched is referred to as the antagonist. The technique involves the submaximal contraction of an agonist while the individual attempts to stretch the antagonist. For example, if the goal were to stretch the hamstrings (Figure 5.17), then the AC technique would involve the submaximal activation of the quadriceps during the stretch. The quadriceps activity should be submaximal because maximal efforts tend to produce cocontraction rather than relaxation of the antagonist (Condon & Hutton, 1987). The rationale for the AC technique is that the agonist activity will produce reciprocal inhibition, and hence relaxation, in the antagonist during the stretch.

The **hold-relax agonist-contraction (HR-AC)** stretch attempts to go one step better by combining the postactivation inhibition of motoneurons with the reciprocal-inhibition reflex (Figure 5.16B), the basis for Kabat's second method of muscle-spasm relaxation. The scheme illustrated in Figure 5.16 represents some of the neuronal connections related to an agonist-antagonist muscle set, in this case the hamstrings and quadriceps femoris. The somas for the various neural elements (alpha and gamma motoneurons, Ia inhibitory interneuron, and Renshaw cell) are located in the spinal cord. The efferent input to the muscle (axons from the alpha and gamma motoneurons) and the afferent output from the muscle (axons from the spindle and tendon organ) traverse from the spinal cord to the muscle together in a nerve. The reciprocal-inhibition reflex, for example, is shown as an inhibitory effect from the hamstrings muscle spindles onto the quadriceps alpha motoneurons (Figure 5.16B). This effect is mediated by the Ia inhibitory interneuron. The AC and HR-AC techniques supposedly capitalize on this circuit by having the Ia inhibitory interneuron related to the quadriceps group exert an inhibitory effect on the hamstring alpha motoneurons while the hamstring muscle is being stretched.

The AC and HR-AC exercises supposedly promote relaxation of the muscle being stretched by activating the reciprocal-inhibition reflex. For example, suppose an individual was attempting to stretch the hamstring muscle group (Figure 5.17). These techniques propose that while the hamstrings are being stretched, the quadriceps muscles should be isometrically activated. Such activation will result in the sending of commands from the supraspinal centers (brain) to the quadriceps alpha and gamma motoneurons and Ia-inhibitory interneurons. The next effect of this input would be to relax the hamstrings by activating the reciprocal-inhibition response through the Ia inhibitory interneuron (Figure 5.16C). Thus *the HR (post-activation motoneuron inhibition), AC (reciprocal*

inhibition), and HR-AC techniques are designed to capitalize upon neural effects.

In a comparison of the ballistic and HR techniques, Wallin, Ekblom, Grahn, and Nordenborg (1985) found that HR led to greater improvements in flexibility. This distinction, however, has not always proven obvious. Moore and Hutton (1980) compared the static, HR, and HR-AC methods and found that (a) there was substantial variability in the responses, (b) HR-AC tended to produce the greatest increase in hip flexibility, and (c) there was no difference between the gains obtained with the static and HR methods. In contrast, Etnyre and Abraham (1986) found that the change in range of motion for soleus was greatest for HR-AC, intermediate for HR, and least for a static stretch. However, Condon and Hutton (1987) reported no differences among the HR-AC, AC, HR, and static techniques in increasing soleus range of motion. Taken together, these observations suggest that there is no clearly superior flexibility-training technique.

One significant observation, however, that did emerge from these studies (Condon & Hutton, 1987; Moore & Hutton, 1980) was that the HR-AC was associated with the most pain, and, *rather than causing inhibition (reciprocal) of the muscle being stretched* (the hamstrings in Figure 5.17), *HR-AC caused cocontraction*. This latter observation underscores the complexity of neural interactions and the danger of designing procedures based on oversimplified constructs (Kudina, 1980). For example, the AC- and HR-AC-induced cocontractions suggest that the major effect of contracting the quadriceps during a hamstrings stretch is *not* the elicitation of the reciprocal-inhibition reflex with relaxation of the hamstrings. Instead, confounding this connection (reciprocal inhibition) are the inhibitory interactions of the Renshaw cell. Alpha-motoneuron activation of Renshaw cells through recurrent collaterals (recurrent inhibition) results in inhibitory local-graded potentials in, at least, alpha motoneurons and Ia inhibitory interneurons. That is, supraspinal drive onto quadriceps alpha motoneurons activates recurrent inhibition of the Ia inhibitory interneurons (Figure 5.16D). The cocontraction observed during AC and HR-AC, therefore, could be explained as an overriding of the reciprocal-inhibition reflex by the Ia inhibitory interneuron (i.e., the Renshaw cell inhibits the Ia inhibitory interneuron, thus preventing reciprocal inhibition).

What does all this tell us about flexibility training? We know about different flexibility-training techniques (e.g., ballistic, static, dynamic, and PNF-based). There does not appear to be any clear and simple evidence indicating which technique is the most effective. Furthermore, we do not seem to understand the mechanisms involved in altering flexibility. For example, Moore and Hutton (1980) demonstrated that complete muscle relaxation is not necessary for effective flexibility training. A critical assumption often encountered in the discussion of flexibility is the notion that the contractile machinery in muscle represents the limiting element in flexibility. Sapega et al. (1981) suggest that the range of motion about most joints is limited by one or more connective-tissue structures, including those in muscle, rather than the ability to relax the muscle completely. The contribution of the various joint structures to the stiffness of the joint varies among the joints; however, for the metacarpophalangeal joint it was found to be joint capsule 47%, muscle 41%, tendons 10%, and skin 2% (Johns & Wright, 1962). This means that the range of motion (flexibility) of the metacarpophalangeal joint was determined by the passive properties of these tissues in this proportion. As a consequence, these observations suggest that *the target of stretching exercises for flexibility should be to induce plastic changes in connective tissue when the muscle is as relaxed as possible.*

To achieve this goal, flexibility exercises should cause plastic rather than elastic changes in connective tissue, because plastic changes cause more permanent changes in tissue length. The relative proportions of plasticity and elasticity within a stretch are influenced by the amount and duration of the applied force and the tissue temperature. The low-force, long-duration stretch optimizes the plastic changes—this is a trade-off between tissue elongation and weakening. It should be emphasized that *whenever plastic changes are induced in tissue this causes a weakening of the tissue.* However, this stress stimulates the tissue to adapt, and, provided the stress is not too great, the weakening will only be short term. In reality, flexibility training merely involves the stressing of tissue so that it will adapt to a new length without any long-term loss in strength. The tissue is most extensible when temperature is higher, such as at the end of a workout, and the amount of elongation retained is greatest if stretch is applied while the tissue cools. Some individuals even suggest applying ice packs while stretching. Hence, effective stretching for flexibility should employ low-force, long-duration stretches and be performed at the end of a workout. This is not to say that stretching exercises should not be done at the beginning of a workout since stretching can be used as part of the warm-up as well as for increasing flexibility; that is, a distinction should be maintained between stretching for flexibility and stretching as part of a warm-up.

Neural Integration

The performance of a movement requires the activation of the motor system, those elements of the nervous system involved in controlling muscles. In general, motor systems must be capable of three basic requirements in order to produce useful movements: (a) information from sensory receptors must be channeled to motoneurons; that is, sensory information from the different parts of the body must affect the operation of the appropriate muscles. For example, if you touch a hot object, you would rather have your hand withdrawn rapidly than for a muscle in your face to become activated—the latter can come later; (b) the nervous system must be able to control accurately the level of force exerted by a muscle—this involves an interaction between the control of motor-unit activity and feedback from muscle receptors; and (c) the activity of different muscles must be coordinated.

The study of reflexes has, at least since the time of Sherrington (1857-1952), provided a dominant focus in the study of motor control. In this scheme, the motoneuron is represented as the central element to which afferent and supraspinal input is directed (Figure 5.18A). Although the motoneuron is still thought of as the **final common pathway**—the route through which the commands are issued to muscles—accumulating evidence suggests that the motoneuron is not the major integrating element that it was once thought to be. There are millions of synaptic connections within the spinal cord that form the basis of the interactions among the neural elements. These interactions are based upon the summation of excitatory and inhibitory local-graded potentials. It appears that the interneuron (Figure 5.18B), rather than the motoneuron, serves as the focal point for this integration (Baldissera, Hultborn, & Illert, 1981; see also Figure 5.15B). Figure 5.18B shows that afferent and supraspinal input converges on a number of different interneurons rather than going directly to the motoneurons. As a consequence, the input (e.g., Ia input caused by muscle stretch) can

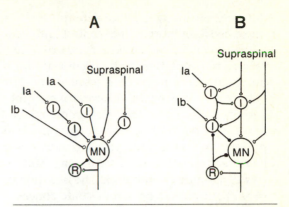

Figure 5.18. Schemes for the convergence of input in the spinal cord. (A) Motoneuron focus. (B) Interneuron focus. I = interneuron, Ia = afferent from muscle spindle, Ib = afferent from tendon organ, MN = motoneuron, R = Renshaw cell, o = excitatory, ● = inhibitory. *Note.* From ''Integration of Sensory Information and Motor Commands in the Spinal Cord'' by R.E. Burke, 1985, in P.S.G. Stein (organizer), *Motor Control: From Movement Trajectories to Neural Mechanisms* (pp. 47, 53), Class at the Society for Neuroscience, Washington, DC. Adapted by permission.

be altered before it is transmitted to the motoneurons. One effect of this arrangement is that input-output relationships (e.g., reflexes) can vary depending on the nature of the other input converging on the interneurons. The main advantage of this scheme for the system is that it allows greater flexibility in terms of input-output coupling.

This shift in focus to the interneuron largely came about because of technical developments and because of the systematic study of spinal-cord connectivity. These studies have revealed a number of interesting features of nervous-system operation (Stuart 1987a, 1987b): (a) Reflex circuitry involves alternate pathways, an idea emphasizing that afferents (e.g., spindle Ia) have alternative excitatory and inhibitory pathways to motoneurons; (b) there appear to be considerable differences among muscle systems, such as those between muscles that control limb, respiration, and head-neck movement (e.g., reciprocal inhibition only occurs in limb muscles); and (c) the connections that occur between interneurons appear to be quite sophisticated in that they are responsible for organizing most of the movements that we perform. With the advance of technology we have been able to record neural activity under less constrained conditions. These opportunities have caused us to reevaluate concepts and have generated unforeseen dilemmas.

For example, experimental work from the first half of this century established a clear distinction between muscle spindles and tendon organs; however, recent work from more natural conditions shows that spindle and tendon organ responses from the same active muscle are quite similar. In addition, much of our understanding of the role of afferentation has been derived from the study of postural reflexes. Such developments emphasize that much remains to be determined about the role of afferentation during movement (Hasan & Stuart, in press).

Problems

5.1. The motor unit is described as the basic functional unit of the simple joint system. What does this idea mean?

5.2. What does the innervation ratio suggest about the control of muscle force?

5.3. Why is the decline in force during a twitch represented with the measure one-half relaxation time rather than the total relaxation time?

5.4. If a motor unit had a peak twitch force of 15.2 mN and a twitch-tetanus ratio of 1:8, how much force could it exert during a fused tetanus?

5.5. What two physiological measurements are used to separate motor units into different types?

5.6. Three physiological characteristics used to distinguish motor units are
   a. innervation ratio, fatigability, and oxidative enzymes.
   b. oxidative enzymes, contraction speed, and fatigability.
   c. contraction speed, force, and innervation ratio.
   d. fatigability, contraction speed, and force.
   e. tetanus, twitch, and one-half relaxation time.

5.7. Suppose a Type S motor unit exerted a peak twitch force of 5.0 mN and had an innervation ratio of 1:300. What was the average force exerted by each muscle fiber belonging to the motor unit?

5.8. If a motor unit in a human biceps brachii muscle had a twitch contraction time of 42 ms and a fatigue index of 0.80, what type of motor unit would it be?

5.9.   Many people use the Type S-FR-FF and Type I-IIa-IIb classification systems interchangeably. What are the objections to this practice?

5.10. For an FF motor unit that had a peak tetanic force of 52 mN and a fatigue index of 0.14, how much force would it exert at the end of the fatigue test?

5.11. Which statement about the resting membrane potential is incorrect?

   a. The four most important ions in maintaining the resting membrane potential are A^-, Na^+, K^+, and Cl^-.
   b. The inside of the membrane is negative with respect to the outside.
   c. The two forces acting on the ions are the electrical and chemical gradients.
   d. The Na^+-K^+ pump is always active.
   e. K^+ has a higher concentration outside the cell.

5.12. The potential that exists across an excitable membrane is due to the distribution of ions.

   a. Which ions are involved in maintaining a resting membrane potential?
   b. What two forces are exerted on each of these ions?
   c. If one type of positive ion enters the cell and another type of positive ion leaves the cell, the net change in charge is zero. Since an action potential is basically due to positive ions' entering (influx) and leaving (efflux) the cell, why does the membrane potential change during an action potential?

5.13. The various phases of the action potential are referred to as depolarization, repolarization, and afterhyperpolarization. What is the role of polarity (e.g., de*polar*ization) in this scheme?

5.14. What is meant by the phrase *voltage-gated change in conductance*?

   a. Changes in permeability that depend on membrane potential.
   b. A shift of ions across a membrane.
   c. The initiation of a local-graded potential, such as at the neuromuscular junction.
   d. The generation of an action potential when the membrane potential reaches threshold.
   e. The temporal effect in the change in g_{Na} and g_K (sodium and potassium conductance, respectively).

5.15. Which of the following is not associated with exocytosis?

   a. Afterhyperpolarization
   b. Neurotransmitter
   c. Vesicles
   d. Synaptic cleft
   e. Chemical process

5.16. Local-graded potentials can be excitatory or inhibitory. Is this true for the motor end-plate potential?

5.17. Action potentials are physically represented as ionic shifts across an excitable membrane. We have considered selected features of an axonal action potential.

   a. Describe the ion shifts that underlie a muscle action potential.

   b. Sketch two diagrams of this event: an intracellularly recorded voltage-time graph and an extracellularly recorded voltage-time graph. (Hint: What is a synonym for *extracellular voltage-time* record?)

5.18. Why would a researcher be interested in rectifying an EMG signal?

5.19. When a command is issued from the brain down to motoneurons in the spinal cord, motoneurons plus their associated muscle fibers (i.e., motor units) are activated.

   a. Indicate in this sequence of events where action potentials versus local-graded potentials are used.

   b. Similarly, where in this sequence of events are voltage- and chemical-gated changes in conductance used?

5.20. How does a neural action potential (an electrical event) cause the release of neurotransmitter (a chemical event)?

5.21. In the process of muscle contraction, which substance was described as a disinhibitor and why?

5.22. Excitation-contraction coupling refers to

   a. attachment, rotation, and detachment of the crossbridge.

   b. connection of the muscle action potential to the sarcoplasmic reticulum through the triad.

   c. Ca^{++}-based disinhibition.

   d. conversion of the neural action potential (electrical) to neurotransmitter (chemical) and finally to a muscle action potential (electrical).

   e. sliding filament theory of muscle contraction.

5.23. In severe cases of starvation and after death, muscles go into rigor mortis. What is this and why does it occur?

5.24. Which statements (a-e) about reflexes are *correct*? Both parts (i-v) of each statement need to be correct.

   i.   A reflex can be defined as a constant input-output relationship.

   ii. Not all reflexes involve a sensory receptor.

   iii. A reflex need not involve a signal's passing through the spinal cord.

   iv. Reflex responses are thought to represent the simplest neural circuits.

   v.   Reflexes can be transmitted between limbs.

   a. i, v

   b. iv, iii

   c. v, iv

   d. ii, i

   e. iii, i

5.25. One central reflex action of muscle spindles and tendon organs is to minimize the stimulus that led to their activation. Use the stretch reflex to describe what is meant by this statement.

5.26. Consider a simple reflex, such as the stretch reflex. Which phases of this response are controlled by local-graded potentials and which by action potential? (Hint: Kandel, 1985, p. 20).

5.27. The effect of negative feedback is to generate activity that
a. diminishes the stimulus.
b. enhances the stimulus.
c. reroutes the stimulus.

5.28. Does the reciprocal-inhibition response occur between limbs or between an agonist-antagonist muscle set?

5.29. As with most neurons, the Renshaw cell makes a variety of connections. Two of these connections are of interest: that with the motoneuron that gives rise to the collateral, and that with the Ia inhibitory interneuron. Consider either of these connections and comment on its functional significance.

5.30. Which statements (a-e) about stretching for flexibility are correct? Both parts (i-v) of each statement need to be correct.
i. Muscle tissue is largely responsible for limiting the range of motion at a joint.
ii. The HR stretch is based upon reciprocal inhibition.
iii. The term PNF does not describe stretching procedures.
iv. Reflex responses during movements (e.g., stretching) are not well understood.
v. Flexibility training does not damage any of the tissues in the simple joint system.
a. iv, iii
b. i, iv
c. v, ii
d. ii, iii
e. v, i

5.31. What is the significance of the shift in ideas about the focal point in spinal cord connections (i.e., the change from the motoneuron to the interneuron focus)?

Summary—Part II

The goal of Part II (chapters 4 and 5) has been to define a biological model, the simple joint system, and to describe the interactions among its elements. At this stage you should be familiar with the following features and concepts related to the simple joint system:

- Observe that the morphological and mechanical features of the simple-joint-system elements are largely determined by the functions they serve.
- Note the structural features of the five elements of the simple joint system.
- Understand why an explanation of the control of movement can be studied with a model that comprises these five ele-

ments. That is, what is the role of each of these elements in the simple joint system?
- Realize that the motor unit is the basic functional unit of the system and be able to describe its features.
- Conceive of the means by which information is transmitted rapidly throughout the system.
- Understand the mechanism that links the neural signal with muscle, resulting in its activation.
- Comprehend the basic features of afferent feedback, including simple reflex circuits and the prominent role of interneurons in processing information.

Movement: A System-Surround Interaction

The objective of this discourse is the study of human motion. To accomplish this goal, the text has been organized into three parts: Part I considers the relationship between force and motion and the approaches used to analyze the latter; Part II defines the characteristics and operation of the elements of a simple biological model that can be used for the study of motion; and finally, Part III combines the concepts developed in the first two parts to examine the role of the nervous system and various muscle properties in controlling the force exerted by muscle. The focus of Part III is the force exerted by muscle because it is the relationship between this muscle force and the load acting on the simple joint system (i.e., the effect of the surrounding environment) that determines the nature of the accompanying movement.

Objectives

The goal of this text is to describe movement as the interaction of a biological model (a simplified version of us) with the physical world in which we live. In this scheme, the nervous system determines and sends out to the simple joint system a set of commands for the elaboration of a movement. What happens, however, depends on the mechanical state of the system and the mechanical interaction between the system and its surrounding environment. Part III focuses on the system-surround interaction. Specific objectives include the following:

- To examine the role of the nervous system in controlling muscle force.
- To define the mechanical characteristics of the force-generating units.
- To describe the design effects of different arrangements of the force-generating units.
- To establish the concept that movements require different control strategies.
- To deduce net muscle activity based on kinematic and kinetic descriptions of a movement.
- To evaluate performance on the basis of the base parameters: strength, power, and fatigue.

6

Control of Muscle Force

There are many factors that affect the force a muscle exerts. In this chapter, these factors have been divided into two categories: the excitation of the force-generating units and the characteristics of the force-generating units.

Excitation Factors

The transformation of a muscle action potential into muscle force is referred to as excitation-contraction coupling. In this process, the electrical events that accompany the action potential provide the excitation for the muscle contraction. In a broader context, however, the muscle action potential is a product of nervous-system input; consequently, *the topic of excitation factors concerns the role of the nervous system in controlling muscle force.*

In Part II ("The Simple Joint System"), we developed the concept that the motor unit represents the operational unit by which the simple joint system modulates muscle force. The nervous system has two available options for varying muscle force. The force that a muscle exerts depends on (a) the number of active motor units and (b) the rate at which each of the active motor units generates action potentials. These two alternatives are typically referred to as **motor-unit recruitment** (the process of motor-unit activation) and **rate coding** (action potential frequency), respectively.

Motor-Unit Recruitment

In 1938, Denny-Brown and Pennybacker reported that the performance of a particular movement always appeared to be accomplished by the activation of motor units in a set sequence. This organization of motor-unit activation has been called **orderly recruitment**. As the force exerted by a muscle increases (up to 10% of the maximum in Figure 6.1), additional motor units are activated or recruited. Once a motor unit is recruited, it remains active until the force declines. Thus, in Figure 6.1, Motor Unit 1 is recruited first and remains active as long as the force does not decrease. The increase in force is accomplished by continuing to recruit motor units (four more in Figure 6.1). The force reaches a plateau value when additional motor units cease to be recruited. As the force is reduced, motor units are sequentially inactivated or **derecruited**. Motor-unit derecruitment occurs

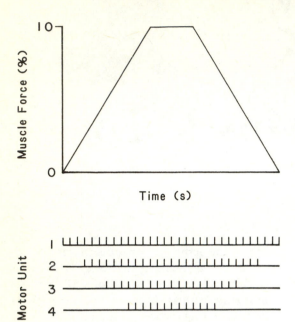

Figure 6.1. Idealized variation in muscle force due to the orderly recruitment and derecruitment of motor units. The motor-unit records represent the action potentials generated by each motor unit as muscle force varies.

mann, 1981). The increase in muscle force beyond that due to motor-unit recruitment reflects the effects of rate coding, a topic that will be addressed later.

Although orderly recruitment is a robust phenomenon that has been demonstrated in a wide variety of muscle groups and animal species, its physiological mechanism remains undetermined. Several hypotheses have been proposed to account for orderly recruitment, but there is no agreement on a single mechanism (Stuart & Enoka, 1983). Of the alternatives, the most popular is the **size principle**, a proposal made in 1957 by Henneman (Enoka & Stuart, 1984; Henneman, 1957). *The size principle suggests that the orderly recruitment of motor units is due to variations in motoneuron size*; the motor unit with the smallest motoneuron is recruited first and the motor unit with the largest motoneuron is recruited last (Henneman, 1979). This organization is thought to exist among the motoneurons that serve one particular muscle. Such a group of motoneurons is referred to as a **motoneuron pool**. For example, the human muscle tibialis anterior is innervated by approximately 445 alpha motoneurons; this represents the size of the motoneuron pool for that muscle. The size principle suggests that, within a motoneuron pool, the motoneurons are functionally organized according to their size, where motoneuron size is defined as the surface area of the soma and dendrites. When the muscle is required to exert a force, the smallest motoneuron in the pool is recruited first and the largest is recruited last. For example, in tibialis anterior the largest alpha motoneuron (Number 445) will only be recruited when all the other motoneurons (Numbers 1-444) have been recruited.

It appears that, as the size of the motoneuron varies, so do its various morphological (e.g., number of dendrites, axon diameter) and electrical characteristics (Figure 6.2), such that the smallest motoneurons are

in the reverse order to recruitment; that is, the last motor unit recruited is the first derecruited. It should be emphasized, however, that Figure 6.1 is a special case as it represents the condition in which changes in force are due solely to a variation in the number of active motor units.

The relative contribution of motor-unit recruitment to muscle force varies between muscles. For example, in some muscles (e.g., adductor pollicis) all the motor units are probably recruited when the force reaches a value of about 30% of maximum. Conversely, in other muscles (e.g., biceps brachii) motor-unit recruitment is thought to continue up to 85% of the maximum force (Kukulka & Cla-

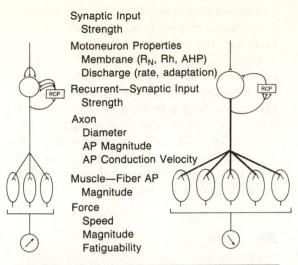

Synaptic Input
   Strength
Motoneuron Properties
   Membrane (R_N, Rh, AHP)
   Discharge (rate, adaptation)
Recurrent—Synaptic Input
   Strength
Axon
   Diameter
   AP Magnitude
   AP Conduction Velocity
Muscle—Fiber AP
   Magnitude
Force
   Speed
   Magnitude
   Fatiguability

Figure 6.2. A model of two motor units (motoneuron and muscle fibers) that illustrates selected morphological and physiological measurements that correlate to varying extents with motoneuron size. Morphological implications of motoneuron size are indicated graphically as variations in the strength of synaptic input, axonal diameter, innervation ratio, and muscle-fiber size. The functional consequences of such variations are examined physiologically by the measurement of the variables indicated in the center of the figure. AHP = afterhyperpolarization, AP = action potential, RCP = Renshaw-cell pool, Rh = rheobase (an index of motoneuron excitability), R_N = input resistance (electrical resistance of a motoneuron to current input), sag = decline in unfused-tetanic force after the initial 4-8 stimuli, strength = amplitude of postsynaptic response. *Note.* From "Henneman's 'Size Principle': Current Issues" by R.M. Enoka and D.G. Stuart, 1984, *Trends in Neurosciences,* **7**, p. 227. Copyright 1984 by Elsevier Science Publications B.V. Reprinted by permission.

the most easily excited. However, the threshold of activation for a motoneuron is not dependent solely on size but is also influenced by other factors. For example, the organization of input onto a motoneuron pool (e.g.,

from muscle spindles, supraspinal structures, skin sensory receptors) may differ depending upon the input system; the recruitment order of motor units due to the activation of skin sensory receptors has been shown to be different from that which is produced by muscle-stretch-receptor input (Kanda, Burke, & Walmsley, 1977). Thus motoneuron size appears to be a significant but not exclusive factor in determining recruitment order (Gustafsson & Pinter, 1985).

The advantage of orderly recruitment is that, when a muscle is commanded to exert a force, the sequence of motor-unit recruitment will have been predetermined. In particular, the supraspinal center (brain) issuing the command does not have to specify which motor units are to be activated. Since recruitment order is predetermined, it is not possible to activate selectively motor units in any order other than that specified by orderly recruitment. Consequently, if the purpose of a training program were to stress only the motor units with the largest motoneurons, this could not be accomplished, according to the size principle, by selectively activating those motor units.

Why might one even contemplate attempting to stress one group of motor units? It appears that, in general, the small motoneurons belong to Type S motor units and that the largest motoneurons innervate Type FF motor units. The Type S motor units are slow-contracting, low-force, and fatigue-resistant whereas the Type FF units possess the converse characteristics (i.e., fast-contracting, high-force, and fatigable); thus it is conceivable that an individual may wish to train one set of motor units for a particular event. For example, endurance athletes (e.g., long-distance runners, skiers, and cyclists) tend to prefer units that are fatigue-resistant whereas power athletes (e.g., weight lifters, sprinters) may be more concerned with high-force capabilities.

Figure 6.3 represents a hypothetical model of the relationship between recruitment order and the power demands of an activity. For example, jogging at a slow speed represents an activity in which the muscle-power requirements are minimal. The model indicates that jogging can be accomplished by recruiting only the Type S and FR motor units. In this scheme *recruitment order is fixed, beginning with the Type S motor units and progressing to the Type FR and FF units as the power demands increase.* For high-power events, such as a maximum vertical jump, all the motor units are recruited, again in the sequence that is specified by orderly recruitment (i.e., S, FR, then FF). This means that, for high-power activities, Type S motor units are recruited along with the high-force-producing Type FF units. Why then do only the Type FR and FF motor units adapt (e.g., Schmidtbleicher & Haralambie, 1981) to the stress imposed in high-power training? We will answer this question in chapter 8.

It is necessary to emphasize one of the major shortcomings of the Figure 6.3 model.

The motor-unit types do not exist as discrete populations relative to their activation threshold (i.e., the force at which a motor unit is activated). Instead there is considerable overlap between the groups, especially Type S and FR units. In other words, it does not appear possible to activate a muscle such that only Type S motor units are recruited without any Type FR units. By extension, therefore, it does not seem possible to activate only slow-twitch muscle fibers and no fast-twitch fibers (Stuart & Enoka, 1983).

Rate Coding

The force exerted by a muscle is due, in part, to variable combinations of the number of active motor units and the rate at which these motor units discharge action potentials. The relationship between muscle force and action-potential rate (frequency) is not linear; the increase in force due to increasing action-potential rate from 5 to 10 Hz is not the same as that due to increasing the rate from 20 to 25 Hz, although there is a difference of 5 Hz in each case. The force-action potential rate relationship is sigmoidal (S-shaped) rather than linear (Figure 6.4), with the greatest increase in force (steepest slope) occurring at the lower action-potential rates (3-10 Hz). The actual relationship depicted in Figure 6.4 depends upon muscle length; the curve shifts to the left for longer muscle lengths and to the right for shorter lengths (Rack & Westbury, 1969). Although the relationship remains sigmoidal, the frequency for effecting the greatest changes in force (i.e., the steepest part of the curve) becomes 3-7 Hz for long muscle lengths and 10-20 Hz for short muscle lengths.

One group of investigators has explored the differences between motor units in their discharge (action-potential rate) characteristics and has proposed that, based on the re-

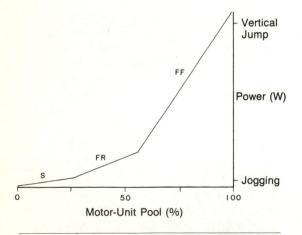

Figure 6.3. Hypothetical model of the motor-unit-recruitment requirements as dependent upon the muscle-power demands of the activity.

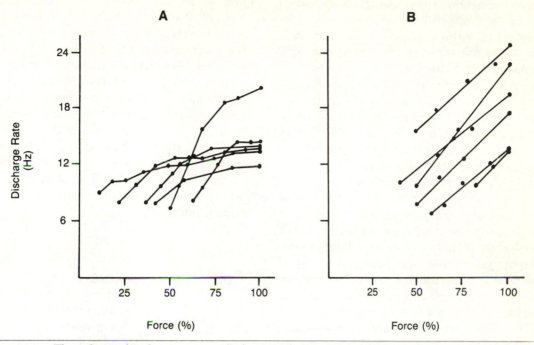

Figure 6.4. The relationship between muscle force and action-potential rate of motor units for a muscle held at constant length. Gydikov and Kosarov (1973, 1974) report that human motor units display either of two characteristics: (A) ramp and plateau, or (B) linear relationship. *Note.* From "Some Features of Different Motor Units in Human Biceps Brachii" by A. Gydikov and D. Kosarov, 1974, *Pflügers Archiv,* **347**, p. 79. Copyright 1974 by Springer-Verlag, Inc. Adapted by permission.

lation between discharge characteristics and muscle force, there are two types of motor units: tonic and phasic (Gydikov & Kosarov, 1973, 1974). One obvious difference between the two types is the relationship between muscle force and action-potential rate (viz., Figure 6.4). For tonic motor units, the relationship is a ramp and a plateau; discharge rate increases as muscle force increases at low levels, but at high forces the discharge rate remains constant. In contrast, the discharge rate of phasic motor units increases over the entire range of muscle forces (i.e., a linear relationship). In addition, the tonic motor units generate smaller action potentials, are recruited at lower muscle forces, and are less

fatigable. The phasic motor units seem to be important for dynamic conditions and contribute more to muscle force than do the tonic units. It is not known, however, how this tonic-phasic classification relates to the FF-FR-S system.

As is the case for motor-unit recruitment, the extent of rate coding appears to be muscle dependent. If motor-unit recruitment for a particular muscle is complete by 30% of the maximum force (e.g., adductor pollicis), then subsequent increases in force (i.e., 31%-100%) must be due to rate coding. This also means that whenever that muscle is used at greater than 30% of maximum all the motor units are recruited. In contrast, for muscles in which recruitment continues until 85% of the maximum force, rate coding assumes a somewhat lesser role. In this case, all the motor units are not recruited until forces greater than 85% are achieved. However, it should be emphasized that *increases in muscle force are not due to exclusive increases in either recruitment or rate coding since the two are undoubtedly concurrent processes* (e.g., Monster & Chan, 1977; Person & Kudina, 1972). It has been suggested that the relative contribution of recruitment and rate coding to the generation of muscle force depends upon the distribution of motor-unit mechanical properties (Harrison, 1983).

In addition to discharge rate (frequency of action potentials), another aspect of rate coding that affects force production is **temporal patterning**. This concept refers to *the relationship in time between an action potential and other action potentials generated by the same and other motor units*—that is, intra- and intermotor unit relationships. With respect to action potentials generated by a single motor unit, the discharge of two action potentials (a **doublet**) with a short interval of time between them (e.g., 10 ms) results in a substantial increase in the force exerted by the motor unit (Burke, Rudomin, & Zajac, 1976). This phenomenon is called the **catch** property of muscle. Doublets have been observed in human low- and high-threshold units, particularly in slower muscle contractions (Bawa & Calancie, 1983). Furthermore, since doublets represent a rate-coding effect, their occurrence probably varies from muscle to muscle and may even depend on the task, such as concentric versus eccentric conditions (Gydikov, Kossev, Kosarov, & Kostov, 1987).

In a similar vein, the temporal relationship between action potentials of different motor units is also thought to affect muscle force. Normally the action potentials of different motor units are assumed to be discharged at different instants in time (i.e., asynchro-

nously). However, Milner-Brown, Stein, and Lee (1975) found that the motor units of a muscle that had been subjected to a strength-training program tended to discharge action potentials **synchronously** (i.e., at similar instants in time). Since this observation, it has been assumed, though never proven, that an increase in motor-unit synchronization will result in a greater muscle force. If this proved to be true, then it would mean that one way of increasing the force exerted by muscle is to coordinate the activation of motor units within the muscle—this represents a rate-coding effect.

Contraction Factors

In addition to the excitation from the nervous system, the force that a muscle exerts depends on two contraction factors. The first factor, an area of study known as *muscle mechanics*, represents a group of effects that depend on the characteristics of the force-generating units in muscle. The second factor, *muscle architecture*, refers to effects due to different arrangements of these force-generating units within muscle.

Muscle Mechanics

An action potential in a muscle fiber is an all-or-none event. However, the force exerted by a muscle fiber following a muscle action potential is not always the same. The force depends on internal factors, such as the history of previous action potentials, and on external factors, such as muscle fiber length and the speed of movement. Muscle mechanics is the study of the interdependence of the *external* mechanical variables (e.g., length, velocity, power, force) given the *internal* contractile state (e.g., rate of occurrence of action potentials, availability of Ca^{++}) of muscle.

Muscle Length. The sliding-filament theory is a generally accepted concept that states that the exertion of a force by muscle is accompanied by the sliding of thick and thin filaments past one another. Although the actual mechanism causing this sliding is unknown (Pollack, 1983), there are three classes of theories that attempt to provide an explanation; these are the filament-shortening, electrostatic, and independent-force-generator theories. The most popular alternative, the crossbridge theory, belongs to the latter class. Essentially the crossbridge theory suggests that crossbridges extending from thick filaments are able to attach to the thin filaments and then undergo a structural-chemical transition (i.e., rotation of S1 as the muscle shortens) that exerts a tensile force. After the transition, the crossbridges detach and are able to repeat the cycle.

According to this scheme, the development of force is dependent upon these crossbridge attach-detach cycles; the greater the number of cycles, the greater the force (Figure 6.5). Further, as force exertion occurs only during the attachment phase, the thick and thin filaments must be close enough to each other for the attachment to occur and thus a force exerted. As the **length** of a muscle changes and the thick and thin filaments slide past one another, the number of thin-filament binding sites available for the crossbridges will change. Actually, *the tension varies as the amount of overlap between thick and thin filaments within a sarcomere varies*. The tension-striation spacing graph (Figure 6.5) represents the tension produced with six different amounts of myofilament overlap; these six positions of the thick and thin filaments are indicated below the graph. Position 1 represents the condition of maximum stretch in which there is

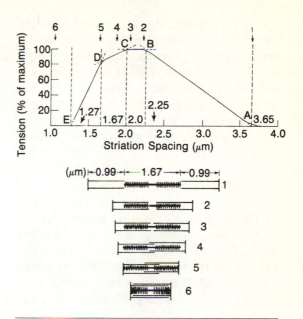

Figure 6.5. Relationship between contractile force, sarcomere length, and filament overlap. *Note.* From T.A. McMahon, *Muscles, Reflexes, and Locomotion.* Copyright © 1984 by Thomas A. McMahon. Published by Princeton University Press. Figure 3.7 reprinted with permission of Princeton University Press.

no overlap of the thick and thin filaments. Positions 2 and 3 indicate conditions of maximum overlap between the S1 extensions and the binding sites on the thin filaments. As the filaments slide further over one another, the amount of **overlap** (i.e., the possibility of interaction between the S1 heads and the thin filaments) decreases through to Position 6. The net result of this change in the potential number of crossbridge attachments (due to variation in muscle length) is that the force that the muscle can exert will also vary with muscle length.

However, the force exerted by muscle is not solely dependent upon the **active** process of crossbridge cycling. In addition, muscle includes a substantial amount of connective tissue (e.g., sarcolemma, endomysium, perimysium, epimysium, tendon), which behaves something like a stiff elastic band. When stretched, these connective-tissue structures exert a *passive* force that combines with the active contribution due to crossbridge activity to produce the total force exerted by the muscle. Figure 6.6 illustrates the contribution of the active and passive components to total-muscle force as muscle length varies. At the shorter lengths, all the force is due to crossbridge activity, whereas at the longer lengths most of the total muscle force is due to the passive elements. The profile for the active component indicates that the greatest overlap of the thick and thin filaments occurs at

a muscle length that is about midway between the minimal and maximal lengths— this is typically the resting length of the muscle (l_o).

Recall, however, that although the force that a muscle exerts may change with muscle length, human movement is primarily due to rotary forces (i.e., torques). Consequently, it is of interest to consider the relationship between muscle torque and length. However, the translation of the force-length to a torque-length relationship is confounded by at least three factors that may alter the length effect. *First*, the movement of most body segments (rigid links in our simple joint system) is controlled by groups of muscles rather than by a single muscle. Often the fibers of each muscle in such a group are arranged differently (e.g., fusiform, pinnate, bipinnate), which means that at any joint position the fibers within the different muscles will probably be at different positions on their force-length curves. *Second*, since a number of muscles (e.g., rectus femoris, semitendinosus, gastrocnemius) act across more than one joint, the length of these muscles, and therefore the force they exert, is not influenced solely by the position of one joint. For example, the knee extensor group includes a two-joint bipinnate muscle (rectus femoris), two single-joint pinnate muscles (vastus lateralis and vastus medialis), and a single-joint fusiform muscle (vastus intermedius). *Third*, variations in muscle force may not be reflected as similar changes in muscle torque because torque is defined as the product of two variables, force and moment arm. In determining muscle torque, the moment arm is measured as the perpendicular distance from the line of action of the muscle-force vector to the axis of rotation (i.e., the joint). Since the distance is known to change with joint position (e.g., Table 2.3), variations in muscle torque represent the interaction of moment-arm and muscle-length effects.

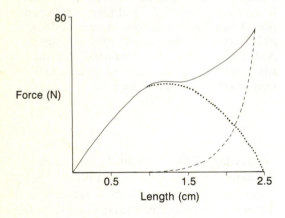

Figure 6.6. Contributions of the active (dotted line) and passive (dashed line) elements to the total-muscle (solid line) isometric force-length relationship for the forearm flexors. The range of muscle length values represents the minimum contracted length and the maximum stretched length. *Note.* From "Mechanics of Human Isolated Voluntary Muscle" by H.J. Ralston, V.T. Inman, L.A. Strait, and M.D. Shaffrath, 1947, *American Journal of Physiology*, **151**, p. 615. Copyright by the American Physiological Society. Adapted by permission.

As a consequence of these three influences (fiber arrangements, number of joints, and moment arm), *the torque-length relationship may be similar to that between muscle length and the active component of muscle force* (Figure 6.6), *or it may take one of two other forms* (Kulig, Andrews, & Hay, 1984). These effects are characterized in Figure 6.7 where variations in muscle length are represented as changes in joint angle; thus our interest is in translating a force-length graph to a torque-angle relationship. In general the torque-angle graph (Figure 6.7) can have one of three forms: ascending, descending, or ascending-descending. In the ascending version (e.g., knee flexors, hip adductors), torque increases as joint angle increases; torque decreases and joint angle decreases in the descending relationship (e.g., hip abductors). In contrast, the ascending-descending form (e.g., elbow extensors and flexors, knee extensors) is qualitatively similar to the force-length relationship. For the muscle groups that belong to this latter category, the greatest torque occurs when the joint is in a midrange position. This affects the position in which the joint should be placed when maximum torque is required. For example, since the knee extensors exert their greatest torque at a knee angle of about 1.75 rad (Komi, 1979), the knee of the driving leg should be at about this position in the crouch start at the beginning of a 100-m sprint.

Once a muscle has been activated and begins to exert a torque, the tendency is for the filaments to slide past one another and for the muscle to shorten its length. However, whether or not the length of the active muscle changes depends upon the magnitude of the torque exerted by the muscle relative to that due to the load (Figure 6.8). This quotient (muscle/load) can have three distinct values: less than one, equal to one, or greater than one. If the quotient has a value equal to one, then the muscle and load torques are equivalent and the muscle length will not change; this condition is referred to as an **isometric** contraction. Conversely, if the two torques are not equal (i.e., less than or greater than one) then muscle length will change. When the muscle torque is greater, the quotient will exceed one and the muscle will shorten its length; this is called a **concentric** contraction. Alternatively, when the torque

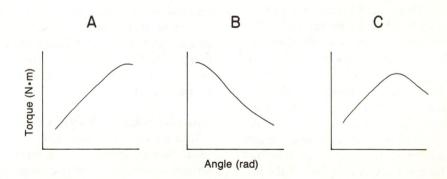

Figure 6.7. Three common forms of the torque-angle relationship: (A) ascending, (B) descending, (C) ascending-descending. *Note.* From Kulig, K., Andrews, J.G., & Hay, J.G., 1984, ''Human strength curves.'' In Terjung, R.L. (Ed.), *Exercise and Sport Science Reviews*, Volume 12, page 422. New York: Macmillan Publishing Company, 1984.

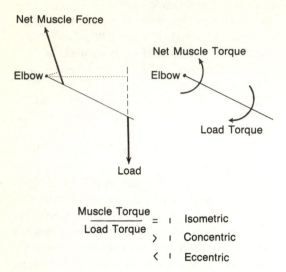

Figure 6.8. The relationship between the net muscle torque and the torque due to a load (which includes system weight) will determine whether the lengths of the active muscles shorten (concentric), lengthen (eccentric), or remain unchanged (isometric).

due to the load is greater than the muscle torque, the quotient will be less than one and the muscle will be lengthened (while it is active), which is known as an **eccentric** contraction. Often these conditions (isometric, concentric, and eccentric) are referred to as types of contractions. Unfortunately, *this is a misnomer because these conditions merely represent differences in the muscle/load quotient and not the manner in which the muscle is contracting.* For example, the nervous system cannot command a muscle to contract eccentrically but rather it can activate the muscle to a lesser degree than the torque exerted by the load and thus the muscle will lengthen while it is being activated (i.e., perform an eccentric contraction). Therefore, the term **contraction** refers to the state of activation in which a muscle actively exerts a force, whether or not muscle length changes.

The torque-angle relationships shown in Figure 6.7 have been examined with isometric, concentric, and eccentric contractions (Kulig et al., 1984). Several investigators have shown that the shape of a particular torque-angle relationship remains the same regardless of whether it has been obtained by isometric, concentric, or eccentric measurements; rather, the general effect of these measurements is to shift the relationship up and down the vertical axis such that the greatest torques are exerted eccentrically, the least concentrically, and intermediate values isometrically at any given joint angle.

Suppose you were asked to go to the laboratory to obtain an isometric torque-angle curve. How would you do it? This would be done, say for the knee joint, by seating a subject on a bench, attaching a cuff around the subject's ankle, and connecting the cuff to a force transducer. You could alter the length of the connection between the cuff and the transducer so that the knee joint could be rotated throughout its range of motion. You would then set the connection to a number of different lengths (i.e., different knee angles) and measure a maximum isometric torque at each length. The result would be a set of isometric torque-angle data. Investigators have found that the concentric and eccentric curves lie below and above, respectively, the isometric curve. How would these curves appear in a graph? Figure 6.9 shows one possibility. How could the concentric and eccentric curves be measured?

Rate of Change of Muscle Length (Velocity). When the muscle torque does not equal the load torque, there is a change in muscle length. The torque that the muscle can exert under these conditions depends on the magnitude and direction of the rate of change in length—the **velocity** of the muscle contraction. When the muscle shortens it performs a concentric contraction, a mode of activity

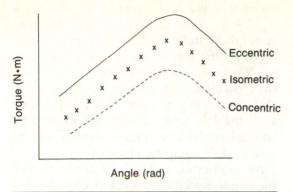

Figure 6.9. Idealized isometric, eccentric, and concentric torque-angle relationships.

the three conditions varies as eccentric is greater than isometric, which is greater than concentric. It must be emphasized, however, that the relationships depicted in Figure 6.10 represent a simplified version of the velocity effects, particularly with respect to the eccentric component of the graph. This can best be demonstrated by explaining how the measurements were made for Figure 6.10. Although the torque-velocity relationships are shown as continuous lines, the data for the graph are actually a number of torque-velocity points. Each data point represents a measurement of torque for a given value of velocity; that is, torque is the dependent variable. The measurement of torque for each data point was made from a single contraction (concentric or eccentric) over a 1.6-rad range of motion. For example, a single measurement of torque was made from a contraction that went from an initial angle of 0.8 rad to a final angle of 2.4 rad at a speed of 3

that is associated with a lesser muscle torque than for an isometric (velocity = 0) contraction; thus, during maximum concentric contractions, the torque exerted by the muscle is less than that for a maximum isometric contraction. In addition, as the velocity of shortening increases, the amount of torque that the muscle can exert decreases (Figure 6.10). Although the rate of crossbridge attachment-detachment increases as the shortening speed increases, the average force exerted by each crossbridge decreases, and there may be fewer crossbridges formed as the muscle shortens more quickly. Since the energy used by the muscle increases (due to increased crossbridge detachment) with shortening speed while the torque exerted decreases, the muscle becomes less **efficient** (work output/energy input) with increases in the discrepancy between the muscle and load torques.

When the muscle torque is less than the load torque, the muscle lengthens. The maximum torque that a muscle can exert when performing an eccentric contraction is greater than that which the muscle can exert isometrically or concentrically. In fact, according to Figure 6.10, *the maximum torque under*

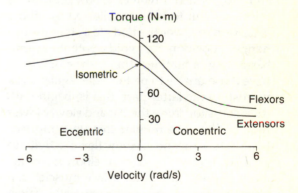

Figure 6.10. The maximum torque exerted by the elbow flexors and extensors at an elbow angle of 1.57 rad as the angular velocity of the forearm-hand segment is varied. *Note.* From ''Force-Velocity Relationship in Human Elbow Flexors and Extensors'' by K. Jorgensen. In *Biomechanics V-A* (p. 147) by P.V. Komi (Ed.), 1976. Baltimore: University Park Press. Copyright 1976 by University Park Press. Adapted by permission.

rad•s^{-1}. The next measurement involved the same conditions but with a different speed, and so on. Furthermore, since the force that a muscle can exert varies with its length, the torque measurement was made at the same elbow angle (1.57 rad) in each case. In effect, then, the torque-velocity relationships shown in Figure 6.10 were obtained under constant-velocity conditions. This distinction is emphasized because it it known that muscle force varies in a complicated way when an active muscle goes from an isometric to an eccentric contraction in which velocity increases (Rack & Westbury, 1974).

Despite these restrictions, the relationships among the maximum torque for the three conditions can often be exploited in the prescription of exercise. For example, suppose as part of an exercise program it is desirable to have a class perform chin-ups. In many groups (e.g., physical education classes, adult-fitness groups), a number of individuals will be unable to perform a conventional chin-up, which involves elbow flexion to raise the chin to the bar followed by elbow extension to lower the body to a straight-arm hanging position. To avoid a potentially embarrassing situation, the instructor could have those unable to perform the regular chin-up just do the latter part, that is, begin with their chins touching the bar and slowly lower their bodies. The regular chin-up comprises two parts: concentric elbow flexor activity to raise the body and eccentric elbow flexor activity to lower the body. Since muscles can exert a greater torque eccentrically, most people are able to accomplish the lowering part of the exercise. However, the greatest torque that a muscle can generate eccentrically occurs at lower constant velocities, at about 2.0 rad•s^{-1}, so that to reap the benefits of eccentric contractions the movement must be done slowly. Fortunately, the stress that a muscle experiences when it is exercised seems to induce similar adaptations whether the muscle is active eccentrically or concentrically (Komi & Buskirk, 1972). Thus any strength an individual gains by performing the eccentric part of the chin-up is also accessible in concentric contractions. Therefore, the individual who is unable to do a regular chin-up and begins a period of conditioning with the lowering chin-up will eventually strengthen the appropriate muscles and be able to do a complete chin-up.

As another example of the application of the torque-velocity relationship, consider two individuals as they perform chin-ups; one individual can do 20 chin-ups, and the other can only do 2. Suppose they both did as many chin-ups as they could and as fast as they could. Intuition would tell us that the 20-chin-up individual would do the first chin-up much faster than the other person. Why is this? An explanation can be given on the basis of the torque-velocity relationship. To do this let us make some simplifying assumptions that will not affect the essence of the explanation: Both individuals weigh the same, the prime movers are the elbow flexors, and just the concentric phase is considered. Because of differences in strength, as indicated by the isometric torque in Figure 6.11, the 20-chin-up person can generate the necessary torque (the horizontal line in Figure 6.11) at a higher velocity. In this example, velocity represents the speed of flexion at the elbow joint. Thus, the first chin-up, before the effects of fatigue, can be done faster by the stronger individual.

Why can a muscle exert a greater torque eccentrically than concentrically? The answer to this question is unknown. One possibility may be that the force required to break a crossbridge is greater than that required to hold an isometric contraction. The typical account given of crossbridge cycling is that the globular heads (S1) attach to actin-binding sites and then undergo a conformational change, which is depicted as rotation of S1

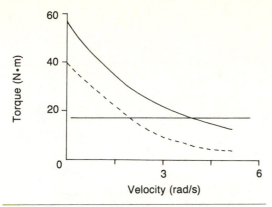

Figure 6.11. Torque-velocity relationships for the elbow flexor muscles of a 20-chin-up (solid line) and a 2-chin-up (dashed line) person. The 20-chin-up person is stronger, as noted by the greater isometric torque. The horizontal line represents the elbow flexor torque that must be exerted by each individual (same body weights) to complete the concentric (up) phase of a chin-up.

(Figure 5.14). Crossbridge activity during an eccentric contraction probably does not involve this sequence in that the S1 component, rather than rotating toward its HMM fragment, may well be rotating the opposite direction as the muscle is lengthened. Under these two conditions, *the mechanism responsible for crossbridge detachment may well differ,* thus altering the duration of the attachment phase and presumably the force exerted by the crossbridge. In addition, a second possibility for the superiority of the eccentric activity may involve an enhancement of the contractile-machinery activity by either *increasing the quantity of Ca^{++} released* or by *stretching the less completely activated sarcomeres within each myofibril* (Hoyle, 1983).

As a consequence of comparing the effects of concentric- and eccentric-training programs, several investigators (Armstrong, Ogilvie, & Schwane, 1983; Komi & Buskirk,

1972) have concluded that the eccentric activation of muscle is closely associated with the **muscle soreness** that occurs 24-48 hr after exercise. There is no agreement on the cause of this delayed postexercise pain. The two theories most commonly cited to account for the soreness are the muscle-spasm and structural-damage theories. The muscle-spasm theory (de Vries, 1966) suggests that exercise-induced ischemia allows the transfer of substance P across the muscle-cell membrane and into the tissue fluid. Once in the extracellular fluid, the substance P is thought to activate pain-nerve endings that elicit reflex activity in the form of a muscle spasm. In general, however, there is minimal evidence to support increased postexercise EMG activity (Abraham, 1977).

The alternative to the muscle-spasm theory proposes that activity induces structural damage that is translated into muscle soreness. The damage sites appear diffuse and may include connective tissue (Abraham, 1977), muscle fibers (Kuipers, Drukker, Frederik, Geurten, & v. Kranenburg, 1983), and the activation of sensory neurons due to the accumulation of metabolites (Armstrong, 1984). *Eccentric contractions are thought to enhance structural damage.* However, the mechanism by which such damage is sensed as painful is unknown and will undoubtedly be difficult to determine since muscle soreness is a subjective and therefore a physiologically elusive localized discomfort.

Muscle Power.   When a muscle shortens and the force it exerts causes an object to move, the muscle is described as doing positive work; that is, work is done by the muscle on the object. Conversely, a muscle does negative work, or has work done to it, when it lengthens while exerting a force on the object that is moved. We encountered these concepts in chapter 3 when we discussed the example of the elbow extension-flexion movement in the horizontal plane. Since work is defined as the product of force and distance, when an object is not moved, as in an isometric contraction, no work is done. Recall from Part I, however, the relationship between work and energy: The amount of work done was determined by the change in energy that occurred. In the case of an isometric contraction, such as holding a heavy suitcase, since the suitcase does not move, its energy (kinetic and potential) does not change, and thus no work has been done in a mechanical sense. However, for the suitcase to be held, the muscles that flex the fingers must be activated. As we have mentioned previously, the activation of muscle involves the expenditure of energy (ATP). In this example of holding the heavy suitcase, the fact that the muscles are doing work becomes quite apparent because after a period of time the muscles tire and are unable to lift the suitcase. If no work were being done then it would be possible to hold the suitcase indefinitely. Consequently, although the suitcase experiences no work, the finger flexor muscles must do work to lift the suitcase. To distinguish between the two, we could say that the suitcase experiences no mechanical work, but the muscles do metabolic work to hold the suitcase in place.

The rate of doing work is referred to as **power**. *The rate of positive work or work done by the muscle is indicated as power production.* Alternatively, the term *power absorption describes the rate of doing work on muscle.* Consider an individual performing a squat exercise with a barbell (Figure 6.12). This exercise relies primarily on the knee extensor muscles. In going from the standing position to a squat, the knee extensors lengthen as they assist in lowering the body. In this instance the knee extensors are active eccentrically and are described as doing negative work: work is done on the muscles by the weight of the barbell and the athlete. When work is done on a

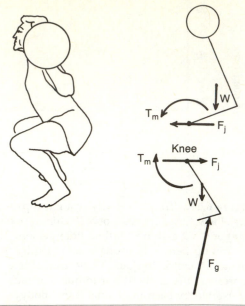

Figure 6.12. The squat exercise. The free-body diagram isolates the net activity about the knee joint. The knee extensors are largely responsible for the execution of the movement.

muscle we say that the muscle absorbs power. When an individual rises from the squat, the knee extensors perform positive work and hence produce power. *Power production is limited by the rate at which energy is supplied for the muscle contraction* (i.e., ATP production) *and the rate at which the myofilaments can convert chemical energy into mechanical work* (Weis-Fogh & Alexander, 1977). Power production is often thought to limit human performance, especially if the event is of short duration (Enoka, in press).

Power is determined as the product of the force and velocity of the muscle contraction. Let us examine the relationship graphically with the aid of some data from an isolated-muscle preparation. Figure 6.13 illustrates how the force that a muscle can exert declines as the speed of the shortening contraction increases. The curve contacts the axes at the

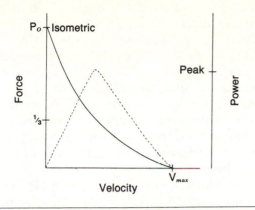

Figure 6.13. The force-velocity relationship based on data from an isolated-muscle preparation. The power curve (right-hand vertical axis) is derived from the product of force and velocity.

two ends of this graph. At one end, velocity has a value of zero, and so the force value represents isometric force. At the other end, velocity has its highest value (known as v_{max}), and the force is equal to zero. Figure 6.13 also shows how the power produced by the muscle varies as the velocity changes. Perhaps the most important feature of the power graph is that it has a bell shape with maximum values in the midrange. That is, power is defined as the product of force and velocity. At the extremes of the force-velocity relationship the product is zero because either velocity or force (and hence the product) has a value of zero. Because both velocity and force are nonzero, power production varies between these two limits depending on the product of force and velocity. It turns out that *maximum power occurs when the force being exerted is about one-third of the maximum isometric force.*

As an example of the interplay between the force-velocity relationship and power, let us consider the changes that occur in these parameters when riding a bicycle. First, it is necessary to draw a free-body diagram to

represent the situation. Suppose we define as the system the bicycle and rider and then indicate with arrows (vector representation of forces) how the system interacts with its environment. Figure 6.14A shows that a bicycle traveling along level ground experiences three major interactions with its environment; these are system weight, air resistance, and ground reaction force. The latter force represents the response of the ground to the forces exerted by the wheels, which are mainly determined by the forces the rider exerts on the pedals and system weight. The speed of the bicycle-rider system depends on the net force acting in the direction the bicycle is traveling (propulsive force). When the bicycle is on level ground, this net driving force is equal to the horizontal component of the ground reaction force minus the effect of air resistance. When the cyclist goes up a hill (Figure 6.14B), the net driving force is also opposed by the tangential component of the system-weight vector. That is, for the same ground reaction force on the

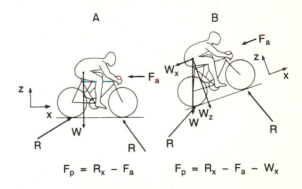

Figure 6.14. Free-body diagram of a bicycle-rider system. (A) The system traveling along level ground experiences system weight (**W**), air resistance (**F**$_a$), and a ground reaction force (**R**). The net driving force (**F**$_p$; propulsive force) acts in the direction the cyclist is progressing. (B) The system now going up a hill.

level and going up hill, the net driving force is less when going up the hill because of the added opposition of a component of the system weight.

Given this free-body diagram, we can now proceed to consider the interactions among force, velocity, and power. Figure 6.15A shows that the force applied to the pedals decreased as the rate at which the crank rotated was increased; this is analogous to the right-hand side of the torque-velocity curve (Figure 6.10) and the force-velocity graph for isolated muscle (Figure 6.13). In this instance, we can take the force applied to the pedals to be a fair approximation of the propulsive force (i.e., let us consider air resistance to be negligible in this example). It is clear from Figure 6.15B that, although this force decreases as crank velocity increases, the two variables combine to produce an increase in power up to a crank velocity of 110 rpm (11.52 rad•s⁻¹). If the cyclist changed gears on the bicycle so that crank velocity was slowed down (e.g., to 80 rpm), then intuitively we know that the speed of the cyclist would decrease if the pedal force remained constant.

This effect can be seen in Figure 6.15B by a decline in power produced by the cyclist—the power would go from the peak to a lesser value to the left. This decline, of course, would occur because of the decrease in the product of force and velocity. Notice also, that if the gear ratio were changed so that crank velocity increased, the effect would be the same in that power production would decline (i.e., move to the right on Figure 6.15B), and the cyclist would slow down.

The situation shown in Figure 6.14B is a more complicated example of these same relationships. Suppose a cyclist were traveling along level ground with a crank velocity of 110 rpm and a pedal force (propulsive force) of 0.5 kN. When the cyclist goes up a hill, the net driving force will decrease because now a component of the system weight (W_x) opposes the motion (Figure 6.14). If crank velocity remains constant then the product of the two (i.e., power) will decrease. For example, suppose an individual is cycling along level ground with the force and crank-velocity conditions represented by the asterisk in Figure 6.15A. When the cyclist reaches

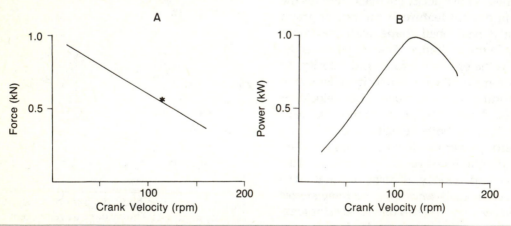

Figure 6.15. Effect of crank velocity (rpm—revolutions per minute) on the peak force and power applied to the pedals during cycling. *Note.* From ''Measurement of Maximal Short-Term (Anaerobic) Power Output During Cycling'' by A.J. Sargeant and A. Boreham, 1981, in J. Borms, M. Hebbelinck, & A. Venerando (Eds.), *Women and Sport*, p. 122. Basel: S. Karger AG. Copyright 1981 by S. Karger AG, Basel. Adapted by permission.

the hill, the force (driving force) will decline (the asterisk will move vertically downward on the graph), and the product of force and velocity (i.e., power) will also decline. The force and velocity conditions indicated by the asterisk coincide with the peak of the power curve (Figure 6.15B). Consequently, the decline in force will result in a decline in the peak power. One way to increase power, given that force declines, would be to increase velocity. This provides the rationale for bicycles having gears; they allow the cyclist to manipulate crank velocity and therefore to optimize power output. A similar rationale applies to a cyclist who is riding into a gusting head wind. As the air resistance changes, the cyclist instinctively changes gears so that optimum power output can be delivered to the pedals.

Inasmuch as power is influenced by both force and velocity, any effect on the latter two variables will also alter power. *Muscle temperature is one such variable and predominately affects contraction speed*. For example, Davies and Young (1983) found that increasing muscle temperature by 3.1 °C caused a decrease in both contraction time and one-half relaxation time by 7% and 22%, respectively, but did not affect twitch or tetanic tension. In contrast, decreasing muscle temperature by 8.4 °C (by immersing the leg in an ice bath) produced an increase in both contraction time (38%) and one-half relaxation time (93%). From these types of observations, it is apparent that relaxation rather than force development is more dependent on muscle temperature. In terms of the force-velocity relationship, changes in temperature within the physiological range affect the maximum velocity of shortening (12%•°C^{-1}) but not the maximum isometric force (Binkhorst, Hoofd, & Vissers, 1977). Given that a particular muscle group has a certain force-velocity relationship, the effect of changing muscle temperature in Figure 6.13 will be (a) not to alter

the isometric force (i.e., velocity = 0), and (b) to shift the maximum velocity of shortening (v_{max}) to the right by 12% for each degree (°C) increase in temperature (Figure 6.16).

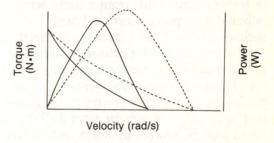

Figure 6.16. Idealized effect of a change in temperature (e.g., due to a warm-up) on the torque-velocity and power production of muscle. The increased-temperature condition is represented by the dashed lines. The power curves are bell-shaped, and the force-velocity relationship is shown by the parabolas.

Although temperature is generally regarded not to affect the maximum isometric force, there can be a minimal effect over a reasonable change in temperature. For example, Bergh and Ekblom (1979) report a change in maximum isometric torque of the knee extensors from 262 N•m at 30.4 °C to 312 N•m at 38.5 °C (2•4%•°C^{-1}), with the temperature measured in the vastus lateralis muscle. However, although muscle temperature primarily affects contractile speed, *changes in temperature also influence the peak power production* (approx 4%•°C^{-1}; Sargeant, 1983) in such activities as cycling and vertical jump. Bergh and Ekblom (1979), for example, changed the temperature of the vastus lateralis muscle from 30.4 °C to 38.5 °C and found that subjects could increase their vertical jump height by 44% (17 cm) and their maximum power production in cycling by 32% (316 W).

Ingjer and Strømme (1979) report that the best strategy for inducing changes in muscle temperature, as measured by performance in a maximum effort 4-min treadmill run, is by doing an active-related warm-up (see also Shellock, 1986; Shellock & Prentice, 1985). An active warm-up is one in which the changes in temperature result from muscle activity rather than a passive external heat source, such as a warm bath. Similarly, in a related warm-up, the muscles activated during the warm-up are subsequently used in the event. Ingjer and Strømme (1979) were able to raise the intramuscular temperature of the lateral part of quadriceps femoris from 35.9 °C to about 38.4 °C with both active and passive techniques but argued in favor of active warm-up because of superior performance by the subjects during a 4-min maximum aerobic treadmill run. In short, a greater part of the total energy expenditure is provided by aerobic processes when the work is preceded by an active warm-up. These authors further suggest that the duration of the warm-up should be greater than 5 min and done at an intensity equivalent to a 7.5-min-mi pace for a trained athlete or sufficient to cause perspiration and an increase in heart rate in an untrained individual. The increase in muscle temperature from such activities will be lost by about 15 min after the warm-up; therefore, there should be no longer than 15 min between the warm-up and the event. In addition, a warm-up is probably only necessary if the speed of the task requires it and the environmental temperature is low.

Architecture

The basic functional unit of muscle is the sarcomere. The effect that a muscle exerts on a rigid link depends on how the sarcomeres are arranged within the muscle.

Arrangement of Force-Generating Units. The maximum force or torque that a muscle can exert and its maximum velocity of shortening are typically used to characterize the performance of a muscle. However, these variables, which reflect the intrinsic properties of the force-generating units within myofilaments, are further modified by the organization of the muscle fibers within the muscle, that is, the architectural or design features of muscle. The three major architectural influences are the average number of sarcomeres per muscle fiber (i.e., arranged end to end; the **in-series** effect), the number of fibers in parallel (i.e., lying side by side; the **in-parallel** effect), and the angle at which the fibers are oriented relative to the line of pull of the muscle (i.e., the degree of pinnation). We can examine the consequences of these effects by representing each force-generating unit with an appropriate mechanical model. Since this model has three components, it is called a three-component model—we shall consider this model in more detail in chapter 7. Figure 6.17 shows three of these models arranged end to end (A) and three side by side (B).

A myofibril was previously described as a series of sarcomeres. Variations in myofibril length are generally due to differing numbers of sarcomeres in series; the length of each sarcomere within a myofibril is not thought to change much. If each sarcomere or force-generating unit is represented as a three-component mechanical model, the resting-myofibril length can be changed by altering the number of units in the chain (Figure 6.17A). When an action potential propagates along a muscle fiber, all of the sarcomeres within a myofibril experience more or less the same degree of excitation, and therefore each sarcomere will undergo about the same change in length (Δl). As a consequence, the *greater the number of sarcomeres (n) in series, the greater will be the change of length* of the myofibril (ΔL) to a given stimulus, since $\Delta L = n(\Delta l)$. Because a myofibril can change its length by one-third, the greater

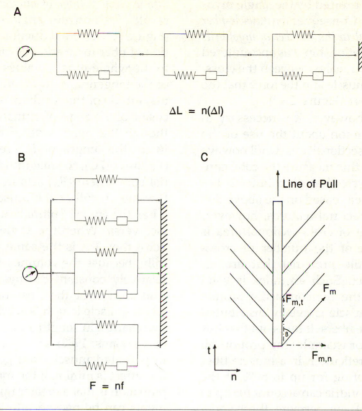

Figure 6.17. Architectural features of muscle. (A) An in-series arrangement of sarcomeres. (B) An in-parallel arrangement of sarcomeres. (C) The effect of pinnation on the contribution of each muscle fiber to whole-muscle force and velocity of shortening. β = angle of pinnation; F_m = muscle force or velocity vector; $F_{m,n}$ = normal component; $F_{m,t}$ = tangential component.

its length, the greater its absolute change in length. For example, a 100-sarcomere myofibril will experience a ΔL of 50 μm if each sarcomere produces a 0.5-μm change in length in response to a stimulus. In contrast, under the same conditions a 1,000-sarcomere myofibril will undergo a 500-μm length change.

Another feature of the in-series arrangement is the effect of shortening on the velocity. The rate of change in length (velocity) of the myofibril is determined as the product of the number of sarcomeres and the average velocity of each sarcomere. The greater the

number of sarcomeres in series, the greater is the change in myofibril length and the rate of change in myofibril length in response to a given stimulus; thus, $\Delta V = n(\Delta v)$.

In contrast, if each myofibril comprised a single sarcomere, and three such myofibrils were arranged in parallel (Figure 6.17B), the change in myofibril length would be equivalent to that experienced by the single sarcomere. However, in this configuration, the forces exerted by each sarcomere combine so that the muscle-fiber force (F) is equal to the product of the number of myofibrils (n) and the average force exerted by the single myo-fibrils (f): F = nf. Consequently, *muscle-fiber force is proportional to the number of myofibrils in parallel.* This relationship was encountered earlier as a proportionality between the cross-sectional area of muscle and the force that the muscle could exert (Figure 2.19).

At this point, however, it is necessary to add a note of caution about the use of the measure of cross-sectional area. Until now we have included in this measure the total contents of the muscle that contribute to the cross-sectional area. Based on the above discussion on architectural features, however, the measurement of cross-sectional area is merely an index of the number of cross-bridges (contractile proteins) that are arranged in parallel. Such an index is valid if, and only if, the noncontractile protein content of the muscle is evenly distributed among the muscle fibers. It turns out that this is not the case; for example, the proportion of sarcoplasmic reticulum in a muscle fiber can vary, accounting for up to 60% of the area, and mitochondria can account for up to 50% (Hoyle, 1983). Furthermore, these variations appear to be related to muscle-fiber type. Consequently, the measurement of cross-sectional area, which includes all the intramuscular material, can be used only as a rough estimate of the force capabilities of the muscle; in fact, this source of error probably contributes to the variation in the reported values for specific tension (Part I).

The effects of design features on muscle function, however, are not limited to simple in-series or in-parallel alternatives. Instead, the effect of the alignment of the force-producing units is further modified by a deviation of the orientation of the muscle fiber from the line of pull of the muscle. This deviation is referred to as the angle of **pinnation** and usually varies from 0 to 0.4 rad. *The advantage of pinnation is that a greater number of fibers and thus sarcomeres in parallel can be packed*

into a given volume of muscle. However, the result of a nonzero angle of pinnation (β) (Figure 6.17C) is a reduction in the contribution of fiber force and velocity of shortening to the whole-muscle values; the magnitude of the tangential component is less than the magnitude of the resultant and varies as the cosine of the angle of pinnation ($\cos \beta$). Even though the magnitude of the muscle-fiber force (the length of F_m) remains constant (Figure 6.17C), the magnitude of the tangential component ($F_{m,t}$ acts in the direction of the line of pull of the muscle) gets smaller when the angle of pinnation gets larger, and vice versa. When the angle of pinnation is zero, then $F_{m,t}$ is the same as F_m. Paradoxically, because the volume of a fiber remains relatively constant during contraction, the contribution of the fiber to the change in whole-muscle length is actually greater than the change in length that the fiber experiences (Gans, 1982). However, because fibers in pinnated muscles are generally shorter, this effect is minimal; the main advantage of pinnation is that a greater number of myofilaments can be packed into a given volume.

Whole-Muscle Effects. Muscles can have fibers arranged with a common angle of pinnation (unipinnate), with two sets of fibers at different pinnation angles (bipinnate), or with many sets of fibers at a variety of angles (multipinnate). Muscle fibers aligned with a zero angle of pinnation are usually described as having fusiform or parallel arrangement. The morphological types of muscle, based upon their general form and fascicular architecture, are shown in Figure 6.18. However, this kind of diagram is only a guide since it focuses on the organization of the fascicles rather than the muscle fibers. In fact, studies on the fiber arrangement in muscles have revealed a rather complex arrangement (Figure 6.19).

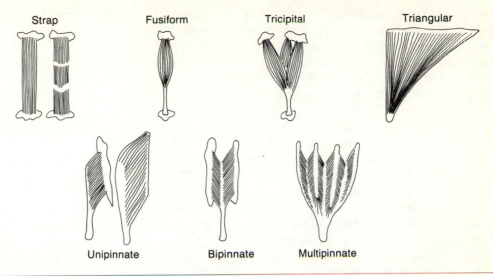

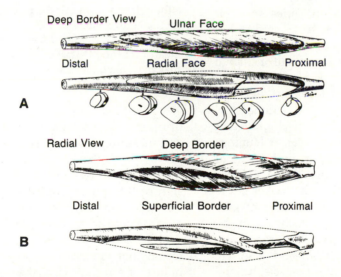

Figure 6.18. Traditionally, muscles are separated into a number of different types based on their general form and fascicular organization. *Note.* From *Gray's Anatomy*, 36th ed. (p. 524), P.L. Williams and R. Warwick (Eds.), 1980, Edinburgh: Churchill Livingstone. Copyright 1980 by Longman Group Ltd. Adapted by permission.

Figure 6.19. Two diagrammatic views (A = ulnar, B = superficial) of the flexor carpi radialis muscle. Each view shows the muscle-fiber orientation (top diagram) and the organization of the tendon and connective tissue (bottom diagram) within the muscle. *Note.* From "Morphological and Histochemical Organization of the Flexor Carpi Radialis Muscle in the Cat" by W.J. Gonyea and G.C. Ericson, 1977, *American Journal of Anatomy*, **148**, p. 333. Copyright 1977 by Alan R. Liss, Inc. Reprinted by permission.

A muscle fiber consists of myofibrils arranged in parallel, and a myofibril represents a series arrangement of sarcomeres; therefore, muscle fibers actually comprise an in-series and an in-parallel collection of force-generating units. Consequently, *a long, small-diameter muscle fiber represents a dominant in-series effect and, conversely, a short, large-diameter fiber mainly exhibits in-parallel characteristics*. Muscles are designed to capitalize on these distinctions. For example, muscles that support an upright posture (e.g., knee extensors, ankle plantarflexors), the antigravity muscles, are generally considered to be twice as strong as their antagonists. This would imply that the physiological cross-sectional area of the antigravity muscles be twice as large. Indeed, the data in Table 6.1 indicate that the cross-sectional area of the quadriceps is about double that for the hamstrings, and that for the plantarflexors is substantially larger ($8\times$) than the dorsiflexors. However, the greater number of sarcomeres in series in each muscle fiber for the hamstrings and dorsiflexors indicate that they have a greater capability for change of length and rate of change in length (Table 6.1).

Table 6.2 extends these ideas further based upon some measurements on human cadavers and some mathematical modeling techniques (Woittiez, Rozendal, & Huijing, 1985). Specifically, a comparison is made of the architectural and physiological features of the muscles comprising the triceps surae complex (soleus, and medial and lateral gastrocnemius). Several conclusions can be made from these data: (a) the greater the number of sarcomeres, the longer the muscle fiber; (b) soleus is the longest muscle, has the greatest volume, and has the largest physiological cross-sectional area; (c) the angle of pinnation is quite large for all three muscles; (d) the range of motion and maximum velocity vary according to fiber length; and (e) maximum power, which occurs at about one-third v_{max}, varies in the order of the

Table 6.1. In-Series (Number of Sarcomeres) and In-Parallel (Cross-Sectional Area) Characteristics of Human Lower-Extremity Muscle Groups

	Number of sarcomeres ($\times 10^3$)	Cross-sectional area[a] (cm²)
Quadriceps	31.2	87
Hamstrings	43.0	38
Plantarflexors	15.2	139
Dorsiflexors	29.3	17

Note. Data from Wickiewicz, Roy, Powell, and Edgerton (1983).

[a]Physiological cross-sectional area considers fiber length and angle of pinnation; this is a more appropriate estimate of the number of sarcomeres in parallel than the measurement of the absolute cross-sectional area. Thus, although the plantarflexor physiological cross-sectional area value of 139 cm² is larger than the 87 cm² for the quadriceps, this does not mean that the plantarflexors are larger, just that they have more sarcomeres in parallel.

product of physiological cross-sectional area and maximum velocity. The data in Table 6.2 serve to emphasize that muscle function (physiology) is profoundly affected by the design of the muscle (architecture).

In addition to these whole-muscle effects of sarcomere arrangement, at least two other design factors are known to influence the torque that a muscle can exert. These are the points of attachment of the muscle relative to the joint and the proportion of whole-muscle length that contains contractile protein. The angle of pull of the muscle (α in Figure 6.20), and hence the proportion of muscle force that contributes to rotation, depends on the distances c and q (Figure 6.20) and the joint angle.

Table 6.2. Architectural and Physiological Features of the Human Triceps Surae Complex

	Lateral gastrocnemiuis	Medial gastrocnemius	Soleus
Architecture			
Number of sarcomeres[a]	21,400	18,400	—
Fiber length (mm)[b]	55.7	47.8	37.8
Muscle length (mm)[b]	175.8	202.1	239.6
Volume (cm³)	104	199	250
Physiological cross-sectional area (cm²)	18.7	41.6	66.1
Pinnation angle (rad)	0.35	0.35	0.44
Physiology			
Range of motion (mm)	51.8	43.4	34.8
Maximum velocity (mm/s)[c]	523.4	449.2	353.5
Maximum power (W)	36.9	69.3	69.4

Note. From ''The Functional Significance of Architecture of the Human Triceps Surae Muscle'' by R.D. Woittiez et al., 1983, in D.A. Winter et al. (Eds.), *Biomechanics IX-A* (p. 22), Champaign, IL: Human Kinetics. Copyright 1985 by Human Kinetics Publishers, Inc. Adapted by permission.

[a]Number of sarcomeres per muscle fiber. [b]Lengths measured with the knee = 1.31 rad and ankle = 1.48 rad (complete extension = 0 rad). [c]Right-hand limit of the force-velocity relationship (Figure 6.13).

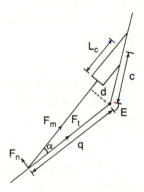

Figure 6.20. The geometry of a single-joint muscle. α = angle of pull, c = distance from proximal muscle attachment to joint, d = moment arm, E = joint angle, **F** = pulling force exerted by the muscle on the distal segment, L_c = proportion of whole-muscle length containing contractile protein, n = normal component of **F**, q = distance from distal muscle attachment to joint, t = tangential component of **F**. *Note.* From ''Attachment and Composition of Skeletal Muscles in Relation to Their Function'' by H. van Mameren and J. Drukker, 1979, *Journal of Biomechanics*, **12**, p. 860. Copyright 1979 by Pergamon Journals, Ltd. Adapted by permission.

The major effects of varying the parameters c, q, L_c, and E on the torque exerted by a muscle include the following (van Mameren & Drukker, 1979):

1. The torque-angle relationship has a sharper peak when c and q are equal. When either c or q is much greater than the other parameter, the peak is much broader; that is, the maximum torque values are attainable over a greater range of joint angles.
2. Peak torque is reached closer to full extension when c and q are equal but closer to the midrange position (e.g., elbow angle = 1.57 rad) when c and q are quite different.
3. The maximum torque exerted by the muscle is greater when c and q are different and when L_c is greater for a given c-q relationship. This interaction is readily apparent anatomically in that muscles with a c/q quotient near 1 always have a high L_c value whereas muscles with c/q quotients of a lot less than 1 generally have long tendons (low L_c value).
4. Muscles that have a c/q quotient quite different from 1 do not gain much torque by increasing L_c.

As an example of these effects, consider the interactions of two major elbow flexor muscles, brachialis and brachioradialis. The brachialis muscle, considered the major elbow flexor muscle, contains a substantial variation in c/q quotients and L_c values throughout the muscle; the deeper part has c/q quotients near 1 and high L_c values, whereas the superficial part has c/q values far from 1 and low L_c values. Thus the different parts possess distinct features, and, as a consequence, the muscle contributes over the entire range of motion (Basmajian & Latif, 1957). In contrast, brachioradialis has a lesser variety of c/q quotients and L_c values, and the muscle tends to be active only against a load or in instances of quick flexion movements.

Problems

6.1. The following statements were made by experts in a roundtable discussion on strength (*National Strength and Conditioning Association Journal*, 1985). Which of these statements are incorrect?

a. ''When a motor unit (the motor nerve and the muscle fibers it innervates) is stimulated, all of the muscle fibers of that unit contract maximally. A muscle fiber contracts maximally (100%) or not at all; this is the 'all or none principle' '' (p. 10).

b. ''There is some evidence that one can increase the probability of two or more units being activated in a synchronous manner. This has been referred to as synchronizing motor unit excitation. It is not clear why, or if this necessarily leads to improved strength'' (p. 12).

c. ''Motor recruitment can be thought of in four ways: (1) fiber type recruitment (FT or ST), (2) number of motor units recruited, (3) order of recruitment with regard to type I, IIA, IIB, and (4) frequency of motor unit contraction'' (p. 15).

d. "The number of impulses is regulated mainly by the muscle spindles which monitor tension (static length, change in length and pressure) on the muscle" (p. 15).

e. "The motor unit recruitment pattern depends upon the type of physical stimulus being placed on that motor unit. The pattern will be one of mainly slow twitch fibers with a few fast twitch fibers when aerobic, endurance type activity is done, requiring low force output. The situation will be reversed for an activity requiring a high force output" (p. 16).

6.2.   Which of the following statements (a-e) about motor-unit recruitment are correct? Both parts (i-v) of a-e have to be correct for the statement to be correct.

   i.   The size principle is a proposed mechanism to account for orderly recruitment.
   ii. Motor-unit recruitment and rate coding are concurrent processes.
   iii. Muscle-fiber size is not thought to be correlated with motoneuron size.
   iv. Evidence has shown that Type S motor units are always recruited first, even for high-power tasks.
   v.   Orderly recruitment is a concept that applies to the motor units belonging to a single muscle.

   a. i, iii
   b. ii, v
   c. iv, iii
   d. v, iv
   e. ii, i

6.3.   The size principle suggests that motor-unit recruitment order is based upon differences in motoneuron size.

   a. What is meant by motoneuron size?
   b. What morphological features of the motor unit seem to be related to motoneuron size?
   c. What types of synaptic input onto the motoneuron also seem to vary according to size?

6.4.   The relationship between action potential rate and force is known to be sigmoidal.

   a. Qualitatively, what is the difference between sigmoidal and linear relationships?
   b. How does muscle length affect the relationship?
   c. Similarly, the relationship for individual motor units seems to depend on twitch contraction time. What is this effect and why might it exist (Hint: tetanus)?

6.5.   Identify the *incorrect* statement(s) about motor-unit activity.

   a. Rate coding refers to the discharge of action potentials.
   b. Recruitment continues up to 85% of the maximum force for all muscles.
   c. Recruitment and rate coding can be concurrent.
   d. Synchronization is known to increase the force exerted by the active units.
   e. All slow-twitch units are recruited before any fast-twitch units.

6.6.   The force that a muscle can exert comprises two components—one due to active processes and the other due to passive properties.

   a. What features of muscle function contribute to the active processes?
   b. What are the passive properties?
   c. Does the moment arm (muscle-force vector to joint) contribute to the active or the passive elements?
   d. Will the rate of crossbridge cycling affect the magnitude of the force?

6.7.   Muscle torque-angle relationships typically have one of three forms: ascending, descending, or ascending-descending.

   a. What does ascending-descending mean?
   b. Suppose the following graph represents the most common form of the torque-angle relationship, such as for the elbow flexors. If the force exerted by the elbow flexor muscles remained constant at 3.5 kN over this range of motion, what would be the minimum and maximum values for the moment arm?

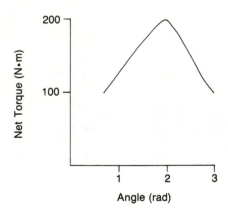

   c. Draw a free-body diagram to show the moment arm referred to in b.
   d. If the graph shown in b was obtained under conditions of a maximum voluntary contraction, is it reasonable to expect that the shape of the graph is mainly due to variation in the moment arm?

6.8. The terms *isometric*, *concentric*, and *eccentric* refer to differences in the mechanical conditions and not to different types of muscle contractions.

   a. What is the mechanical distinction between these terms?

   b. Can there be different types of muscle contractions? Explain your answer.

   c. The term *isotonic* means constant muscle tension. Why does this not occur under natural conditions, even when lifting a constant load?

6.9. From Part I, the first law of thermodynamics is

$$\Delta C = \Delta H + W$$

where C = chemical energy, H = heat or thermal energy, and W = work. We know that, as the shortening velocity of a muscle contraction increases, the muscle becomes less efficient (work output/energy input). If the amount of ATP used remains the same, what happens to the heat generated by the muscles as velocity increases? What happens to the work done by the muscle?

6.10. Why does the torque that a muscle can exert decrease as angular velocity increases?

   a. Decrease in muscle efficiency.

   b. Changes in the moment arm.

   c. Reduction in the number of crossbridges contributing to the force.

   d. Decrease in the average force exerted by each crossbridge.

   e. Increase in the quantity of Ca^{++} released.

6.11. From the work-energy relationship, we know that the work done is equal to the amount of energy used.

   a. What are the SI units of measurement for work and energy?

   b. What are the mechanical sources of energy for work?

   c. Physiologically, we distinguish positive and negative work. Mechanically, we describe positive work as involving the flow of energy from a system to its environment and negative work as involving flow in the reverse direction. What does this mean?

6.12. Imagine that you are holding a heavy briefcase by the handle while waiting for a bus. Although no mechanical work is done on the briefcase, why is it not possible to hold the briefcase indefinitely?

6.13. A warm-up has been shown to increase muscle temperature and subsequently to enhance power production. Why is this?

   a. Stretching exercises increase flexibility.

   b. The v_{max} value increases.

   c. Twitch force does not decrease.

   d. One-half relaxation time becomes longer.

   e. Contraction time decreases.

6.14. The way in which sarcomeres and muscle fibers are arranged in muscle can affect the force that a muscle exerts. Identify the incorrect statements about muscle architecture.

   a. The myofibril is described as an in-series arrangement of myofilaments.
   b. An average fiber in the human quadriceps femoris muscle group has about 30 sarcomeres in series.
   c. Pinnation results in a greater number of fibers being squeezed into a given volume.
   d. The in-parallel arrangement of thick and thin filaments is reflected in the measurement of cross-sectional area.
   e. Antigravity muscles are generally stronger than their antagonists.

6.15. Use the three-component model of muscle to account for the difference between twitch and tetanic force.

6.16. Which of the following statements (a-e) about muscle architecture are correct? Only one part (i-v) of a-e has to be wrong for the statement to be incorrect.

   i. The in-series arrangement of sarcomeres enhances the velocity of myofibril shortening.
   ii. Muscle-fiber force is proportional to the number of sarcomeres in series.
   iii. Maximum pinnation angles are about 1.57 rad.
   iv. The specific tension of muscle varies with its cross-sectional area.
   v. Fibers in pinnated muscles are generally shorter.

   a. ii, iv
   b. i, iii
   c. iv, v
   d. i, v
   e. iii, v

6.17. If each sarcomere produces a 0.5-μm change in length and there are 31.2 $\times 10^3$ sarcomeres in a muscle fiber, how much could the muscle fiber maximally change its length?

6.18. For a specific tension of 30 N/cm², what is the maximum force that the four muscle groups in Table 6.1 could exert?

CHAPTER 7

Patterns of Muscle Activation

Muscle can be described as an effector organ because it translates neural commands into force. As we have noted previously, the interaction between this muscle force and the forces exerted by the surroundings determine the nature of the ensuing movement. Until now, we have paid scant attention to the origin of the neural commands. In dealing with the topic of muscle-activation patterns, however, we will begin by considering an overview of the major neural interactions associated with the performance of a movement. Figure 7.1 represents such an overview and depicts four general aspects to movement: motivation, ideation, programming, and execution. We will focus largely on the latter two aspects.

The limbic system concerns emotional needs and behavior that are based on such biological drives as hunger, thirst, reproduction, maternal behavior, and socialization. In addition, it is crucial to our ability to learn from experience. The limbic system exerts its effects on the sensorimotor system, which transforms the motivation into an idea and initiates the supraspinal interactions that result in a command to execute a movement

(see Brooks, 1986, for more detail on these systems). The limbic system refers to a functional unit that includes a set of forebrain structures that are interconnected with the hypothalamus and parts of the midbrain. The hypothalamus is central to this system and regulates many vital factors, such as body temperature, heart rate, blood pressure, and water and food intake. The demands expressed by the limbic system are analyzed and integrated into ideas by the association cortex (e.g., prefrontal, parietal, and temporal lobes); these ideas project onto the sensorimotor cortex, cerebellum, part of the basal ganglia, and associated subcortical nuclei (Brooks, 1986).

The process of *programming* occurs in supraspinal centers and involves the conversion of an idea into the proper strength and pattern of muscle activity necessary for a desired movement. The neural output that emerges from this process is known as the **central command** and is transmitted to lower neural centers (brainstem and spinal cord). *Execution* involves two components: (a) the central-command activation of the lower neural centers, which in turn issue signals that

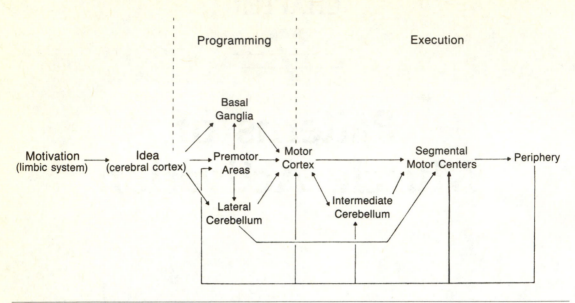

Figure 7.1. Flow chart of major neural interactions associated with the performance of a movement. The four aspects of this function include motivation, ideation, programming, and execution. *Note.* From "Role of Cerebral Cortex in Voluntary Movements. A Review" by P.D. Cheney, 1985, reprinted from *Physical Therapy* (Vol. 65, p. 625, 1985) with the permission of the American Physical Therapy Association.

determine the sequence of activity in different muscles; and (b) the modification of movements due to feedback from sensory receptors (e.g., muscle spindle, tendon organ, joint receptors, visual system, vestibular system).

Although the execution phase of movement performance (**motor control**) has these two components (neural command and feedback modification), movements can occur without the need for or use of feedback. To underscore this distinction we talk about closed- and open-loop modes of control. **Closed-loop** control involves the use of sensory feedback signals (e.g., muscle spindles, joint receptors, cutaneous receptors) to guide the movement continuously. **Open-loop** control refers to movements or responses controlled entirely by the neural command—

such movements are often called *preprogrammed* movements and are described as being under feedforward control. For example, rapid movements can be made so quickly that sensory feedback has no chance to have an effect before the movement is completed; consequently, these movements can be said to be predetermined. Alternatively, we all know that heart rate increases when we exercise. The increase occurs in two stages: before we begin the activity and while we are doing the activity. The increase before exercise (i.e., in anticipation of the exercise) represents open-loop control whereas the changes in heart rate during exercise occur due to closed-loop control.

Movements come in all shapes and sizes. This means that the commands that generate them must similarly be quite variable.

Presumably, the execution of different types of movements involves the generation of different central commands. Part of the programming process, therefore, must involve the selection of the appropriate motor control **strategy**—that is, the organization of a central command that will produce the desired movement. Although we do not have a standardized way of distinguishing control strategies, movements may be classified according to a number of criteria (Cheney, 1985):

1. Speed—slow or rapid
2. Number of joints involved—simple (one joint) or compound (two or more joints)
3. Type of feedback guidance—somesthetic, vestibular, auditory, visual, some combination of these, or none
4. Complexity—the number of phases
5. Termination mechanism—whether the movement is stopped by the individual or by some external means (e.g., a mechanical stop)
6. Accuracy—absolute, relative, or none
7. Degree of learning—the most automatic or stereotyped (e.g., locomotion, writing) through to the least automatic (e.g., exploratory activity with the hands)

The suggestion, therefore, is that a change in any of these variables will be accompanied by a change in both the control strategy and the associated pattern of muscle activity. In general, movements are designed to accomplish some goal, and they emerge as events that are realized within constraints imposed by the morphology of the system and the forces due to the surrounding environment.

Roberts (1976) considered these different criteria and suggested that these effects allow us to distinguish six different modes of motor control, each of which requires a different strategy of command. Roberts defined his six modes in the following manner:

1. Set. A part of the body is moved freely from one position to another without encountering resistance (e.g., rotating the head about a vertical axis).
2. Hold. A part of the body resists displacement due to external forces (e.g., holding a cup that is being filled).
3. Drive. A limb segment is shifted in position, despite an opposing resistance, by exerting sufficient force to overcome the resistance (e.g., thrusting a hand into a glove).
4. Punch. A limb segment acquires momentum due to forces much greater than are necessary to move the limb from one position to another. Some of the momentum of the limb is transferred to an object as the result of an impact (e.g., hitting a punch bag, kicking a football).
5. Catch. The muscles of a limb perform negative work and absorb power from an external agent (e.g., catching a ball, landing from a drop).
6. Throw. The muscles of a limb perform positive work on the limb segment, including some object that may be held; subsequently, the muscles do negative work to slow down the limb (e.g., when throwing a ball, momentum is imparted to the arm as well as to the ball, but the arm momentum is absorbed after ball release).

These modes of motor control are delightful in their simplicity yet instructive as to how they might be accomplished. For example, the set mode implies that the movement, which encounters no unexpected loads, can be performed with open-loop control. In contrast, the hold mode requires continual adjustment of the muscle activity, and this is probably accomplished with sensory-feedback effects. At the other end of the spectrum, the throw mode is reminiscent of the three-burst pattern of EMG that we encountered in chapter 1 (Figure 1.5). Roberts (1976) suggests that all movements can be accounted for by various combinations of these motor-control modes.

Muscle Organization

In terms of the focus used throughout this text, a major consequence of these modes of motor control is the form of the central command that is delivered to the simple joint system. More generally, however, muscle-activity patterns represent a combined effect of the type of movement desired and the way in which our bodies are put together (i.e., functional and structural constraints). By structural constraints we mean the way in which muscles are organized around joints.

In our simplified view of movement, the human body comprises a series of segments. These rigid links are connected by joints, the structures of which vary throughout the body. *The structure of the joint largely determines the quality of motion that can occur between two segments.* For example, some joints are designed so that only the flexion-extension movement can occur (e.g., elbow). In other joints the design also allows abduction-adduction (e.g., wrist) and rotation (e.g., pronation-supination at the radio-ulnar joint, internal-external rotation of the hip). The number of movements (flexion-extension, abduction-adduction, rotation) that a joint permits defines the **degrees of freedom** of the joint. Movable joints will possess a minimum of one (e.g., elbow) and a maximum of three (e.g., hip, shoulder) degrees of freedom.

Since muscles can only pull and not push, a minimum of one pair of muscles must cross a joint to control each degree of freedom. For example, the elbow needs at least one muscle to control flexion and one to control exten-

sion. Often, however, the arrangement of muscles is not this simple, and we usually have several muscles contributing to the same action. The primary elbow flexors, for example, include biceps brachii, brachialis, and brachioradialis. The main difference between such groups of muscles is the points of attachment, and hence the mechanical action, of the constituent muscles. These points of attachment may vary so that (a) the changes in moment arm distances are maximized for one muscle over one part of the range of motion and for another muscle over another part of the range; for example, the further a muscle attachment is from a joint, the greater the velocity of muscle shortening for a particular angular velocity of the limb but the greater the variation in the moment arm; (b) muscles can contribute to different actions; for example, as well as contributing to elbow flexion along with brachialis and brachioradialis, biceps brachii assists with supination of the forearm-hand due to the location of its attachment site on the tuberosity of the radius; and (c) one muscle in a group may be more ideally located to assist with the maintenance of posture; for example, muscles involved with maintaining our upright posture tend to be closer to the long bone of the segment (Lexell, Henriksson-Larsén, & Sjöström, 1983).

One common variation in the points of attachment is the number of joints that a muscle spans. A significant number of muscles, for example, span two joints and hence are referred to as **two-joint muscles** (e.g., biceps brachii, rectus femoris). It is typically argued that *two-joint muscles simplify the control of movement* for the central nervous system (Arsenault & Chapman, 1974; Fujiwara & Basmajian, 1975; Mussa-Ivaldi, Hogan, & Bizzi, 1985). For example, biceps brachii crosses both the elbow and the shoulder joints and thus contributes to both elbow and shoulder flexion. Since these two movements are concurrent in many of our activities, it is useful to have a muscle that contributes to both actions. In addition, two-joint muscles can be relatively independent of moment-arm effects; both joints that the two-joint muscle spans can change so that the changes in the moment arm are small.

These comments serve to remind us that the simple joint system we described in Part II is, in reality, not that simple. However, so that we may proceed, at least on a conceptual basis, we shall confine our consideration to the effects of generic muscles; namely, muscles controlling knee extension shall be referred to as knee extensors, those controlling hip abduction as hip abductors, and so on.

Net Muscle Activity

In previous chapters, our consideration of movement has assumed a mechanical focus in which we have been concerned with the net effect of muscle activation rather than with the muscle activity itself. We can, however, monitor the electrical activity of a muscle (EMG) and tell whether or not the muscle is active during a movement. Under some circumstances it is even possible to estimate how much force a muscle is exerting based on a record of its EMG activity (Hof & Van den Berg, 1981a, 1981b, 1981c, 1981d). We have not adopted this approach but rather have quantified the mechanical effect of muscular activity by the terms *resultant muscle force* and *resultant muscle torque*.

Shortly, we shall extend this approach to deduce the net muscular activity based on the mechanics of the movement. Before we proceed, though, it is worth emphasizing two limitations of our concept of resultant muscle torque: its mode of determination and nonmuscular contributions. With the Newtonian

approach to the study of motion, we use the following relationships:

$$\sum F = ma$$
$$\sum M_g = I_g \alpha$$

From these expressions, *the resultant muscle torque is calculated as the residual moment*. A free-body diagram is drawn and set equal to a mass acceleration diagram (chapter 3, "Force-Mass-Acceleration: Dynamic Analysis"). The analysis begins by identifying the moments of force (Figure 7.2).

$$(W_b \times a) + (W_u \times b) - (F_i \times c) - (F_m \times d) = I_{LS}\alpha$$

As was indicated when this analysis was presented earlier (Figure 3.6), values for all the terms are known except for the resultant

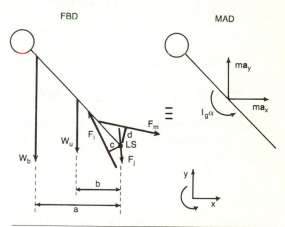

Figure 7.2. Free-body diagram (FBD) and mass-acceleration diagram (MAD) of the upper body of a weight lifter performing the clean. W_b = 1003 N = weight of the barbell; W_u = 525 N = weight of the upper body; F_i = 1250 N = intraabdominal pressure; a, b, c = moment arms; F_m = resultant muscle force; LS = lumbosacral joint; F_j = joint reaction force; $I_{LS}\alpha$ = inertia torque; ma_x and ma_y = inertia force.

muscle torque ($F_m \times d$), and so the expression is rearranged to solve for the unknown.

$$(F_m \times d) =$$
$$(W_b \times a) + (W_u \times b) - (F_i \times c) - I_{LS}\alpha$$

($F_m \times d$) is called *residual moment* because the kinematic effect ($I_{LS}\alpha$) is known and some of the moments of force (W_b, W_u, F_i) are known, and so the difference (i.e., what is left over) is attributed to the ($F_m \times d$). There are at least two limitations associated with this procedure. First, there are other structures (e.g., ligaments, joint capsule) besides muscle that can contribute to the residual torque (Andrews, 1982; Williams & Cavanagh, 1983). Second, the ($F_m \times d$) term does not represent the absolute quantity of muscle activity.

In what follows we shall consider an example that addresses the magnitude of the discrepancy between the net effect and the absolute value, and then we shall extend our mechanical focus to deduce the patterns of net muscle activity.

Bone-on-Bone Force

In Part I we encountered the concept of a joint reaction force, which represents predominantly bone-on-bone forces. In many instances, however, the joint reaction force is a gross underestimation of the contact forces that occur between bones in a joint. The main reason for this difference is associated with this idea of a net effect (e.g., the difference between forces) versus the sum of all contributing elements. In other words, when a muscle is active, the tangential component of the force vector represents the proportion of the muscle activity that stabilizes the joint and contributes to bone-on-bone forces. When a single muscle (or muscle group) is active, the tangential component contributes to the joint reaction force and influences the

magnitude of the bone-on-bone force—other tissues (e.g., ligaments, capsule) and external forces will also affect the contact force. However, *when an opposing set of muscles is coactive, the contribution to the joint reaction force is calculated as the difference between the opposing activity* (tangential components) *whereas the bone-on-bone force must include the sum of the activity* (Figure 7.3). The muscles about the ankle joint can be grouped into those that contribute to a plantarflexor (F_{pf}) torque and those that exert a dorsiflexor (F_{df}) torque (Figure 7.3B). The bone-on-bone force must

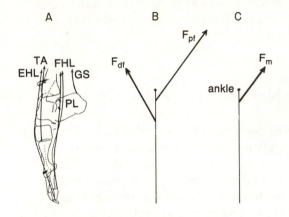

Figure 7.3. Schematic view of the foot on full *pointe* showing the lines of action of the muscles. (A) The major muscles (EHL = extensor hallucis longus, FHL = flexor hallucis longus, GS = gastrocnemius-soleus, PL = peroneus longus, TA = tibialis anterior) and skeletal structure about the ankle joint. (B) Separation of the muscular effects into those that exert dorsiflexor (F_{df}) torque and those that exert plantarflexor (F_{pf}) torque. (C) The net muscle activity (F_m). *Note.* From "Bone-on-Bone Forces at the Ankle Joint During a Rapid Dynamic Movement" by V. Galea and R.W. Norman, 1985, in D.A. Winter et al. (Eds.), *Biomechanics IX-A* (p. 72), Champaign, IL: Human Kinetics. Copyright 1985 by Human Kinetics. Adapted by permission.

include the tangential component of the F_{pf} vector *plus* the tangential component of the F_{df} vector. In the calculation of the resultant muscle force (F_m), however, F_m is determined as the net effect, that is, F_{pf} *minus* F_{df} (Figure 7.3C).

In the human movement literature, there is little information about bone-on-bone forces. As was indicated in Part I, we have kinematic and kinetic techniques with which to estimate joint reaction forces. However, calculation of bone-on-bone forces requires that we be able to measure the force exerted by individual muscles. As you can imagine, this has proven to be rather difficult to perform in human subjects. One technique that some researchers have used is based on an association between the change in length of a muscle, its electrical activity (EMG), and the force that it can exert (Hof, 1984; Hof & Van den Berg, 1981a, 1981b, 1981c, 1981d). An interesting example of this approach is provided by Galea and Norman (1985) in a study of the bone-on-bone forces at the ankle joint during a rapid ballet movement, a spring from flat feet onto the toes. The model used to perform these calculations (Figure 7.3) takes into account the major muscles crossing the ankle joint and therefore those that will contribute to the bone-on-bone force: These include extensor hallucis longus (EHL), tibialis anterior (TA), flexor hallucis longus (FHL), peroneus longus (PL), and gastrocnemius/soleus (G/S). The model takes into account the length of the muscle, its velocity, and its EMG in determining the force exerted by each muscle.

Once Galea and Norman identified the force for each muscle, they inserted these values into a dynamic analysis (chapter 3, "Force-Mass-Acceleration: Dynamic Analysis"). For one subject, the peak bone-on-bone force based on net muscle force averaged 732 N during the movement and the peak

bone-on-bone force based on absolute muscle forces averaged 6,068 N. In this case there was a substantial difference between the two measures, the absolute and the net effects. Incidentally, values for bone failure in compression stress range between 14 and 28 kN/cm^2, which is well above the bone-on-bone forces reported by Galea and Norman (1985).

Muscle Activity and Movement

Despite this discrepancy between absolute and net effects, it is still instructive to consider the mechanics of movement and deduce the net muscle activity. Consider a person lying supine on a bench and performing forearm curls (elbow flexion-extension movements) with a 120-N weight (Figure 7.4). If the individual executes a *slow* movement throughout the full range of motion, what is the net muscle activity as the arm moves from Position 1 through Position 4? Which muscle group (elbow flexors or extensors) is primarily responsible for the movement? Is it active concentrically or eccentrically? Also, what provides the load and about what point is it acting?

The load against which the muscle group is acting is the weight held in the person's hand plus the weight of the forearm-hand segment. The appropriate free-body diagram indicates that the axis of rotation is the elbow joint (Figure 7.4B). The analysis concerns the torques that are acting about the elbow joint, and the free-body diagram can be simplified as shown in Figure 7.4C. In this simplification, the load torque represents the effects of the system weight ($W_s + W_h$). The direction of the weight vectors is obtained by the right-hand-thumb rule; the fingers of the right hand are curled in the direction that each force (resultant muscle force and resultant load force) will cause the system to rotate,

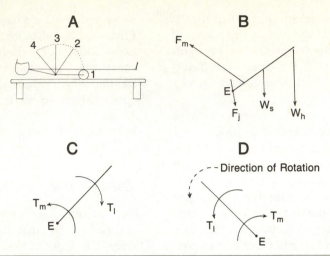

Figure 7.4. Determination of the pattern of net muscle activity for a slow movement. (A) A supine elbow flexion-extension movement with a dumbbell. (B) Free-body diagram isolating the elbow musculature: E = elbow joint, W_h = weight held in the hand, F_j = joint reaction force, F_m = resultant muscle force, W_s = forearm-hand segment weight. (C) Resultant muscle (T_m) and load (T_l) torques. (D) The net muscle activity is based on a comparison of the directions of the T_m and the movement.

and the right-hand thumb is extended. If the thumb extends out from the page (as opposed to into the page), the torque vector is drawn in a counterclockwise direction.

From these diagrams we can determine the muscle group mainly responsible for the movement and the direction of its change in length (concentric or eccentric). The appropriate steps involve drawing

1. the body segment in the approximate position,
2. the load-torque (T_l) vector,
3. the resultant-muscle-torque (T_m) vector in the opposite direction of the load-torque vector, and
4. the direction of rotation of the body segment.

For example, consider the movement of the forearm-hand segment in the above example

from Position 3 to Position 4. Note that the body segment is drawn not at either Position 3 or Position 4 but rather midway between the two positions (Figure 7.4D). From this diagram, we can deduce the direction of the resultant-muscle-torque vector and determine whether the net muscle activity is concentric or eccentric. For *slow* movements, *the direction of the resultant-muscle-torque vector is opposite that of the load-torque vector.* To determine which muscle group the resultant-muscle-torque vector represents, imagine that there are no other forces or torques acting on the system and that the segment rotates in the same direction indicated by the resultant-muscle-torque vector. *If this direction is one of extension, then the responsible muscle group is the extensors; and if the resultant-muscle-torque vector produces flexion, then the vector represents the flexor muscles.* Alternatively, recall that muscles can only exert a pulling force so that when the resultant-muscle-force ($\mathbf{F}_m$) vector is drawn on the free-body diagram, it is possible to determine which muscles (e.g., flexors or extensors) would exert such a force. In the above example, a clockwise torque indicates the elbow extensors and counterclockwise represents the elbow flexors (i.e., $\mathbf{T}_m$ represents an elbow extensor torque).

By comparing the directions of the resultant-muscle-torque vector and the segment rotation, we can determine whether the net muscle activity is concentric or eccentric. If the directions of the resultant-muscle-torque vector and the segment rotation are the same, then the muscle group is experiencing a concentric contraction. If the segment rotation and the resultant muscle torque are not acting in the same direction (as in the movement from Position 3 to 4), then the net muscle activity is an eccentric contraction. Thus the movement from Position 3 to Position 4 is controlled by an eccentric contraction of the elbow extensors. In general, if an extensor muscle group produces extension or a flexor group causes flexion, the net muscle activity is concentric. In contrast, flexion controlled by an extensor group or extension by a flexor group represents net eccentric activity.

By using these procedures it is possible to address the entire range of motion for such slow movements as the forearm-curl example:

This particular example of the forearm-curl exercise with a supine subject emphasizes an important feature of the way in which we use our muscles. Suppose that the individual now moves from the supine position to upright posture and performs a similar exercise of raising and lowering an extended arm between Positions 1 and 2 (Figure 7.5). What patterns of net muscle activity are necessary to complete this movement? If we answered this question by going through the procedure that has just been described, we would find that, in going from both Position 1 to 2 and Position 2 to 1, the movement is controlled by the elbow flexors. The muscle activity is concentric going up (Position 1 to 2) and eccentric coming down. The difference in the patterns of activity between the supine and upright postures has to do with *the orientation of the individual (and hence the movement) relative to the direction of gravity.* Our existence in a gravitational environment has a major effect on the pattern of muscle activation. For example, in both the upright standing and the supine examples, imagine a vertical line (gravity) that passes through the axis of rotation (shoulder and elbow, respectively). The major qualitative difference is that the movement never crosses this line in the upright exercise whereas it does in the supine exercise. For *slow* exercises, crossing this line means changing the muscle group that controls the movement.

Movement	1 → 2	2 → 3	3 → 4	4 → 3	3 → 2	2 → 1
Elbow flexors	C	C			E	E
Elbow extensors			E	C		

C = concentric, E = eccentric

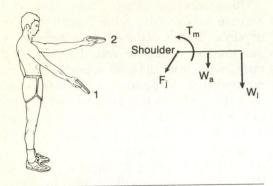

Figure 7.5. A shoulder flexion-extension movement. Since the load torque ($W_a + W_l$) acts in the same direction throughout the movement, the direction of the resultant muscle torque (T_m) is constant over the course of the movement.

It should be emphasized, however, that the analysis just employed applies only to conditions that we might call **quasistatic**: those instances that are almost static and in which the acceleration of the system and its various parts is quite small (Miller, 1980). Under quasistatic conditions we can approximate the mechanical state of the muscle by doing a static analysis (i.e., $\Sigma F = 0$). There is no agreement among researchers on the actual boundary that separates the condition when a quasistatic state can be assumed and the condition when it cannot. Alexander and Vernon (1975), for example, have used a version of the quasistatic approach to calculate the resultant muscle torques about the ankle and knee joints during the stance phase of a jog. Others, however, have felt it necessary to perform a complete dynamic analysis (i.e., $\Sigma F = ma$) for such conditions (Mann, 1981; Miller & Munro, 1985).

Certainly a dynamic analysis is necessary for more vigorous activities, such as kicking. For example (Miller, 1980), consider the pattern of muscle activity about the knee joint during the execution of a soccer toe kick

(Figure 7.6). The position of the kicking leg (the one with the filled-in shoe) from Figure 7.6 is superimposed onto one stick figure, first relative to the hip joint and then with respect to the knee joint (Figure 7.7).

Next, let us perform a quasistatic analysis, as we did with the forearm-curl example, to determine the pattern of net muscle activity about the knee joint during the kick. Since the movement (Position 1 to 4) never crosses the vertical line that passes through the axis of rotation (knee), the load-torque vector, and therefore the resultant-muscle-torque vector, acts in the same direction throughout the movement.

Movement	1 → 2	2 → 3	3 → 4
Knee flexors	C	C	E
Knee extensors			

C = concentric, E = eccentric

On the basis of this quasistatic rationale, the motion about the knee joint during the toe kick (Figure 7.6) is supposedly controlled by the knee-flexor muscles. Our intuition tells us that we would be hard-pressed to convince anybody that the knee flexors were primarily responsible for this kicking movement. The obvious shortcoming of this analysis is the assumption that the movement is slow. In chapter 2 we considered the different types of contact forces that are commonly encountered in human movement: joint reaction, ground reaction, fluid resistance, elastic, inertial, and muscle forces. Recall that inertial forces were effects that occurred due to the motion of the object or segment. *In fast movements these forces become quite substantial and drastically alter the pattern of muscle activity that is necessary to control the movement.* Indeed, for an event such as a strong kick, it

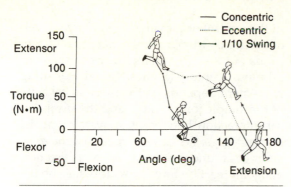

Figure 7.6. Resultant muscle torque about the knee joint of the kicking leg as a function of knee angle during the swing preceding ball contact in a fast soccer toe kick. The total time for the swing was 170 ms, 17 ms between each of the large dots. To interpret the graph, begin at the bottom right-hand corner and proceed in a counterclockwise direction from Position 1 to 4. *Note.* From "Body Segment Contributions to Sport Skill Performance: Two Contrasting Approaches" by D.I. Miller, 1980, *Research Quarterly for Exercise and Sport,* **51**, p. 225. Copyright 1980 by the American Alliance for Health, Physical Education, Recreation, and Dance. Reprinted by permission of the American Alliance for Health, Physical Education, Recreation, and Dance, 1900 Association Drive, Reston, VA 22091.

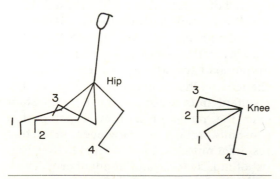

Figure 7.7. Angular displacement of the lower leg (shank) relative to the knee during a kick.

even becomes necessary to consider the way in which the motion of the shank will affect the thigh and, conversely, how thigh motion will affect the shank (Putnam, 1983).

The magnitude of the inertial effects can be seen by comparing the resultant muscle torque about the knee joint in Figure 7.6 with that deduced above by the quasistatic approach. Interpretation of the torque-angle graph (Figure 7.6) begins in the lower right-hand corner and progresses in a counterclockwise direction. The graph indicates several interesting features: (a) except for the first part of the kick, the resultant muscle torque is due to the extensors and not the flexors, as suggested by the quasistatic analysis; (b) most of the movement from Position 1 to Position 3, during which knee angle decreases, is controlled by eccentric extensor activity; (c) from Position 3 to contact with the ball the net activity is a concentric extensor effect; and (d) the peak resultant muscle torque occurs at the change from eccentric to concentric activity. These observations indicate that a quasistatic analysis, which ignores the effects due to acceleration, is inappropriate to reveal the pattern of net muscle activity in this instance (a rapid kicking motion).

A good way to derive the information shown in Figure 7.6 is to perform a temporal alignment of the resultant-muscle-torque and angular-velocity graphs. To illustrate this procedure, let us return to the example of horizontal extension-flexion at the elbow joint (Figure 3.11). Half of the movement involves extension and half involves flexion. The change in direction occurs when velocity is zero. Each displacement epoch (i.e., extension, then flexion) is accomplished by net extensor and flexor muscle activity. For the first part of the movement, extension is produced by a net extensor torque, hence the extensors are active concentrically. The rest of the extension movement, however, is accomplished by net flexor activity, which means that the flexors are being actively lengthened (i.e., an eccentric contraction). By similar reasoning, the flexion phase of the movement is controlled first by concentric flexor activity and then by an eccentric extensor phase (Figure 7.8). We arrived at this same pattern of net muscle activity by other means in chapter 1 (Figure 1.5).

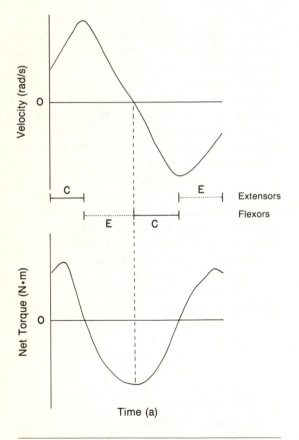

Figure 7.8. Deduction of the net muscle activity responsible for a horizontal elbow extension-flexion movement. Positive velocity represents extension at the elbow joint. Positive net torque indicates a resultant extensor muscle torque. *Note.* C = concentric, E = eccentric.

Patterns of EMG Activity

In the control of movement, we have developed the concept that the nervous system sends out a set of commands from segmental motor centers (Figure 7.1); the ensuing movement depends on the mechanical state of the simple joint system and the mechanical interaction between the system and its surroundings. We have learned that the measures of ground reaction force, air resistance, and joint reaction force provide details on the system-surround interaction whereas the concept of a resultant muscle torque represents the mechanical output of the system. In addition to these two approaches, considerable attention has been directed toward understanding the control of movement by measuring the commands sent out by the nervous system to the simple joint system. This is normally done by measuring the electromyogram (EMG). We shall briefly consider some of the ideas that have emerged from these endeavors by examining three topics: moment-arm effects, the three-burst pattern, and cocontraction.

In Part I (Table 2.3), we encountered the notion that, as a muscle is moved through its range of motion, the *moment arm* from the muscle-force vector to the axis of rotation (joint) changes. For the elbow flexors, the moment arm is greatest in a midrange position (elbow angle about 1.57 rad) and least at full extension and full flexion. Based on this relationship, we would expect that the muscle force necessary to support a constant-torque load would vary inversely with the changes in the moment arm. That is, the resultant muscle torque must be constant over the range of motion to support a constant-torque load. However, recall that resultant muscle torque is equal to the product of muscle force and moment arm. Thus, if the moment arm changes, then muscle force must change in an inverse manner to maintain a constant product. This relationship is difficult to assess directly because both moment arm and muscle force are difficult quantities to measure. Instead, Hasan and Enoka (1985) examined the EMG and found that it varied in the manner that we would expect of muscle force (Figure 7.9).

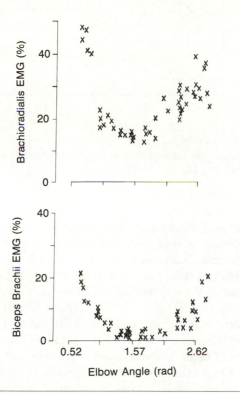

Figure 7.9. EMG activity necessary for two concurrently active elbow flexors (biceps brachii and brachioradialis) to support a constant-torque load over a substantial range of motion of the elbow joint. EMG was measured as the average voltage level needed to support the load. *Note.* From ''Isometric Torque-Angle Relationship and Movement-Related Activity of Human Elbow Flexors: Implications for the Equilibrium-Point Hypothesis'' by Z. Hasan and R.M. Enoka, 1985, *Experimental Brain Research*, **59**, p. 447. Copyright 1985 by Springer-Verlag, Inc. Adapted by permission.

The relationship between muscle force and EMG is complex (Hof & Van den Berg, 1981a, 1981b, 1981c, 1981d; Perry & Bekey, 1981). However, it appears that under isometric conditions EMG is related to force in a fairly predictable manner (Bigland & Lippold, 1954). The data in Figure 7.9 were obtained under isometric conditions; consequently, the interpretation that the EMG-angle relationship is inversely related to the changes in moment arm seems reasonable.

The *three-burst pattern* of EMG activity was first mentioned in chapter 1 when we discussed the elbow extension-flexion movement in a horizontal plane (Figure 1.5). That example involved a biphasic movement (i.e., an extension phase, then a flexion phase). The extension phase comprised an agonist burst (elbow extensors) to initiate the movement and then an antagonist burst (elbow flexion) to brake the movement. Similarly, the flexion phase comprised an agonist (elbow flexors) and an antagonist (elbow extensors) sequence. Taken together, the EMG pattern appeared as an extensor-flexor-extensor sequence.

The three-burst of EMG is also seen for unidirectional movements (Wachholder & Altenburger, 1926). The pattern involves an initial agonist burst, an antagonist burst, and a second agonist burst (Figure 7.10). This sequence has been referred to as an ABC set, where A = action burst, B = braking burst, and C = clamping burst (Hannaford & Stark, 1985). The action burst accelerates the limb toward the target position, the braking burst slows down the limb as it approaches the target position, and the clamping burst fixes the limb in the target position. One feature of the three-burst pattern that is often not appreciated is its variability. For example, the timing of the antagonist activity is highly variable and depends on such features of the movement as speed, amplitude, and load (Karst & Hasan, 1987). In fact, the antagonist is not

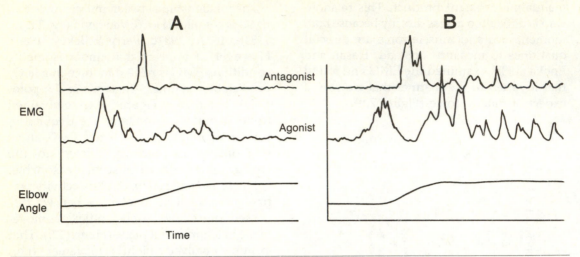

Figure 7.10. The three-burst pattern of EMG activity for an elbow-flexion movement. The EMG data is rectified and filtered. (A) A distinct sequence. (B) A movement displaying cocontraction at the termination of the movement. *Note.* Data from Karst and Hasan, 1987.

even activated for many movements performed in a vertical plane (Figure 7.9). Furthermore, the activity of the muscle set (agonist-antagonist pair) can have varying levels of cocontraction as the target position is approached.

Although the presence of a three-burst pattern of EMG for unidirectional movements has been known for a number of years, no unifying hypothesis has been formulated to account for the variety of observations (reviewed in Hasan et al., 1985). There is no doubt that the three-burst pattern concerns stopping a movement at a targeted position, but the control strategy adopted by the central nervous system has not yet been determined. For example, many investigators have attempted to determine which parts of the sequence are under open-loop control and which can be altered by closed-loop control. Two major limitations, however, have prevented a complete understanding of this EMG sequence: (a) The three-burst pattern is drastically affected by the features of move-

ment, including the instructions given to the subject, and to systematically control all the variables has proven difficult (Karst & Hasan, 1987); and (b) not enough attention has been paid to the mechanical conditions, such as the orientation of the subject (plane in which the movement is performed) and the fact that the agonist (or antagonist) for a particular movement often includes more than one muscle.

One of the observations made by Karst and Hasan (1987) concerning the three-burst pattern was the variability in the degree of *cocontraction* at the end of the movement. Cocontraction refers to concurrent activity in the muscles comprising an agonist-antagonist set. There is surprisingly little information available on cocontraction. In particular, conditions under which we use cocontraction have been largely unexplained. Cocontraction has the mechanical effect of making a joint stiffer (i.e., movement becomes more difficult). This would seem like a useful feature when we learn novel tasks or when we perform a movement that requires a high degree of accuracy. For example, Person (1958) monitored the EMG of biceps and triceps brachii while training subjects over a 2-week period to file and cut with a chisel. Over the course of the training, it was quite evident that the commands sent out by the low-level controller changed from a high level of cocontraction to complete reciprocal activity (i.e., no cocontraction).

This example is not meant to imply that skilled movements do not include cocontraction. Enoka (1983), for example, found that skilled weight lifters performing the movement outlined in Figure 1.4 used cocontraction of vastus lateralis and biceps femoris throughout the movement (Figure 7.11). Furthermore, Hasan (1986) has argued that under certain conditions cocontraction will actually decrease the cost of performing the movement in terms of the effort involved in the task—some empirical observations support this suggestion (Engelhorn, 1983). It also appears that the neural strategy involved in performing cocontraction is different from that of more normal activities, such as supporting a load (Gydikov, Kossev, Radicheva, & Tankov, 1981). Thus, although the presence and absence of cocontraction appear to be two distinct strategies used by the central nervous system, we do not understand the rules that determine the option that is selected.

These three examples (moment-arm effects, three-burst pattern, and cocontraction) provide an overview of the ways in which we try to understand the signals sent out by segmental motor centers (Figure 7.1) for the elaboration of a movement. The interpretation of the EMG signals is difficult because the ensuing movement is largely determined by the mechanical conditions onto which the EMG signals are overlaid.

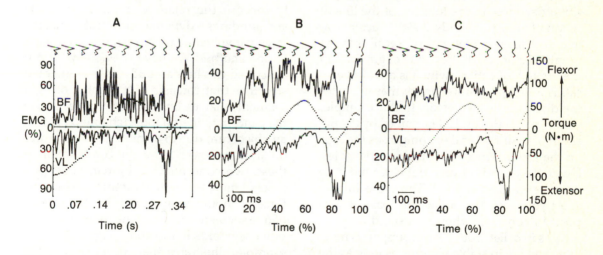

Figure 7.11. Resultant muscle torque (dotted line) and EMG records (solid line) about the knee joint during the clean in weight lifting. The kinematics for the movement are shown in Figure 1.4. The EMG information for biceps femoris (BF) and vastus lateralis (VL) were rectified, filtered, and expressed as a percentage of their respective maximum values. (A) The profiles for one trial. (B) The mean profile for 6 trials for one subject. (C) The mean profile of 15 trials for three subjects. *Note.* From ''Muscular Control of a Learned Movement: The Speed Control System Hypothesis'' by R.M. Enoka, 1983, *Experimental Brain Research*, **51**, p. 140. Copyright 1983 by Springer-Verlag, Inc. Reprinted by permission.

Posture

It has been known for some time that the execution of a movement is accompanied by the need to maintain postural stability. This association was aptly described by Sherrington (1931): Posture accompanies movement like a shadow (Martin, 1977). Posture is a mechanical state that concerns the maintenance of equilibrium. Postural activities, in general, fall into two categories: static and dynamic. Static postural activities are those associated with the maintenance of an upright standing posture. In contrast, dynamic postural activities are those involved with maintaining your balance during movement.

Postural Requirements

Let us consider the static example in more detail. Your ability to remain in an upright position depends on the location of the line of action of your total-body weight vector relative to your base of support. Recall that the weight vector acts at the center of gravity and that its line of action, which is always vertical, is a line of infinite length that indicates the direction of the vector. In this example, your base of support is determined by the position of your feet and encompasses the area on the ground from the outside of your left foot to the outside of your right foot and from your heels to your toes. Thus, the further apart your feet, the larger your base of support. In contrast, when you stand on your toes, as in ballet, your base of support is minimal. You are in stable position as long as the line of action of your weight vector passes through your base of support.

When we stand in an upright position, our bodies sway backward and forward. The muscular activity that prevents us from swaying too far forward or backward represents static postural control. Imagine, for example,

an individual's swaying forward such that there is dorsiflexion at the ankle joint. In this instance, the calf muscles (gastrocnemius and soleus) are stretched. If you recall the discussion in chapter 5 (Figure 5.15) of the neural connections involved in some reflexes, you should realize that stretching these muscles will excite some sensory receptors (probably muscle spindles) located in the muscles. This excitation will be transmitted over afferent pathways back to the spinal cord where it may excite motoneurons that are connected to these same muscles. The net response is that the stretch of the calf muscles will cause their subsequent contraction; this sequence of events is known as the stretch reflex. Thus we suspect that the stretch reflex is a neural mechanism that enables us to maintain this upright position.

The other type of postural control concerns the maintenance of equilibrium during movement. Whereas static postural activities largely concern the relation of the body to its surroundings, dynamic postural concerns largely involve the relation of the body parts to one another. We have previously (Part I) described the human body as a segmented structure that consists of a number of rigid segments that are linked together. Recall also the concept of inertia force (chapter 2) in that an object can, due to its motion, exert a force on another object. With the combination of these two concepts, the human body as a linked, multisegment structure and inertia force, it should be apparent that the motion of one segment can affect the motion of most other segments in the body. Figure 2.18, for example, illustrates that the motion of the thigh during the swing phase of running can affect the motion of the leg.

Consider the movement shown in Figure 7.12A. The subject is asked to shake rapidly the forearm and hand in a forward-backward movement while keeping the upper arm essentially horizontal. This is done by alternately activating the elbow flexor and elbow extensor muscles. In addition, however, the task will require substantial activation of muscles that cross the shoulder joint (Hoy, Zernicke, & Smith, 1985). This is necessary to stabilize the upper arm and to minimize the inertial effects of the forearm motion on other body segments. Similarly, suppose an individual standing upright is asked to raise his arm as rapidly as possible to a horizontal position (Figure 7.12B). This is a reaction-time task in which the movement is done rapidly following a signal to begin. The anterior deltoid muscle is a prime mover for the task. The fastest a muscle can be activated (the minimum reaction time) following a signal is about 120 ms, which is true for anterior deltoid activity in this task. However, about 50 ms before the anterior deltoid activity, the hamstrings on the same side of the body are activated (Belen'kii, Gurfinkel', & Pal'tsev, 1967). The activity in the leg muscles probably represented a stabilization against the inertial effects of the ensuing arm movement.

Adaptability of Postural Responses

Previously (Figure 5.16), we encountered the idea of a reflex as a simple, input-output relationship. For example, we talked about how the stretch of a muscle (the input) will result in a contraction of the same muscle (the output); we have called this particular input-output relationship the stretch reflex. However, a number of investigators have demonstrated that such relationships are not fixed but depend on what the individual is doing at the time that the reflex is elicited. Because of this adaptability, we describe reflexes as being state- and phase-dependent responses. This means that the reflex depends on the state (e.g., standing or walking) and the phase (e.g., stance or swing) of the subject's activity.

One clear example of the adaptability of rapid, automatic responses is shown in Figure 7.13. Nashner has constructed a paradigm in which a subject stands upright on a platform (level with the floor) that is capable of being moved in a number of directions by a hydraulic control system (Nashner, 1982; Nashner & McCollum, 1985). In Figure 7.13A, the platform is translated rapidly backward. This causes the subject to sway forward, which stretches the calf muscles (gastrocnemius and soleus) and elicits a stretch response (EMG records) in these muscles. The effect of the stretch response is

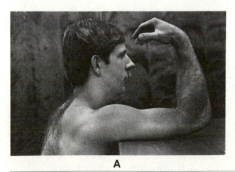
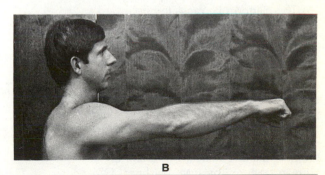

Figure 7.12. (A) The subject performs a rapid elbow flexion-extension movement while keeping the upper arm horizontal. (B) Once a begin signal is given, the subject raises his right arm from his side to a horizontal position as rapidly as possible. Photo by Peter B. Worden.

to cause the body to return to the upright position; that is, it assists with the maintenance of stability. Over four trials, the stretch response occurs earlier, and its magnitude increases so that it minimizes the sway associated with the backward motion of the platform. In contrast, consider the situation in Figure 7.13B in which a toes-up rotation of

the platform also stretches the calf muscles. In this instance, the subject does not sway from the upright vertical position, and so a stretch response is unnecessary. In fact, a stretch response will cause the subject to fall backward. As shown by the EMG records (Figure 7.13B), the subject can learn, after only four trials, to reduce the response and thus prevent the destabilization.

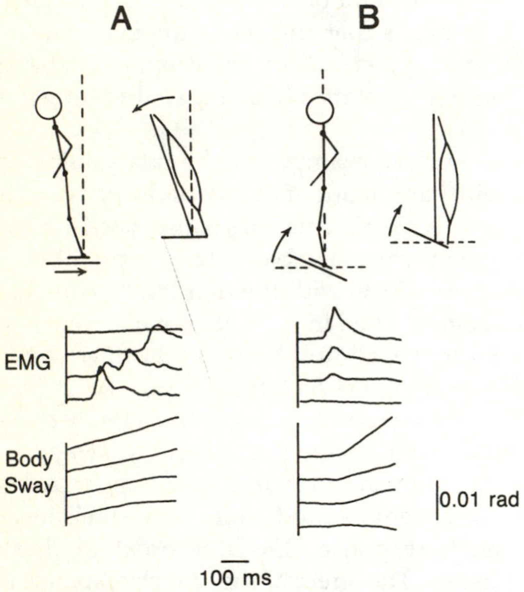

Eccentric-Concentric Contractions

It seems that a common pattern of muscle activation, particularly during high-performance tasks, is to employ eccentric-concentric sequences. Such a pattern is also referred to as "the stretch-shorten cycle." There is much discussion, however, of mechanisms underlying this phenomenon.

Three-Component Model

The behavior of muscle can, to a first approximation (see Hatze, 1981a, for a more detailed account), be represented by a **three-component model** (Figure 7.14). In this

Figure 7.13. Postural responses of a subject to movement of the base of support (platform). (A) The platform is translated backward and elicits a stretch response in the calf muscles. The response is measured as the integrated EMG, the effect of which is shown relative to the sway experienced by the subject. (B) The platform is rotated toes-up and again elicits a stretch response in the calf muscles. The subject is able to (A) enhance or (B) diminish the stretch response, depending upon its appropriateness for the maintenance of stability. *Note.* From "Adapting Reflexes Controlling the Human Posture" by L.M. Nashner, 1976, *Experimental Brain Research*, **26**, pp. 62, 65, 66. Copyright 1976 by Springer-Verlag, Inc. Adapted by permission.

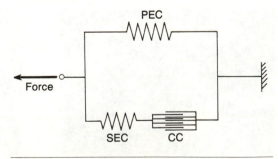

Figure 7.14. A three-component mechanical model of muscle: CC = contractile component, PEC = parallel-elastic component, and SEC = series-elastic component.

scheme, many of the characteristics of muscle can be indicated by three elements: a **parallel-elastic component (PEC)**, a **series-elastic component (SEC)**, and a **contractile component (CC)**. These three elements are intended not to represent specific anatomical structures but to *account for some of the mechanical characteristics of muscle*. The SEC and PEC represent different types of elasticity and are indicated as springs. For example, the length-force relationship of muscle outlined in Figure 6.6 indicates that certain passive structures within muscle (e.g., the sarcolemma of individual fibers and the connective-tissue sheaths of the muscle) will exert a passive force when unstimulated muscle is stretched; the PEC represents this effect. As depicted in Figure 6.6, the contribution of the passive elements (PEC) to total muscle force increases with muscle length, being greatest at the longest muscle lengths. The behavior of active muscle is determined by the characteristics of the CC and the SEC that are connected in series. One consequence of this arrangement in isometric contractions is that, even though whole-muscle length essentially remains constant, CC may shorten significantly while SEC is stretched.

In addition to this elasticity that lies in parallel with the force-exerting sarcomeres, some of the structures that comprise the myofilaments and tendon possess an elasticity that is aligned in series with the force-generating units; this characteristic is identified as the SEC. Within the sarcomere, the thick and thin filaments, crossbridges, and Z bands contribute to the SEC, but the filaments provide the greatest contribution (Blangé, Karemaker, & Kramer, 1972; Suzuki & Sugi, 1983). The SEC, which is only apparent when the muscle is contracting, is much less extensible than the PEC and has a length of about 4%-5% l_o (where l_o refers to the resting length of muscle). The CC represents the force-generating capability of muscle.

The data illustrated in Figure 5.2 indicated, among other observations, that the peak force that a muscle exerts in a twitch response is much less than that exerted in a tetanus. Why does the peak force differ for these two conditions? An explanation can be given with reference to the three-component model (Figure 7.14). The state of activation of the contractile machinery reaches maximum intensity within 4 ms after the action potential and is maintained at maximum for about 30 ms before it begins to decline (Hoyle, 1983). In response to this activation, the CC generates force, but this force is only registered externally by being transmitted through the SEC. That is, since the SEC may be represented as a spring, the slack must be first stretched out of the SEC before it will transmit any force exerted by the CC. The characteristics of the SEC are such that the state of activation of the CC has begun to decline in a twitch (muscle response to a single action potential) before the SEC has been fully stretched. More simplistically, the CC generates a certain quantity of force in response to a single action potential. Some of this force is used to stretch the SEC, and the remainder can be measured externally (Figure 7.14). In contrast, during a tetanus, the SEC becomes fully stretched after the first 5-10 action potentials, and, consequently, all the force exerted by the CC in response to each action potential can be registered externally (Hoyle, 1983).

Storage and Utilization of Elastic Energy

In addition to accounting for the discrepancy in the peak twitch and tetanic forces, the three-component model is also used to explain the phenomenon of the **storage and utilization of elastic energy**. This phenomenon is based on the observation that *a muscle can perform more positive work if it is actively* *stretched* (i.e., stretched while being activated; an eccentric contraction) *before being allowed to shorten* (Cavagna & Citterio, 1974; Fenn, 1924). The result of an eccentric-concentric sequence of muscle activation is that a greater quantity of work is done during the concentric contraction than if the muscle merely experiences a concentric contraction alone. As depicted in Figure 7.15, the positive work done by a muscle from a preceding isometric contraction is less than that done from a preceding eccentric contraction. This is seen in Figure 7.15 by differences in the areas under the force-length graphs for the two conditions. From the work-energy relationship (chapter 3), an increase in the work performed requires an increased expenditure of energy. Where might this additional energy come from? The typical two-part rationale (e.g., Cavagna, 1977) is as follows. First, during the eccentric contraction the load stretches the SEC, which can be envisaged as a transfer of energy from the load to the SEC; this represents the storage of elastic

energy. For example, if an elastic band is held with one end in each hand and then stretched, some of the arm-hand muscle activity involved in stretching the band is stored in the band as elastic energy. And second, once released, the molecular structure of the elastic band will use this stored elastic energy to return to its original shape. Similarly, as the ratio of muscle force to load force changes and the muscle undergoes a concentric contraction, the elastic energy stored in the SEC can be recovered and used to contribute to the shortening contraction (positive work).

This phenomenon can be stated algebraically by using the first law of thermodynamics (chapter 3):

$$W = \Delta H + \Delta C + \Delta E$$

where W = work, H = change in heat or thermal energy, C = change in chemical energy, and E = change in elastic energy. The eccentric-concentric sequence in Figure 7.15 resulted in an increase in the work (W) done during the concentric activity. When muscle is activated, ATP is supplied by a variety of metabolic processes as the essential unit of chemical energy (C). In both the generation and the use of the ATP, some of the energy is degraded as heat (H). From the above equation, if both the chemical energy used and the heat given off remain constant (let E = 0 for now), then the amount of work done will remain the same. But the point of Figure 7.15 was that the work done increased with an eccentric-concentric sequence. One explanation for this is that either C or H changed. The explanation based on the phenomenon of the storage and utilization of elastic energy, however, is that *additional energy (E) beyond that provided by chemical means is made available for the performance of work*. According to this point of view, C and H may vary a little between the concentric and eccentric-concentric modes, but most of

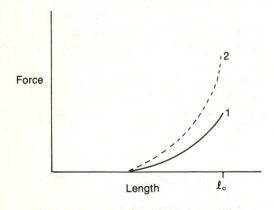

Figure 7.15. The positive work performed during a concentric contraction from a preceding isometric contraction (solid line) compared to that done from a preceding eccentric contraction (dashed line). The work done is represented as the area under the force-length curve.

the extra work can be done because of the elastic-energy contribution.

This ability to use stored elastic energy is affected by three variables: time, magnitude of stretch, and velocity of stretch. Cavagna (1977) has demonstrated that there should be no time delay between the eccentric and concentric contractions; otherwise, some of the stored elastic energy would be lost. Presumably this will occur due to detachment and reattachment of crossbridges during the delay such that, following reattachment, the myofilaments will be under less stretch. In a similar vein, if the magnitude of the lengthening contraction is too great, a lesser number of crossbridges will remain attached following the stretch, and hence less elastic energy will be stored (Edman, Elzinga, & Noble, 1978). Provided the crossbridges remain attached, however, the greater the velocity of stretch, the greater the storage of elastic energy (e.g., Rack & Westbury, 1974).

Despite the widespread use of the phenomenon of the storage and utilization of elastic energy to account for the increased positive work associated with eccentric-concentric contractions, it seems reasonable to suppose that the enhanced positive work might be due to a substantial increase in the amount of available chemical energy. *Perhaps one consequence of an eccentric-concentric sequence is a marked increase in the chemical energy (C) so that now more work can be done* (Jarić, Gavrilović, & Ivančević, 1985). This possibility is called the **preload effect**. For example, in an eccentric-concentric sequence, the force at the beginning of the concentric phase is much greater, due to the preceding eccentric activity, than the initial force had only a concentric contraction been performed (compare Point 2 and Point 1 in Figure 7.15). In other words, the muscle has been preloaded so that the initial force is greater than that needed to maintain posture. This preload effect is similar to what Hochmuth (1968)

called the principle of initial force. In an elaboration of biomechanical principles that dictate the success of a performance, Hochmuth reported that the height an individual could jump varied with the ratio of the braking phase to the propulsion phase of the vertical component of the ground reaction force. (Figure 7.16; analagous to the horizontal braking and propulsion impulses in running, Figure 2.12). The main effect of the interplay between the braking and propulsion phases was interpreted as varying the initial force at the beginning of the propulsion phase.

An estimate of the relative contributions of the elastic-energy and preload effects can be obtained by considering the height that subjects can jump using two types of vertical-jump techniques (Komi & Bosco, 1978). The *squat jump* refers to a vertical jump that is begun from a squat position (knee angle about 2 rad) and simply involves an extension of the knee and ankle joints; the arms are kept stretched overhead to minimize their contribution to the jump. The *countermovement jump* begins from an upright posture and involves, in one continuous movement, squatting down to a knee angle of about 2 rad and then extending the knee and ankle joints as in the squat jump. The major difference between these two techniques is the manner in which the powerful knee extensors are used (they perform about 50% of the work during a maximum vertical jump; Hubley & Wells, 1983); namely, the squat jump involves only a concentric contraction of the knee extensors, whereas a countermovement jump requires an eccentric-concentric sequence.

An example of the vertical component of the ground reaction force and the associated kinematics for a countermovement jump is provided in Figure 7.16 (Miller, 1976). The subject begins from an upright position by lowering the center of gravity by approximately 0.2 m before changing direction (velocity goes from negative to positive values) and moving upward toward the takeoff position. Takeoff is indicated as the time at which the vertical component of the ground reaction forces falls to zero (time = 0.53 s).

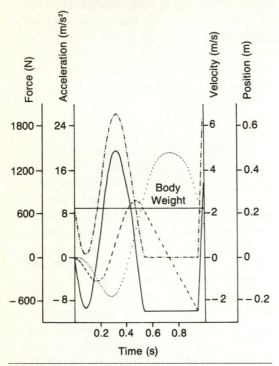

Figure 7.16. The vertical components of the kinematics and kinetics associated with a vertical jump. The position (dotted line), velocity (dashed line), and acceleration (solid line) graphs are for the center of gravity of the jumper. The vertical component of the ground reaction force is indicated with a dash-dot line. The countermovement activities include a downward-upward movement and take about 0.53 s. The subject is in the air (ground reaction force = 0) for about 0.41 s during which time the center of gravity is raised 0.49 m above the starting position. *Note.* From ''A Biomechanical Analysis of the Contribution of the Trunk to Standing Vertical Jump Takeoffs'' by D.I. Miller, 1976, in J. Broekhoff (Ed.), *Physical Education, Sports and the Sciences* (p. 357), Eugene, OR: Microform Publications. Copyright 1976 by Microform Publications. Adapted by permission.

The peak downward velocity (acceleration = 0) occurs about midway during the downward movement (time = 0.19 s), and the peak upward velocity (positive values; acceleration = 0) occurs just prior to takeoff. During the flight phase of the jump, the ground reaction force is zero and the vertical component of acceleration has a value of 9.81 m/s² (i.e., the effect of gravity at the jumper's center of gravity). As noted previously in the context of Newton's law of acceleration, the ground reaction force and the acceleration graphs parallel each other. Finally, consideration of the ground reaction force record relative to the value for body weight indicates Hochmuth's braking and propulsion phases. Initially, the ground reaction force is less than body weight, and this represents the braking phase. The braking impulse can be measured as the area between the ground reaction force and the body-weight lines. Similarly, the propulsive phase refers to the subsequent period when the ground reaction force is greater than body weight; the propulsion impulse refers to the indicated area. Of course, for the subject to perform a vertical jump the propulsion impulse must be greater than the braking impulse.

In contrast to the countermovement jump (Figure 7.16), the squat jump does not include an initial braking impulse. For both types of vertical jump, the net activity of the knee extensors is reflected in the vertical component of the ground reaction force; *the squat jump comprises a concentric contraction and only a propulsion impulse, whereas the countermovement jump includes a net eccentric-concentric sequence of activity and a braking-propulsion sequence in the ground reaction force.*

In addition to this braking-propulsion difference, performing these jumps on either one or two legs will alter the initial magnitude of the knee extensor concentric contractions—that is, *one-legged jumps will generate a preload effect.* This point is illustrated conceptually in Figure 7.17, which shows the torque-angle relationship for two squat jumps. The torque represents the resultant muscle torque about the knee joint for a single leg. The two jumps shown are one-legged (dashed line) and two-legged (solid line) squat jumps, during which the knee angle changes from approximately 2.0 rad through to complete extension at takeoff. The major point of Figure 7.17 is that the initial torque in the one-legged jump is about twice that for the two-legged jump. This is because, in the one-legged jump, the single leg must support the whole body weight, whereas, in the two-legged jump, a single leg need only support one-half of that weight. Because of this difference, the initial load supported by the single leg is much greater in the one-legged jump, and hence we say the limb (particularly the muscles about the knee joint) has been preloaded.

A comparison of the height reached in these different jumps (Table 7.1) was used to examine the contribution of the two effects (preload storage and utilization of elastic energy). *Where does the energy come from (chemical or elastic) for the greater work done in countermovement jumps?* A one- versus two-legged comparison gets at the issue of preload (chemical energy), whereas differences between squat and countermovement jumps include both effects (chemical and elastic). The differences in height jumped with these four combinations illustrate three features of muscle use. First, for both the one- and two-legged jumps, the subjects reached a greater height with the countermovement jump than with the squat jump, supporting the superiority of the eccentric-concentric sequence over the single concentric contraction. Second, the heights attained with the two-legged jumps were greater than those attained with the one-legged jumps due to the greater muscle mass available (and hence chemical energy) to the former. Third, the height jumped in the two-legged situations, however, was not twice that jumped in the one-legged jumps despite the fact that twice the leg mass is available. That is, in the two-legged squat jump the subjects jumped, on average, 10.3 cm higher than in the one-legged squat jump. If the difference between

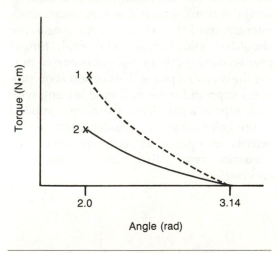

Figure 7.17. Idealized resultant muscle torque-angle relationship about one knee joint during one-legged (dashed line) and two-legged (solid line) squat jumps.

Table 7.1 The Vertical Heights Attained With One- and Two-Legged Squat and Countermovement Jumps

	Squat	Countermovement
One-legged	22.1 ± 5.9[a]	24.0 ± 6.6
Two-legged	32.4 ± 9.1	36.4 ± 8.5

[a]The values are mean ± SD in centimeters for 44 subjects.

the two jumps were simply the quantity of muscle mass involved (chemical energy), then we would expect the subjects to have jumped 16.2 cm (1/2 of 32.4 cm) in the one-legged jump. However, because the height reached in the one-legged jump was greater than what we expected, then the difference must be due to some feature of muscle performance, that is, preload for the squat jump and preload plus elastic energy for the countermovement jump. It appears, therefore, that both energy sources (storage and utilization of elastic energy and preload) account for the enhancement of positive work in the eccentric-concentric sequence. Somewhat similar reservations about the elastic-energy mechanism have been expressed by van Ingen Schenau (1984).

Many human movements have evolved to capitalize on this eccentric-concentric phenomenon. For example, the normal mode of performing the vertical jump (e.g., in basketball and volleyball) is the countermovement style, which, as demonstrated above, maximizes the height that can be reached. This eccentric-concentric pattern of muscle activation is also readily apparent in many other activities, such as kicking (Figure 7.6). Similarly, during running, when the foot is first placed on the ground, the knee flexes and then extends (Figure 1.8) as the total-body center of gravity passes over the foot. This pattern of knee flexion-extension is accomplished by an eccentric-concentric sequence of knee extensor activity. However, it appears that this mode of activity does not always enhance the ensuing positive work;

Cavagna (1977) has estimated that the elastic energy recovered in running makes significant contributions to the power generated by the muscles only at running speeds greater than about 6.5 $m \cdot s^{-1}$. The same type of observation has been made for the takeoff in the long and triple jumps (Luhtanen & Komi, 1980).

As a final example, consider the experimental situation in which a barbell is suspended from the ceiling so that it is horizontal and located at shoulder height. The subject is asked to position himself under the barbell so that it touches his shoulders, but not to support its weight, and to grasp the ends of the barbell, one with each hand. Once in this position, the subject is given a signal to rotate the barbell in the horizontal plane by approximately 1.57 rad as rapidly as possible. How might the subject accomplish this task? Grieve (1969) performed this experiment and found that subjects first rotated the hips in the desired direction while the shoulders and barbell were briefly rotated in the opposite direction. This action had the effect of actively stretching (eccentric contraction) the trunk muscles, which were subsequently used concentrically to rotate the shoulders and barbell. The peak torque exerted during this movement occurred during the eccentric phase. This observation provides support for the notion of leading with your hips in a golf drive; the torque applied to the golf club will be greater if the muscle activity comprises an eccentric-concentric sequence rather than just a concentric contraction.

Problems

7.1.   The central command is issued from which nervous-system structure?
    a. Motor cortex
    b. Limbic system

c. Cerebellum

d. Basal ganglia

e. Brain stem

7.2. The term *degrees of freedom* refers to

a. the motor control strategy.

b. one of Roberts' modes of motor control.

c. the type of feedback control used during a movement.

d. the number of movements that a joint permits.

e. the number of joints over which a muscle exerts an effect.

7.3. The resultant muscle torque is calculated as the residual moment. What does this mean?

7.4. Which of the following statements (a-e) about the bone-on-bone force are correct? Both parts (i-v) of each statement need to be correct.

    i. It is greater than the joint reaction force.

    ii. It is not affected by cocontraction.

    iii. It will not be different for static and dynamic conditions.

    iv. It can be calculated if all the muscle forces crossing the joint are known.

    v. It is not usually close to the value that causes bone failure due to compression.

a. iii, v

b. i, iv

c. ii, v

d. iii, i

e. v, iv

7.5. An individual (body weight = 586 N) performs an exercise that involves raising and lowering the straight legs between Positions 1 and 2.

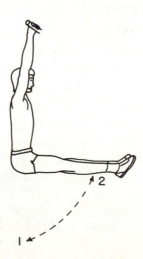

a. Suppose you wanted to determine the torque exerted by the muscles at the hip joint during this exercise. Draw and label the appropriate free-body diagram.
b. Describe the pattern of net muscle activity (hip flexors and extensors) during one complete slow repetition (raise and lower legs) of this exercise.
c. Given the following dimensions:

leg length (hip joint to ankle) = 72 cm
weight of both legs   = 30% of body weight
CG location (hip to ankle)   = 43.4% of leg length from the hip

calculate the resultant muscle torque required for the individual to *maintain* the legs in Position 2 (the legs are horizontal).

7.6.   An athlete recovering from knee surgery performs a slow knee extension exercise with a light load.

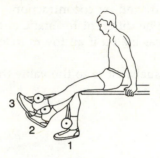

a. Identify the net pattern of muscle activity for one *slow* repetition of the exercise.

	1 →2	2 →3	3 → 2	2 → 1
Knee extensors				
Knee flexors				

C = concentric, E = eccentric

b. If the limb were held stationary at Positions 1, 2, then 3, which of the positions would require the

greatest torque to maintain? _____

least torque to maintain? _____

c. Calculate the resultant muscle torque about the knee joint that the athlete must exert to hold the leg in Position 3. In this position, the leg is 0.21 rad below the horizontal. The following system dimensions apply:

body weight   = 758 N
leg length (knee to ankle) = 42 cm
load   = 172 N

load acts perpendicular to the leg, 37 cm from the knee
limb (leg + foot) CG   = 41.3% of leg length from the knee
limb (leg + foot) weight = 0.045 BW − 1.75 (BW = body weight)

Draw a free-body diagram before you attempt to solve the problem.

7.7.   The performance of a particular movement is associated with the following hip joint velocity-time relationship:

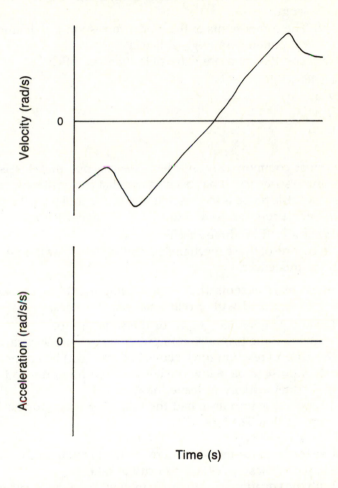

a. From the velocity-time graph, derive the acceleration-time graph as we did earlier (Figure 1.3).
b. Since acceleration is proportional to force (Newton's law of acceleration), the acceleration-time graph will also represent the profile of the resultant muscle torque about the hip joint. Assume that positive velocity indicates extension and positive acceleration (torque) represents a net flexor torque; deduce the pattern of net muscle activity associated with the movement.

7.8. Which of the following statements (a-e) about the three-component model of muscle are incorrect? Only one part (i-v) of a-e has to be wrong for the statement to be incorrect.

    i.   PEC stands for passive-elastic component.

    ii. The model can be used to account for the differences in twitch and tetanic forces.

    iii. In an isometric condition, neither the CC nor the SEC change length.

    iv. The components of the model correspond to distinct morphological parameters (e.g., Z band).

    v. The PEC is more extensible than the SEC.

a. iv, iii

b. v, i

c. i, iv

d. iii, ii

e. ii, v

7.9. The most common way in which we use our muscles is an eccentric-concentric sequence. It has been shown that the positive work done during the concentric phase is increased under such conditions. Three mechanisms have been proposed to account for this phenomenon.

a. What are these three mechanisms?

b. Select one of these mechanisms and explain how it is supposed to produce this effect.

7.10. Figure 7.16 represents the vertical components of the kinematics and kinetics associated with a *countermovement* vertical jump.

a. Draw a comparable graph for the squat jump.

b. Why must the propulsion impulse (area of the vertical component of the ground reaction force above body weight) be larger than the braking impulse (area below the body weight line prior to takeoff) for the individual actually to leave the ground?

c. Suppose the impulses had the following magnitudes:
    propulsion 320 N•s
    braking 82 N•s
Use the impulse-momentum relationship (chapter 3) to determine the jumper's (mass = 64 kg) velocity at takeoff.

d. With the equations for projectile motion (chapter 1), calculate the height of the jump.

7.11. When the torque exerted by an active muscle does not equal the load torque, the length of the muscle changes. Which of the following statements about this relationship are incorrect?

a. Maximum eccentric torque is greater than concentric torque.

b. A muscle becomes less efficient as the speed of a concentric contraction increases.

    c. Maximum power occurs when the force being exerted is about one-third of the maximum isometric force.

    d. Changes in muscle temperature do not affect twitch contraction time or one-half relaxation time.

    e. When a cyclist goes uphill, a component of the weight vector opposes the forward driving force.

7.12. On several occasions throughout the text, we have considered the kinematics and kinetics of a simple elbow extension-flexion movement in the horizontal plane (e.g., Figures 1.5, 3.11, and 7.8).

    a. Describe the net muscle-activation patterns associated with the four phases of the power-time profile.

    b. How would these muscle-activity patterns vary if the movement was done as a flexion-extension task?

    c. Would the muscle-activity patterns change if the extension-flexion movement was done in a vertical plane?

    d. The third phase of the movement represents a power-production phase. Where does the energy come from to produce this power?

CHAPTER

8

Performance Evaluation

Throughout the course of this text, which has focused on the study of movement, we have had to make a number of simplifying assumptions to begin to understand some of the more fundamental features of movement. One of these assumptions has led to the development of a simple joint system. We have used this five-element biological model primarily to examine the way in which the nervous system controls the activity of muscle. As an extension of this approach, our task now is to consider how we might evaluate the state or condition of the simple joint system. Can we identify features of the simple joint system that correlate highly with success in performance? If indeed the simple joint system is a useful model for the study of movement, then it should be possible to use the model to indicate measurements that could be made on an individual to estimate the level of performance for a particular activity.

It should be readily apparent that there are many measurements that could be made as an assessment of an individual's (or a simple joint system's) condition. Several of these measurements would be related to one another in that they would measure either the same or a related feature of the simple joint system. To minimize the effort involved

in such an evaluation, *it is desirable to use only measurements that indicate distinct features*. For example, the SI units of measurement (Appendix A) are separated into two categories: base and derived units. The base units represent the unrelated measurements, whereas the derived units are related to the base units. In a similar manner, this chapter considers the base units of performance for the simple joint system. This is not to suggest that other related (derived) measurements are not useful (e.g., force is derived from mass yet we have made considerable use of the concept of force throughout this text). The idea here is that, if we can identify all the base units of performance, then by various combinations of these and other derived units we should be able to come up with appropriate estimates of performance for different movements. For example, the combination of measurements necessary to evaluate performance in power lifting will certainly be different than that necessary for sprint events.

The focus of this section, however, is to identify not the many base and derived units that might be used in such an evaluation, but the base units of performance. In addition, this section comments on their status in the research literature. The task of elaborating the derived units and the combinations necessary for the evaluation of different activities will be left to others (e.g., Harre, 1982). In this vein, *the base units considered here are strength, power, and fatigue.* Our focus is twofold: (a) What do we know about these measures? (b) What functional features of the simple joint system do these measures represent? Before we proceed with a consideration of these issues, however, it is necessary to digress momentarily and set the scene by considering the principles of training and a model that is useful in the discussion of the neural control of movement.

Principles of Training

Substantial effort, though largely inconclusive, has focused on the study of muscle strength. One outcome of these efforts has been the elaboration of several rules for the prescription of exercise. These rules are often referred to as the principles of training. One such rule is the **overload** principle, which may be stated as follows:

> *To increase the size or functional ability of muscle fibers they must be taxed toward their present capacity to respond.*

This principle implies that *there is a threshold point that must be exceeded before an adaptive response will occur.* Normally the threshold point is expressed as a percentage of maximum. For example, it has been suggested that the threshold for isometric exercises is about 40% of maximum; that is, adaptations will occur only if the force exceeds 40% of maximum. Since the maximum torque that a muscle can exert changes with time due to variations in the level of activity (i.e., training and detraining), so too the absolute load that will exceed threshold changes. This is readily apparent in individuals who train regularly and then experience a period of in-

activity (e.g., having a limb in a cast, being confined to bed for an illness), only to find that they cannot resume training at their pre-inactivity level.

In addition to manipulating the training load relative to maximum capabilities, exercise prescription must match the mode of training to the desired effect. This concern is embodied in the principle of **specificity** (McCafferty & Horvath, 1977):

> *Training adaptations are specific to the cells and their structural and functional elements that are overloaded.*

In other words, *exercise stress is selective in the kind of change it induces.* If an individual constructs a training program that stresses the power-production capability of muscle, then only this characteristic and not others (e.g., endurance) will exhibit an adaptation. Sale and MacDougall (1981) report that adaptations associated with strength training are specific to the movement and the velocity used in training. Similarly, recall that, according to the size principle, motor units are recruited in the order S-FR-FF. When discussing this phenomenon, we posed the question as to why the Type S motor units, although recruited, may not demonstrate any adaptations as a consequence of high-load training. The appropriate answer is based on the specificity principle: Although the Type S motor units are active, none of their features (i.e., low-force, fatigue-resistant) are stressed in this type of training (McDonagh & Davies, 1984).

Finally, the **reversibility** principle formalizes an aspect of exercise-induced adaptation that was mentioned previously:

> *Training effects are transient.*

The change in the functional and structural status of a muscle depends upon the continued use of the overload and specificity principles (Thorstensson, 1977). Once an individual begins a training program, the maximum ability of the muscle(s) will increase as training continues. If the training load is not changed, the load as a percentage of maximum will decrease. Eventually the load will decline to below threshold, and, because this will violate the overload principle, no further adaptations will occur. Rather, the effect of the training program will be to maintain the gains acquired while the load was above threshold. In other words, the stimulus for continued adaptation has been removed. Once the individual became frustrated with the lack of adaptation and stopped training, the increases in function would begin to disappear as the muscle(s) adapted to the new (reduced) demands of usage.

Tripartite Model

The nervous system contains millions of neurons. These cells communicate with one another and with target cells by two means: local-graded potentials and action potentials. We have previously encountered the notion that neural circuits are generally complicated (chapter 5, "Feedback From Proprioceptors") and that input-output relationships are rather complex processes. Fortunately, however, we can reduce this array of complex interactions to a simple, three-component model. This **tripartite model** was largely developed from research on locomotion (Wetzel & Stuart, 1977). The model assumes that the neuromuscular processes associated with movement (e.g., Figure 7.1) belong to one of three compartments (Feldman & Grillner, 1983; Hasan et al., 1985). These compartments represent general functions that the nervous system performs during movement (Figure 8.1).

In terms of performance, the critical element of this model is the interaction between

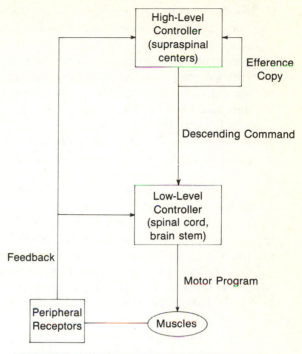

Figure 8.1. A tripartite model for the neural control of movement. *Note.* From "The Interface Between Biomechanics and Neurophysiology in the Study of Movement: Some Recent Approaches" by Z. Hasan et al., 1985, in R.L. Terjung (Ed.), *Exercise and Sport Sciences Reviews*, **13** (p. 175), New York: Macmillan. Copyright 1985 by the American College of Sports Medicine. Reprinted by permission.

the **low-level controller** and the muscles. For different movements, the nervous system activates the appropriate muscles in different sequences. According to Roberts (1976), the nervous system uses six basic modes or strategies of activation: set, hold, drive, punch, catch, and throw. The set of commands sent out by the low-level controller for a particular motor-control strategy (sequence of muscle activity) is known as a **motor program**. The neural circuitry responsible for the motor program comprises collections of motoneurons and interneurons and is located in the low-level controller, which may (depending upon the task) correspond anatomically to the spinal cord and brain stem. The low-level controller is an extremely capable component; for example, the basic features of muscle activation necessary for locomotion are generated not by the brain, but by the low-level controller.

The low-level controller does have surprising capabilities, but it cannot function alone and needs the other two components to provide an on-off switch and an adaptability to a variable environment. The low-level controller is activated and sustained by descending commands (central command) from the high-level controller (supraspinal centers). The central command from the **high-level controller** serves to activate a motor program in the low-level controller. Afferent feedback from **peripheral receptors** (e.g., muscle spindle, tendon organ), can modify the output from both the high- and low-level controllers to adapt to changing conditions.

One additional feature of the tripartite model deserves emphasis. The high-level controller actually represents a complex interaction among many different supraspinal structures (Figure 7.1). A copy of the central command, which represents the output of these interactions, is led back to the high-level controller so that the various structures are made aware of the final output. This copy is referred to as the **efference copy**. It appears that the supraspinal structures determine the effort involved in a particular activity on the basis of this efference copy. Our monitoring of the efference copy for this purpose is known as the **sense of effort**.

As an example of the utility of this tripartite model, let us reconsider the topic of reflexes. In chapter 5, we considered the traditional notion that a reflex is an input-output relationship. The input is provided by some sensory mechanism (e.g., muscle spindle, tendon organ), and the output occurs over the final common pathway, the alpha motoneuron. Between the input and output stages, however, there exist many interneurons (Figure 5.15). Any change in the level of excitation of the interneurons will readily affect the coupling between the input and output stages of a reflex. As shown in Figure 5.15C, many interneurons are under the direct influence of the high-level controller. Consequently, as the output from the high-level controller changes during an activity, the input-output coupling associated with a reflex may also change. It is not surprising, therefore, that we describe reflexes as phase- and state-dependent responses. This simply means that the response depends on the state of excitation within the low-level controller.

Strength

Throughout this text we have adopted the focus that movement occurs due to the interaction between the force exerted by muscle and its external environment. To explore this concept, we defined a biological model, the simple joint system, which enabled us to consider five basic elements involved in the development of muscle force. To characterize the function of this simple joint system, we are interested in measuring its output—muscle force or torque. The measures we call strength and power are used to assess different featues of this output.

As a basis for distinguishing between strength and power, let us return to the force-velocity relationship of muscle. We noted in chapter 6 that the concentric component of the force-velocity characteristic could be represented by the relationship shown in Figure 8.2. Qualitatively, the relationship comprises three distinct regions: (a) when velocity = 0 (isometric or P_o), (b) when force =

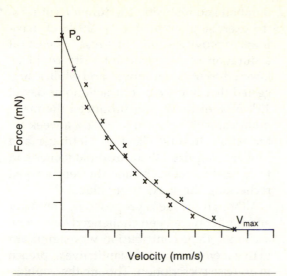

Figure 8.2. The force-velocity relationship of muscle.

0 (v_{max}), and (c) when neither force nor velocity is zero. Region Number 2 (force = 0) never exists for the simple joint system because the muscle always shortens against a load (force), even if it is only the weight of the rigid link to which it is attached. Functionally, therefore, this force-velocity domain of the simple joint system reduces to two distinct regions, one in which velocity is zero and another in which it is not. This distinction forms the basis for the two measures known as strength and power.

Muscle **strength** is defined as *the magnitude of the torque exerted by a muscle (or muscles) in a single maximal isometric contraction of unrestricted duration* (Atha, 1981). However, recall that the measurement of muscle torque does not represent any single intrinsic property of muscle but rather is the consequence of neural (motor-unit recruitment and rate coding), mechanical (moment arm), and muscular (length and cross-sectional area) simple joint system interactions (Howard, Ritchie, Gater, Gater, & Enoka, 1985). Con-

sequently, it is best to think of strength as a complex rather than a simple parameter. By this definition there is only one type of muscle strength—that measured under isometric conditions. Therefore it becomes inappropriate to talk of such things as isotonic or dynamic strength, isokinetic strength, or static strength. Traditionally, people interested in human performance have used the term *static strength* to refer to P_o in Figure 8.2 and *dynamic strength* for measures of torque when velocity was nonzero. This terminology is cumbersome and, to a large extent, responsible for much of the confusion that exists in the strength-training literature. We shall use a narrow definition of strength, one confined to the measure of peak torque under isometric conditions. We shall characterize the nonzero-velocity region by the measure of power.

Strength is defined by the torque rather than the force exerted by the simple joint system for purely pragmatic reasons: It is much easier to measure the torque in human subjects. The measurement of force would involve either the attachment of a force transducer to the muscle tendon or a means of converting the myoelectric activity (EMG) into a measure of force. Neither of these procedures is simple, hence, the choice of torque.

We shall address three issues related to strength: (a) The training techniques often used, (b) the ways in which the load can be made to vary during training, and (c) the adaptations that occur within the simple joint system as a result of strength training.

Training Techniques

According to the crossbridge theory of muscle contraction, once Ca^{++} has inhibited the inhibitory effect of the troponin-tropomyosin complex, myosin crossbridges attach to binding sites on actin and then undergo a conformational change that results in the generation of force. Despite this single-mechanism account of muscle activation, the strength-training literature is largely organized around the different types of muscle contractions. Rather, it seems more appropriate in a discussion of strength training to emphasize variations in the load-muscle torque relationship. For example, the terms isometric, concentric, and eccentric, though typically referred to as different types of contractions, have been used in this text to distinguish between ratios of the muscle torque relative to the load torque (Figure 6.8). Such a focus is employed here in considering the effectiveness of strength-training techniques for achieving increases in muscle strength and work.

Isometric. An **isometric** (*iso* = constant, *metric* = measure of whole-muscle length) contraction was previously defined as a condition in which the torque due to the load is matched by a torque of equal magnitude but opposite direction exerted by the muscle; as a consequence, there is no change in whole-muscle length. In the 1950s, Hettinger and Muller (e.g., Hettinger, 1961) popularized isometric exercises as a fitness activity. This mode of training gained in popularity because these exercises supposedly produced good hypertrophic responses, took little time, and were convenient and economical. The Hettinger and Muller scheme was characterized by *consideration of threshold points, intensity levels, and the systematization of an exercise program.* For example, it was suggested for the elbow flexors that daily exercises at 40%-50% of maximum would produce strength gains, intensity levels of 20%-30% of maximum would maintain the status quo, and less than 20% of maximum would result in a loss of strength. The isometric scheme also proposed a trade-off between exercise duration and intensity; for durations of 1-2 s, the exercise must be done at 100% of maximum to provide sufficient stress, whereas at a duration of 4-6 s the intensity could be lowered to 66%. Hettinger and Muller suggested that one 4-6 s contraction per day at 40%-50% of maximum produced the maximum gains in strength (e.g., 2% a week for the elbow flexors). Finally, Hettinger and Muller recognized that threshold values had to be reset periodically, and they encouraged rechecking the maximum value.

Although the ideas proposed by Hettinger and Muller have been challenged on several accounts, their contribution was significant in that it emphasized a quantitative approach to exercise prescription. Though the popularity of isometric exercises has subsided in recent years, such exercises are still advocated as part of a strength-training program. The East Germans (Harre, 1982), for example, advise that isometric exercises be used as follows: (a) for untrained or trained individuals, daily workouts of 5-8 repetitions per muscle group in which the active muscles exert a force of 40%-50% of maximum; and (b) for elite athletes, performance of exercises at several joint angles with forces of 80%-100% of maximum, each exercise lasting 5-10 s, and 2-5 repetitions per muscle group with 30 s to several minutes between repetitions.

There are, however, at least two major concerns associated with isometric exercises. First, since movements are dominated by concentric and eccentric muscle activity in which muscle length changes, isometric exercises may not be specific to the training goals of the program, a violation of the specificity principle (Lindh, 1979). Second, when the force that a muscle exerts exceeds approximately 64% of maximum, blood vessels are occluded and peripheral resistance to blood flow increases substantially (Barnes, 1980). The net effect of this occlusion is an increase in heart rate and blood pressure (Seals,

Washburn, Hanson, Painter, & Nagle, 1983), a dangerous consequence for some individuals. However, since strength is defined as the torque exerted in a maximal isometric contraction, the most appropriate way to increase strength per se is probably by isometric exercises (due to the principle of specificity, e.g., Kanehisa & Miyashita, 1983). Currently, *the most effective isometric-training regime appears to involve maximal contractions in which the product of contraction duration and number of repetitions is large*, for example, 30 contractions of 3-5 s each per day (McDonagh & Davies, 1984). This protocol may produce maximum gains in isometric strength of 1% per day.

Dynamic. The alternative to the activation condition in which the muscle and load torques are equal (isometric) is the situation in which they are not equal (anisometric). In these circumstances, the muscle activity is often referred to as **dynamic** due to the changes that occur in muscle length because the system (e.g., simple joint system) is not in equilibrium. In contrast, an isometric contraction may be described as a **static** contraction because the system is in equilibrium; that is, the muscle and load torques balance each other. This notion of system equilibrium, of course, stems from our consideration of Newton's laws of motion (chapter 2). However, the term *static* refers to not only isometric conditions but also conditions (e.g., isokinetic) in which the motion of the system remains constant. By definition, isokinetic means constant speed, and under such circumstances a system is described as being in equilibrium because all the forces acting on the system are balanced; that is, $\Sigma F = 0$ for an isokinetic contraction because acceleration is equal to zero. Despite this confusion, the term *dynamic* is typically used to refer to concentric and eccentric contractions.

In the modern era of strength training,

DeLorme (1945) was perhaps the first to use dynamic exercises systematically. The DeLorme technique, which is known as *progressive-resistance exercises*, involves performing three sets of 10 repetitions in which the load is increased for each set. The maximum load is determined by trial and error; the individual experiments with different loads until the load that can be lifted exactly 10x, not 9x or 11x, is known. This load is identified as the 10-RM (RM = repetition maximum) load. The first set of 10 repetitions is done with one-half the 10-RM load, the second set with three-quarters of the 10-RM load, and the final set with the full 10-RM load. The rationale behind this approach is that the first two sets serve as a warm-up for the maximum effort of the third set. During the same time period, the reverse approach was proposed as the basis for the Oxford technique (Zinovieff, 1951), the rationale being that the second (75% 10-RM) and third (50% 10-RM) sets loaded the muscle(s) during fatigue. The Oxford technique suggested that all motor units are activated during the maximum effort (first set) and maximally stressed during the subsequent (second and third) sets due to the effects of fatigue requiring a maximum effort with the lesser loads. This distinction between the DeLorme and the Oxford techniques has been referred to as *ascending- and descending-pyramid loading*, respectively (McDonagh & Davies, 1984).

Since dynamic exercises include both concentric and eccentric muscle activity, it is misleading to suggest that a 10-RM load represents the maximum that can be handled for all phases of each repetition. From the torque-velocity relationship (Figure 6.10), it is apparent that the torque a muscle can exert is greater for an eccentric contraction than for a concentric one. Consequently, in a movement involving alternating concentric-eccentric sequences, it is the concentric component that limits performance, and thus it is the element to which the 10-RM specification refers. In addition, since the amount of exercise stress depends on the magnitude of the load relative to maximum capabilities (overload principle), it is probably the concentric component of a concentric-eccentric sequence that experiences the greater stress and subsequent adaptation.

A popular idea is that, because a greater muscle force can be exerted during an eccentric contraction, such exercises should produce a more intense training stimulus and hence greater strength gains. As stated in the overload principle, however, it is *not the absolute force that determines the quantity of the stimulus but rather the size of the force relative to maximum.* Indeed, the training literature is inconclusive on the relative merits of concentric versus eccentric exercises. Some studies (Johnson, Adamczyk, Tennøe, & Strømme, 1976) report strength gains and enhanced work capabilities that are indistinguishable between the two techniques, whereas others (Komi & Buskirk, 1972) suggest a superiority of eccentric training over concentric and isometric training. However, one point of confusion in the comparison of training effects has been the indiscriminate reference to strength. The rigorous definition of strength used here implies that it can be measured only in an isometric contraction, and hence the assessment of muscle function in concentric or eccentric contractions should be referred to as the capability of muscle to do work and not as its strength. That is, given the definition of strength as the maximum isometric torque, the *correct* way to evaluate the effects of concentric and eccentric training programs on strength is to measure changes in the maximum isometric torque.

The lack of consensus on the effects of concentric versus eccentric exercises serves to illustrate the general state of confusion that exists in the research literature on strength. There are a host of factors that will affect the outcome of a strength-training program; these include such variables as the duration of the training program, the initial state (strength) of the subjects, the type(s) of exercise used, the loading technique, and so on. Failure by investigators to standardize all of these variables complicates the interpretation of the results. For example, Häkkinen (1985) has demonstrated that the effects due to the mode of training (concentric, eccentric, isometric) depend on the length of the training program (Figure 8.3). Häkkinen trained three

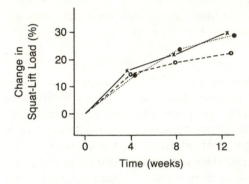

Figure 8.3. Percentage change in maximum performance in the squat lift for three groups of subjects after a 12-week training program with different modes of activity. The concentric group (n = 9; dashed line) used only concentric exercises, the concentric-eccentric group (n = 9; solid line) used 50% concentric and 50% eccentric exercises, and the eccentric-concentric group (n = 9; dotted line) used 75% eccentric and 25% concentric exercises. Loading for the concentric exercises varied progressively from 80% to 100% of the concentric maximum and for the eccentric exercises 100% to 130% of the concentric maximum. *Note.* From "Research Overview: Factors Influencing Trainability of Muscular Strength During Short Term and Prolonged Training" by K. Häkkinen, 1985. Copyright 1985 by the National Strength & Conditioning Association. Adapted by permission, *National Strength and Conditioning Association Journal, 7*(2), 32-37.

groups of subjects: (a) a concentric group used only concentric exercises, (b) a concentric-eccentric group used 50% concentric exercises and 50% eccentric exercises, and (c) an eccentric-concentric group used 75% eccentric and 25% concentric exercises. The effects of the training programs were evaluated by the maximum load each subject could lift in a squat lift. After 8 weeks of training there were no differences among the groups in the increase in squat load (Figure 8.3). At 12 weeks, however, performance was best in those subjects who used a program that combined concentric and eccentric activity.

In addition to the effect of the duration of a training program, the results of a training program are substantially affected by the state of the individual prior to the program. Figure 8.4 illustrates this point by showing the change in performance (squat lift) of two groups of subjects (strength athletes vs. nonathletes) over the course of a training program. The nonathletes were not novices but actually trained individuals who used weight training as part of their programs, but they did not compete in strength events (power lifting, body building). It is apparent from Figure 8.4 that the stronger (greater squat-lift load) strength athletes experienced a lesser absolute change and rate of change (slope of the graph) in performance than the nonathletes. The power-lifting and body-building athletes were stronger at the beginning of the training program; they could lift greater loads. Largely because of this initial condition and their familiarity with the movement, these strength athletes experienced less of an increase in strength, and also the rate (slope of Figure 8.4) at which they increased strength was much less. The initial rapid increase in strength exhibited by the nonathletes (steep curve in Figure 8.4) is thought to be associated with neural aspects of the adaptation to strength training. These points on training-program duration and the initial

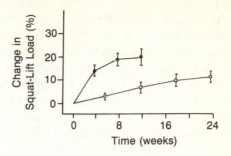

Figure 8.4. Percentage change in maximum performance in the squat lift after a strength-training program. The strength athletes (open circles; power lifters and body builders) had a pretraining maximum squat-lift load of 1,400 N, and the nonathletes (filled circles; conditioned subjects accustomed to weight training) could manage a load of 466 N. Training involved concentric knee extension exercises in which the load varied from 80% to 100% of the concentric maximum. *Note.* From ''Research Overview: Factors Influencing Trainability of Muscular Strength During Short Term and Prolonged Training'' by K. Häkkinen, 1985. Copyright 1985 by the National Strength & Conditioning Association. Adapted by permission, *National Strength and Association Journal,* 7(2), 32-37.

condition of the subjects serve to emphasize that you must take these many factors into consideration when assessing the relative merits of different strength-training programs and equipment. In addition, it is easy to see how researchers might reach different conclusions if they fail to account for these different factors; for example, the effect of training mode is different at 8 weeks than it is at 12 weeks (Figure 8.3).

Accommodation. Exercise machines in which the load is controlled by gear or friction systems (e.g., Cybex) provide an **accommodating** resistance, so named because the device can generate a load equal in magnitude but opposite in direction to the force exerted by the subject. *One consequence of this accommodation (equal but opposite torques) is a movement in which the angular velocity of the displaced body segment is constant*, hence, **isokinetic** for constant speed. An isokinetic contraction, therefore, represents the dynamic condition (because muscle length changes) in which the quotient of muscle torque to load torque is equal to one. A common misconception, however, is that if the muscle and load torques are equal then no movement can occur. Consider a velocity-time graph (Figure 1.2) in which velocity remains constant from one point in time to another (Points 3 and 4 in Figure 1.2). The acceleration is zero for that interval because there is no change in velocity; because force is proportional to acceleration ($\mathbf{F} = m\mathbf{a}$), then there is no *net* force acting on the system. *When the muscle and load torques are equal, the system is either stationary or moving at a constant velocity*, and thus the isokinetic condition can also be described mechanically as static. The advantage of isokinetics is that a muscle group can be stressed differently throughout its range of motion depending upon its capabilities. In rehabilitation settings this accommodation is particularly useful.

Many researchers have used isokinetic devices, particularly the Cybex (Figure 8.5A), to quantify the torque, work, or power output of muscle during activity (Coyle et al., 1981). Typically, this is accomplished by measuring the load provided by the machine ($\mathbf{L}_m$ in Figure 8.5B) and expressing the effort in the selected units. An appropriate free-body diagram of the system (Figure 8.5B), however, indicates that the machine load is not the only factor affecting the load torque; the weight of the limb and the machine lever arm should also be considered. Winter, Wells, and Orr (1981) have demonstrated that neglecting the acceleration components (acceleration due to gravity and the acceleration

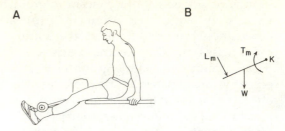

Figure 8.5. A subject performing an isokinetic knee-extension exercise. (A) The Cybex isokinetic dynamometer. (B) A free-body diagram of the forces acting on the lower leg. K = knee joint, $\mathbf{L}_m$ = machine load, $\mathbf{T}_m$ = resultant muscle torque, $\mathbf{W}$ = weight.

of the limb to reach the speed of the machine) can lead to an error of 500% at the highest speeds in determining the amount of work performed by the muscles. However, these acceleration effects can be determined and incorporated into the appropriate calculations to allow more accurate measurements. Without this correction, the torque exerted by the machine (machine load) is not a measure of the resultant muscle torque.

Plyometric. Although isokinetic exercises have proven useful as rehabilitation tools, their applicability as general training techniques is less obvious due to the constraint of a constant limb angular velocity; that is, since few human movements contain phases of constant limb angular velocity, isokinetic exercises violate the specificity principle. In contrast, **plyometrics** has evolved as a training technique in response to the issue of specificity. As was indicated earlier (chapter 7), a majority of human activities involve the condition in which a muscle is first active eccentrically before it contributes concentrically to the task. *Plyometric exercises are designed to stress this eccentric-concentric sequence.*

Recall that such a sequence represents a change in the muscle torque to load torque ratio from less than one to greater than one. The concept of plyometrics, which is also known as depth jumping or rebound training, appears to have originated in Eastern European countries. The exercises involve such activities as starting at the top of a long flight of stairs and jumping down the stairs, one or several at a time (a vertical drop of 50-80 cm), with both feet together.

Although the benefactors of such activity are unknown, they probably include (a) the ability of muscle to *store and utilize elastic energy*, (b) the *preload effect*, and (c) the *stretch reflex*. We have discussed the storage and utilization of elastic energy and the preload phenomena previously in some detail (chapter 7). With regard to the stretch reflex (Figure 5.15A), the idea is that, during the eccentric (lengthening) phase, muscle receptors (e.g., muscle spindle) are activated that, in turn, provide input to homonymous alpha motoneurons that enhances their activity during the subsequent concentric phase. The response known as a stretch reflex (Figure 5.15A) is superimposed on the central command from the high-level controller (Figure 5.15D). However, the relevance of this notion to movement, and this sequence (eccentric-concentric) in particular, remains debatable. Despite this uncertainty regarding the mechanism trained, it is apparent that plyometric exercises do induce a training effect. For example, Blattner and Noble (1979) trained two groups of subjects for 8 weeks, one group on an isokinetic device and the other group with plyometric exercises. The two groups increased their vertical-jump heights by about the same amount (5 cm) as a result of the training. Similarly, Häkkinen, Komi, and Alén (1985) found that jump training caused a minor increase in the maximal knee-extensor isometric force but a substantial increase in the rate of force development and an increase in the area of fast-twitch fibers.

Electromyostimulation. Reports from the Soviet Union in the early 1970s (Elson, 1974) suggested yet another means of strengthening muscle, that of applying electric shocks to the muscle. Such procedures, which are referred to as **electromyostimulation**, involve stimulating the muscle with a complex protocol that is designed to minimize the pain and discomfort associated with this procedure (Moreno-Aranda & Seireg, 1981a, 1981b, 1981c). Electromyostimulation has been used for a number of years in rehabilitation settings (Liberson, Holmquest, Scot, & Dow, 1961), but only recently has been applied to noninjured active athletes. The Soviets reportedly use electromyostimulation with their best athletes in sports where strength is a limiting factor (e.g., weight lifting, wrestling, sprinting, shot put). The intensity of the stimulus is just below the pain threshold, and one muscle is trained per session. The athletes (none younger that 18 years), while tapering their conventional training prior to an important meet, undergo an 18-session stimulation program. The Soviet claims include the following: (a) volleyballers increased vertical-jump height by 10 cm and gymnasts learned an iron cross in 2 weeks, (b) an increase in the number of myofilaments per unit cross-sectional area of muscle (i.e., an increase in the specific tension of muscle), (c) a decrease in subcutaneous fat, and (d) cures for postural abnormalities and sports injuries.

The rationale for electromyostimulation is that individuals are unable to activate a muscle maximally and that electric shocks can stimulate the difference between what an individual can activate and what is available in the muscle. Actually, there is evidence (Belanger & McComas, 1981) that individuals have a greater difficulty fully activating some muscles (e.g., gastrocnemius, soleus) in comparison to others (e.g., tibialis anterior). The extent of the limitation, however, is probably minimal in highly trained individuals. For example, if an individual is asked to exert a maximum knee extensor torque first with the left leg, then with the right leg, and then with both legs together, the sum of the two one-legged torque values is usually greater than that for the two-legged effort (Ohtsuki, 1983; Vandervoort, Sale, & Moroz, 1984). However, for some highly trained athletes such as rowers and weight lifters, there is no difference between the sum of the two one-legged values and the two-legged value (Howard & Enoka, 1987; Secher, 1975). This difference between the two groups of subjects is probably due to differences in the ability of the high-level controller (central command) to activate fully the motor units of a particular muscle group.

Since the application of an artificial electrical stimulus to the muscle bypasses the nervous-system generation of the excitation, another potential advantage of electromyostimulation is that the larger motor units, particularly Type FF, receive a larger training stimulus than they would normally under voluntary conditions.

As with the research on the effects of dynamic training, the evidence for a strength effect with electromyostimulation is mixed. Most investigators (Fahey, Harvey, Schroeder, & Ferguson, 1985; Romero, Sanford, Schroeder, & Fahey, 1982) have demonstrated that electromyostimulation can induce increases in strength. Furthermore, Laughman, Youdas, Garrett, and Chao (1983) have shown that these electromyostimulation-induced changes in strength (22%) are similar to those obtained with isometric training (18%). Other researchers (Davies, Dooley, McDonagh, & White, 1985; Mohr, Carlson, Sulentic, & Landry, 1985) have found no increase in strength with an electromyostimulation-training protocol. As we discussed previously, many different factors could account for this discrepancy: training duration and intensity, initial state of the subjects, the muscle trained, familiarity with the apparatus, and the degree of voluntary activity accompanying the electrical stimulation. For example, most investigators do not monitor the intensity of the effort elicited by the electrical stimulation, which is an important variable given what we know about strength training (but cf. Selkowitz, 1985). It is surprising, given the many anecdotal observations that have been made, that there is no evidence indicating that electromyostimulation provides greater gains in strength than those achieved with voluntary training. There are two factors that may account for this: (a) a failure to have subjects train by imposing electromyostimulation on top of voluntary activation, and (b) the use of subjects who are not elite strength athletes.

As a complex variable, strength is affected by muscular, mechanical, and neural factors, and it is unknown which, if any, of these factors is altered by electromyostimulation. For example, the excitation of muscle fibers by this artificial means is known to occur in the reverse order normally used by the nervous system. The activation of motor units (including muscle fibers) by the nervous system occurs in a manner referred to as orderly recruitment. This orderliness is thought to be due to differences in motoneuron size—the smallest motoneurons are recruited first and the largest are recruited last. When axons and muscle fibers are activated artificially, as in electromyostimulation, the order of activation is from largest to smallest (Gorman & Mortimer, 1983). Thus, although the strength of muscle increases (a maximum contraction), the question remains as to whether electromyostimulation gains are useful for submaximal activities: Are the gains restricted to the largest muscle fibers, which are not used in most activities? Lagasse, Boucher, Samson, and Jacques (1979), for example, found that a 6-week electromyostimulation program did not significantly improve the clean-and-jerk performance of novice weight lifters.

Loading Techniques

There are several issues that should be considered when deciding how to vary the load in order to induce strength gains; these include progressive-resistance techniques—the magnitude of the load, and the way in which the load should vary during a single repetition of an exercise.

Progressive Resistance. In addition to the variety of options available with which to stress muscle (i.e., isometric, dynamic, accommodation, plyometric, and electromyostimulation), the load used in strength training can also be manipulated in a number of ways. DeLorme (1945) was one of the first to address this issue and proposed varying the load according to the technique called **progressive-resistance exercises**. As indicated previously, DeLorme's technique involves three sets of repetitions of an exercise in which the load increases with each set. In conventional weight-training programs, this typically means increasing the weight of the barbell from one set to another. However, the *torque exerted by muscle depends on not only the magnitude of the external load* (the amount of barbell weight) *but also the size of the moment arm.* As a consequence, progressive-resistance exercises can be accomplished without changing the size of the load (barbell weight) but simply by varying moment-arm length. For example, Figure 8.6 illustrates an individual in the middle of a bent-knee sit-up. In the four positions illustrated (Figure 8.6B), the arms move from being at the person's side to being stretched over-

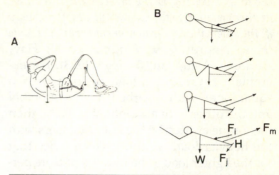

Figure 8.6. Subject performing a bent-knee sit-up. (A) Whole-body figure. (B) The effect of changing arm position on the moment arm of the upper-body weight vector ($\mathbf{W}$) with respect to the hip joint (H) is to increase the required resultant hip-flexion muscle force ($\mathbf{F_m}$) to perform a slow sit-up. $\mathbf{F_i}$ and $\mathbf{F_j}$ represent the intraabdominal pressure and joint reaction force, respectively.

head. The change in arm position does not alter the weight of the upper body, but it does shift the center of gravity toward the head and thus increases the moment arm of the system weight relative to the hip joint (dotted line in Figure 8.6B). The net effect is an increase in the torque that the hip flexors must exert to accomplish the movement.

Magnitude. When defining the concept of progressive-resistance exercises, DeLorme (1945) proposed that each of the three sets should include 10 repetitions. However, most strength-training programs currently advocate using from 1 to 8 repetitions in a set (Kraemer, 1983). In lifting weights, muscles perform work, which is a combination of the size of the load and the distance lifted. If the number of repetitions in a set is decreased, then the load lifted in each repetition should increase (assuming the amount of work done in the two situations remains relatively constant). *When an individual lifts a heavier barbell, the torque exerted by the muscle(s) will increase in direct relation to the increase in load if, and only if, the kinematics of the movement remain the same* (Hay, Andrews, & Vaughan, 1980; Hay, Andrews, Vaughan, & Ueya, 1983). For example, if an individual performed two squats, one with a barbell weight of 500 N and the other with a weight of 1,000 N, then the torque exerted by the knee extensors with the heavier load would be about twice that for the lighter load if the movement were performed in exactly the same way each time. Hay et al. (1983) found that, when subjects lifted loads of 40%, 60%, and 80% of the 4-RM load, the kinematics of the movement were altered (e.g., by flexing more at the hip during a squat) so that the torque exerted by the muscles did not increase in proportion to the load. As a consequence, *the most favored loads for strength training appear to be about 5-6 RM with about four sets of each exercise*; the load remains constant for all four sets (Atha, 1981; McDonagh & Davies, 1984; Sale & MacDougall, 1981). According to Sale and MacDougall (1981), a 5- to 6-RM load would be about 85%-90% of the maximum load (Figure 8.7).

McDonagh and Davies (1984) summarized the effect of load with the following statements, which are based on studies that involved *untrained* individuals: (a) loads less than 66% of maximum do not increase strength even with 150 contractions per day; (b) loads greater than 66% of maximum increase strength from 0.5% to 2.0% each training session; and (c) with loads of greater than 66% of maximum, as few as 10 repetitions per session can increase strength. Harre (1982) and his co-workers further suggested that beginners should use loads of 60%-80% of maximum with 8-10 repetitions in each set, and that elite athletes should use loads of 80%-100% of maximum with 2-5 repetitions per set.

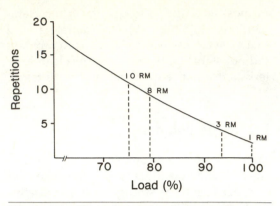

Figure 8.7. The relationship between the number of repetitions in an exercise set (RM = repetition maximum) and the load as a percentage of maximum. *Note.* Reprinted with permission from ''Specificity in Strength Training: A Review for the Coach and Athlete'' by D.G. Sale and D. MacDougall, 1981, *Canadian Journal of Applied Sport Sciences*, **6**(2), p. 90. Copyright 1981 by the Canadian Association of Sport Sciences. Reprinted by permission.

Constant and Variable Loads. With the exception of isometric exercises, strength-training activities involve changing the length of an active muscle over a prescribed range of motion. Since the torque a muscle can exert changes with its length (Figure 6.7), it is necessary to indicate not only the size of the load, as above, but also the way in which the load changes over the range of motion. Millions of dollars have been spent by manufacturers of weight-lifting equipment in addressing this issue. The differences of opinion can be exemplified by the controversy over **constant-** versus **variable-load** training. This is essentially a disagreement between those who advocate the superiority of free weights (i.e., barbells and dumbbells) and those who believe in the superiority of machines (e.g., Nautilus, Universal) in which the load applied to the body segments either remains constant (free weights) or varies (machines) over the range of motion.

For example, consider the forearm-curl exercise that involves alternate flexion-extension of the elbow joint against a load. With free weights (Figure 8.8A), the load held by the individual remains *constant* throughout the exercise and acts vertically downward. The length of the load vector remains constant over the range of motion (Figure 8.8A)—recall that the length of a weight vector indicates the magnitude of the load. With a machine (Figure 8.8B), however, the load moved by the individual *varies*. The load provided by the machine is a torque due to the product of the weight stack and the moment arm of the cam. Although the weight remains constant for a particular exercise, the length of the moment arm (d) from the axis of rotation (O) to the point at which the chain (that connects to the weight stack) leaves the

cam changes throughout the range of motion (Figure 8.8B). This can be seen in the free-body diagram for the machine by the change in length of the load vector over the range of motion.

Another way of distinguishing between constant and variable loads is to notice that in the former the system (free-body diagram in Figure 8.8) works against a force (barbell), whereas in the latter the system works against a torque. For the free-weight condition the load (weight of the barbell) remains constant, whereas for the machine the load (weight stack × cam moment arm) varies. The load applied to the muscles is more variable for the constant-load condition. If we ignore the weight of the limb, the load experienced by the muscles is the product of the external load (barbell or machine torque) and the moment-arm distance (d in Figure 8.9). For the barbell, d varies substantially over the

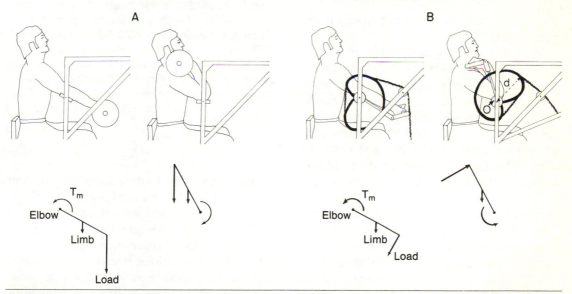

Figure 8.8. Loading conditions associated with (A) constant- and (B) variable-load training. The subject performs a forearm-curl exercise with a barbell (constant load) and with a machine (variable load). The load in the barbell exercise is the weight of the barbell. The load in the machine exercise is the product of the force (weight stack at the end of the chain) and the moment arm (distance d in the second position).

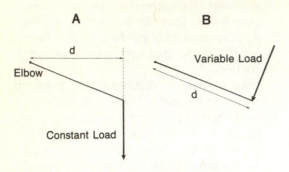

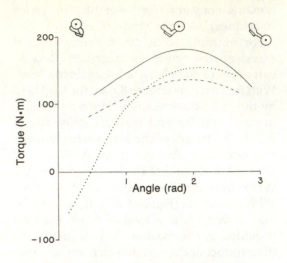

Figure 8.9. The load experienced by the muscles about the elbow joint in response to (A) free weights or (B) a machine load. The load on the muscles is equal to the product of the external load (constant load or variable load) and the moment arm (d). For simplicity, the variable load is shown acting perpendicular to the forearm throughout the range of motion.

Figure 8.10. Resultant muscle torque about the elbow joint during a forearm-curl exercise with a barbell (dotted line) and a Nautilus machine (dashed line) in comparison to the maximum elbow-flexion torque (solid line) that can be exerted over the range of motion. The load employed with both the barbell and the Nautilus exercises was 60% 4 RM. *Note.* From ''Dynamic Variable Resistance and the Universal System'' by F. Smith, 1982. Copyright 1982 by the National Strength & Conditioning Association. Adapted by permission, *National Strength and Conditioning Association Journal,* 4(4), 14-19.

range of motion, much more than for the machine load.

The questions of interest, however, are, How and why does the load change with the machine? The notion of variable load arose from consideration of the torque-angle characteristics of muscle; recall the ascending, descending, and ascending-descending relationships (Figure 6.7). The most common relationship (ascending-descending) depicts the maximum torque as occurring in the middle of the range of motion. Accordingly, *variable-load devices are designed so that the load changes over the range of motion to match the torque-angle relationship of muscle.*

The differences in the stress applied to muscle with constant and variable load is shown in Figure 8.10. The solid line represents the maximum isometric torque-angle relationship for the elbow flexor muscle group. The other two curves indicate the elbow flexion torque required to move a moderate load over the indicated range of

motion for constant- (dotted line) and variable-load (dashed line) conditions. Since the curve associated with the variable load more closely matches (similarity in shape) the maximum capability, some people claim that this loading technique is superior because it *stresses the muscle more evenly over its entire range of motion.* This is but one feature of training protocols, however, and the intent is not to suggest that variable-load devices always provide superior strength-training conditions. For example, although heavier loads can be used with machine training (Hay et al., 1983), the use of free weights also emphasizes the maintenance of balance during maximum efforts. Furthermore, the majority of athletic endeavors do actually involve a constant load so that use of the variable-load devices would seem to violate the specificity principle. Indeed, many athletes, particularly those involved in high-speed movements, argue against variable-load training for this reason.

Simple Joint System Effects

One of the characteristics of biological tissue, as emphasized in chapter 4, is its ability to adapt to the demands of usage. This ability is readily apparent over the spectrum of human activity; for example, body builders use weight-training programs to **hypertrophy** selected muscles, and during spaceflight the muscles of astronauts experience **hypotrophy** due to the reduced-gravity environment.

We have developed the concept that strength is one measure of the output of the simple joint system. We also know that all the components of the simple joint system will adapt to altered use. However, most is known about the adaptations of two elements to strength training, the neural input and the characteristics of muscle (Edström & Grimby, 1986; Hoppeler, 1986; Sale, 1986, 1987).

The probability of a neural adaptation with strength training is generally demonstrated with the use of EMG. Komi, Viitasalo, Rauramaa, and Vihko (1978), for example, found that the quantity of EMG (neural input to the muscle) increased at maximal efforts with strength training. The amount of EMG required to move submaximal loads decreased, indicating an improved efficiency of muscle activation. However, these neural effects seem to be confined to the early stages of a strength-training program in that after

the first 2-3 weeks there are minimal changes in the EMG (Figure 8.4; Häkkinen, Alén, & Komi, 1985; Häkkinen & Komi, 1983; Moritani & de Vries, 1979). At least three mechanisms might be used to account for these changes in EMG. First, one consequence of strength training may be that an individual *learns to generate a greater central command* to drive the motoneurons. Second, since *motoneurons become more excitable* with strength training (Sale, MacDougall, Upton, & McComas, 1983), the same central command may elicit a greater motoneuron command to the muscles. Third, strength training has been shown (Milner-Brown et al., 1975) to be associated with a greater *synchronization of motor-unit discharge* (i.e., an increased likelihood of motor-unit action potentials' occurring at the same point in time). The increased motor-unit synchronization with strength training may result in a greater muscle force.

Another line of evidence supporting a neural adaptation with strength training is based on one- and two-limb strength comparisons (Ohtsuki, 1983; Vandervoort et al., 1984). The data demonstrate that the *sum* of the maximum isometric torques exerted by first the right limb and then the left limb (arm or leg) is greater than the torques exerted when both limbs are activated simultaneously. This *bilateral deficit* is apparent in the measures of both torque and EMG and hence is thought to be neurally based. Furthermore, it appears that this deficit can be overcome with training (Howard & Enoka, 1987; Secher, 1975). However, it is unclear whether this neural effect occurs at the high- or low-level controller (Figure 8.1).

There is even the suggestion that the assessment of strength can be influenced by the previous activity of the simple joint system. We encountered a similar notion in chapter 5 when we talked about the neural basis of flexibility training (i.e., the HR and HR-AC techniques, Figure 5.15). However, unlike the reflex *inhibition* postulated for the PNF-based stretches, *prior antagonist muscle activity appears to enhance the strength and power that a muscle can generate* (Caiozzo, Barnes, Prietto, & McMaster, 1981; Caiozzo, Laird, Chow, Prietto, & McMaster, 1982).

At the muscle-fiber level, increases in strength produce, in addition to an increased maximum-torque capability, an increase in the speed of contraction (contraction time and one-half relaxation time; Schmidtbleicher & Haralambie, 1981; Sale et al., 1983) but a decrease in twitch force (Sale, McComas, MacDougall, & Upton, 1982). Some controversy exists as to whether strength training induces hypertrophy (Gollnick, Parsons, Riedy, & Moore, 1983; Saltin & Gollnick, 1983) or **hyperplasia** (Gonyea, 1980), where hypertrophy denotes an increase in the number of myofibrils per muscle fiber and hyperplasia refers to an increase in the number rather than cross-sectional area of muscle fibers. The existence of hypertrophy as a consequence of heavy-resistance training has been well documented (Etemadi & Hosseini, 1968; MacDougall, Elder, Sale, Moroz, & Sutton, 1980; Taylor & Wilkinson, 1986), but there is also evidence for hyperplasia (Gonyea, Sale, Gonyea, & Mikesky, 1986; Larsson & Tesch, 1986; MacDougall, Sale, Elder, & Sutton, 1982; Tesch & Larsson, 1982). In all probability, both adaptations occur, but the appropriate experiment to distinguish between the two has yet to be done. There are a number of concerns that must be addressed, such as a possible relationship between hyperplasia and the development of satellite cells, standardization of muscle-biopsy sites, interference of anabolic steroids, and differences between species and muscles, before a significant role for hyperplasia is firmly established (Taylor & Wilkinson, 1986).

Although the mechanism essentially responsible for hypertrophy and hyperplasia is an increase in the number of contractile proteins, the net protein accumulation appears to be affected by such variables as *stretch* (e.g., Ashmore & Summers, 1981; Frankeny, Holly, & Ashmore, 1983), *motor-unit rate coding* (Lømo, Westgaard, & Engebretsen, 1980), and *axoplasmic flow* (Hofmann, 1980). The response of muscle to high-load (strength) training may involve hypertrophy or hyperplasia, but at the whole-muscle level *the net effect is an increase in the contractile-protein content of muscle.* MacDougall (1986) reports that 6 months of strength training results in an increase in myofibril area but not density; that is, myofilaments are added to the individual myofibrils without altering the number of myofilaments per unit area. Such an increase represents a net increase in protein synthesis. However, identification of the actual mechanism that causes this increase in response to strength training remains controversial.

Until recently, the effects of exercise on the distribution of motor-unit type were thought to be reasonably well established. The most common opinion was that exercise could induce only conversions between Type FG and FOG muscle fibers (Barnard, Edgerton, & Peter, 1970a, 1970b; Prince, Hikida, & Hagerman, 1976) but not between slow- (SO) and fast-contracting (FG, FOG) muscle fibers. Recent evidence (Howald, 1982; Noble, Dabrowski, & Ianuzzo, 1983), however, suggests that as measurement and experimental techniques become more sophisticated, it will be possible to demonstrate training-induced transformations of slow- to fast-contracting muscle fibers. For example, Green et al. (1984) found in the plantaris and extensor digitorum longus muscles of rats an increase in Type I and IIa fibers as a consequence of an extreme endurance-training program. On the basis of such observations, therefore, it would appear that it may be possible to change the fiber-type proportion of a muscle with training.

At the beginning of this section on strength, we emphasized that the interpretation of strength-training studies can be affected by several different factors. It appears that the fiber-type effect is another of those factors. Previously, we indicated that some investigators (Schmidtbleicher & Haralambie, 1981) reported that the primary effect of a high-load, 8-week training program was limited to the fast-contracting muscle fibers. However, Häkkinen (1985) has shown that the fiber-type effects depend upon the length of training (Figure 8.11A; 8 vs. 16 weeks for the slow-contracting fibers) and the mode of training (Figure 8.11; change in slow-contracting muscle-fiber area for the two training programs). Häkkinen measured strength as the maximum isometric torque exerted by the knee extensors and the fiber area in arbitrary units (au) from a muscle biopsy of vastus lateralis. Figure 8.11 shows the results of strength training for two groups of subjects. For the group that used the same type of training (concentric-eccentric) for 16 weeks, both the slow-twitch (SO) and fast-twitch (FOG and FG) fibers had increased in cross-sectional area at 16 weeks but only the fast-twitch fibers had changed at 8 weeks. In contrast, the group of subjects that varied its training (Figure 8.11B) did not show any change in its slow-twitch fibers over 24 weeks of training. According to the principle of specificity, the first group of subjects must have been doing the exercise in such a way to stress its slow-twitch muscle fibers. However, note also the differences in the initial strength (A = 3.0 kN, B = 3.6 kN) of the two groups of subjects; this difference in strength may have contributed to the differential fiber-type response.

A lot of effort has gone into looking at the changes that strength training causes in muscle; these include such things as the hypertrophy-hyperplasia issue and the fiber-type issue. *In terms of strength, however, the*

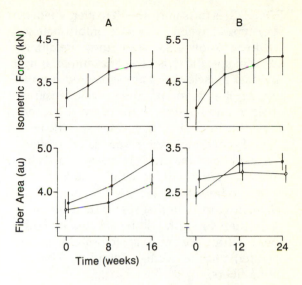

Figure 8.11. Strength and muscle-fiber area effects associated with two training programs. Strength is measured as the maximum isometric force exerted by the knee extensors. The muscle-fiber values were measured for the slow- (open circles) and fast-contracting (filled circles) fibers. (A) The effects of a continuous concentric-eccentric program. (B) The effects of an intermittent concentric and concentric-eccentric program. *Note.* From "Research Overview: Factors Influencing Trainability of Muscular Strength During Short Term and Prolonged Training" by K. Häkkinen, 1985. Copyright 1985 by the National Strength & Conditioning Association. Adapted by permission, *National Strength and Conditioning Association Journal, 7*(2), 32-37.

critical issue is whether or not these adaptations cause any change in specific tension. For example, since the force that a muscle can exert is proportional to its cross-sectional area (crossbridges in parallel), does it matter whether the increase is caused by hyperplasia or hypertrophy? Similarly, if the specific tension of the three muscle-fiber types (SO,

FOG, FG) is the same, does it matter whether fiber-type conversion occurs? Unfortunately, we do not know yet whether there are differences in specific tension. For example, if individual muscle fibers are separated from a muscle, it appears that the specific tensions of slow- and fast-twitch fibers are about the same (Lucas et al., 1987). If the specific tension of individual motor units is calculated, however, it seems that it is greatest for Type FF motor units and least for Type S motor units (Bodine et al., 1985; McDonagh et al., 1980). If it turns out that specific tension does vary, then strength will be affected by both the quantity of muscle (crossbridges in parallel) and the average specific tension of all its fibers.

Power

When we began talking about strength at the beginning of this chapter, we noted that strength and power are measures of the output of the simple joint system. One useful way of distinguishing between these two parameters is in terms of the force-velocity relationship of muscle. In Figure 8.2, for example, the force-velocity relationship was described as comprising three distinct regions: velocity = 0, force = 0, and neither force nor velocity equals zero. Strength has been defined to refer specifically to that point on the curve where velocity is equal to zero. In contrast, power is a measure related to the non-zero force and velocity region.

Many people have traditionally measured human performance by such things as *static strength* and *dynamic strength*. These terms both represent measures of torque, the difference being whether or not muscle length changes. However, it is apparent from Figure 8.2 that the torque that a muscle can exert decreases as velocity increases. In other words, *measures of dynamic strength depend to a great extent on the rate at which muscle length changes*. To avoid this contamination, the measure of peak power represents the combination of force and velocity that produces a maximum mechanical effect.

What features of the simple joint system do strength and power represent? The force that a muscle can exert is known to be proportional to the number of force-generating units in parallel (chapter 5). Consequently, *the measure of strength at least partly reflects the number of in-parallel activated muscle fibers*. At the other end of the force-velocity graph, the maximum speed at which a muscle can shorten (v_{max}) is determined by the enzyme myosin ATPase. This enzyme seems to control the speed at which the interaction between actin and myosin occurs. The physiological factors determining power must lie between these two extremes, cross-sectional area at one end and myosin ATPase at the other end.

In general terms, *the ability of muscle to produce power is limited by the metabolic rate of ATP production or the rate at which the myofilaments can convert energy into mechanical work* (Weis-Fogh & Alexander, 1977). For short duration events, such as a discus throw or a 100-m sprint, the availability of ATP will not be the limiting factor, and hence the power a muscle is able to produce will depend upon how rapidly energy can be converted into mechanical work. In contrast, power production for longer duration events will more likely be limited by the supply of ATP. Events that fall into this latter category generally involve a lesser magnitude of power production.

Power is defined as the rate of doing work, (i.e., the amount of work done per unit of time). However, in Part I we noted that work is equal to the change in energy, and hence power can also be considered in terms of *the rate of change in energy*. We emphasize this point because the change in the energy of the system is not limited to changes in chemical energy (ATP). For example, suppose we reconsider the horizontal elbow extension-flexion movement that we discussed in Part I (Figures 1.5 and 3.11). According to that discussion, the movement was accomplished by a net pattern of muscle activity that proceeded as a concentric-extensor, eccentric-flexor, concentric-flexor, and eccentric-extensor sequence. This sequence of activity was then related to the power-time profile (Figure 3.11) for the movement, and it was mentioned that the periods of power production may not be completely accounted for by the energy flowing from the muscles. In short, during the eccentric-flexor phase, the flexor muscle group is actively lengthened (an eccentric contraction) before performing a concentric contraction. In chapter 7, we considered the possibility that energy may be provided *mechanically* (storage and utilization of elastic energy) or *chemically* (ATP) for the positive work done during the concentric phase. As a consequence of this possibility, the second power-production phase of this movement (Figure 3.11) is affected by the rate of energy conversion from both sources. This possibility applies not to all movements, but only those that contain an eccentric-concentric sequence.

Whereas we have defined strength as a parameter that will assess the isometric torque capabilities of the simple joint system, measurements of power will reveal dynamic features of the system. Recall that power can be calculated as the product of force and velocity and that peak power occurs not at maximum force (velocity = 0) or maximum velocity (force = 0) but somewhere between the maxima (Figure 6.13). As an example of this phenomenon, consider the power delivered to a barbell by a weight lifter during three lifts: (a) the clean, a movement that requires the displacement of the barbell from the floor to a lifter's chest in one continuous rapid motion; (b) the squat, a movement in which a lifter supports a barbell on the shoulders and goes from a standing erect position to a knee-flexed position (thighs parallel to the floor) and then returns to standing; and (c) the bench press, a movement in which the lifter, in a supine position, lowers the barbell from a straight-arm location above the chest down to touch the chest and then raises it back to the initial position. Data have been taken from the literature (clean—Enoka, 1979; squat—McLaughlin, Dillman, & Lardner, 1977; bench press—Madsen & McLaughlin, 1984) to illustrate the differences in power production for three lifts (see Table 8.1).

Table 8.1 Power Delivered to a Barbell During Three Types of Lifts

	Clean	Squat	Bench press
Barbell weight (N)	1,226	3,694	1,815
Peak barbell velocity (m·s^{-1})	2	0.30	1.54
Height (m)	0.30	0.30	0.06
Time to KE_{max} (s)	0.35	1.30	0.70
KE_{max} (J)	250	17	219
PE (J)	368	1,108	109
Power (W)	1,766	865	469

The peak power produced in the three lifts was calculated by determining the rate of change in mechanical energy (Garhammer, 1980). Since the quantity of work done can be determined from the change in energy, and power equals the rate of doing work, then power can be calculated from the rate of change in energy.

$$\text{average power} = \frac{\text{change in energy}}{\text{time}}$$
$$= \frac{KE_{max} + PE}{\text{time}}$$
$$= \frac{1/2\ mv^2 + mgh}{t} \quad (8.1)$$

where KE_{max} refers to the maximum kinetic energy, PE represents potential energy, and time indicates the time to maximum kinetic energy.

These data suggest that the peak power delivered to the barbell is greatest during the clean and least for the bench press. This is interesting because the squat and bench press are two of the three lifts that comprise the sport of power lifting. Indeed, these data suggest that success in the squat and bench press lifts is not determined solely by power production. Furthermore, we could speculate that success in power lifting is more related to strength, as we have defined it.

With regard to training techniques, it appears that the specificity principle also applies to power training. For example, it is known that strength training (isometric) does not affect maximum power (DeKoning, Binkhorst, Vissers, & Vos, 1982). Furthermore, training at different speeds, such as with an isokinetic device, elicits differential power effects (Caiozzo, Perrine, & Edgerton, 1981; Coyle et al., 1981); for example, training at fast speeds increases power production at those speeds. This effect can be seen in Figure 8.12, where it is shown that training with a high-force, low-velocity combination will affect the force-velocity curve in that region; the low-

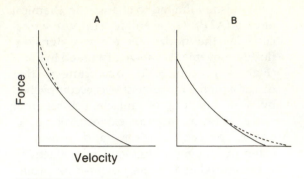

Figure 8.12. Idealized changes in the force-velocity relationship are specific to the training technique. Dashed line represents the training-induced adaptation. (A) High-force, low-velocity effect. (B) Low-force, high-velocity effect.

force, high-velocity combination is similarly specific.

DeKoning et al. (1985) examined the torque-angular velocity relationship for three groups of subjects (15-36 years): untrained females, untrained males, and arm-trained males (i.e., track-and-field athletes, rowers, weight lifters, body builders, handball players, karate exponents, and tug-of-war competitors). Figure 8.13 shows that the torque-velocity curves for the elbow flexors are different for the three groups of subjects. The strength (P_o = isometric torque) varies as you would expect: arm-trained males greater than untrained males greater than untrained females. There was, however, only a small difference in the maximum angular velocity (ω_{max}) among the groups (see Table 8.2).

From these torque-angular velocity data, DeKoning, Binkhorst, Vos, & van't Hof (1985) were able to calculate the maximum power each group of athletes could produce. Again, the maximum power varied in the order you would expect. Although these data may not reflect training adaptations, they do demonstrate the existence of differences among individuals.

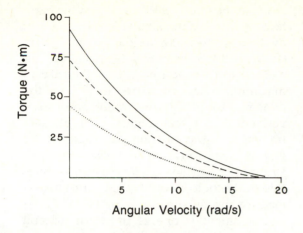

Figure 8.13. Relationships between torque and angular velocity for the elbow flexor muscles of three groups of subjects (solid line = arm-trained male athletes, dashed line = untrained males, dotted line = untrained females). *Note.* From ''The Force-Velocity Relationship of Arm Flexion in Untrained Males and Females and Arm-Trained Athletes'' by F.L. DeKoning et al., 1985, *European Journal of Applied Physiology,* **54**, p. 92. Copyright 1985 by Springer-Verlag, Inc. Adapted by permission.

Of interest to us, however, is which of these types of adaptations will have the greatest effect on power. To this end, Pedemonte (1983) emphasized that the goal of power training should be the maintenance of maximal lifting speed. To accomplish this Pedemonte proposed the following individualized training protocol:

$3 \times X_1$ seconds with 30% load and Y_1 repetitions

$3 \times X_2$ seconds with 40% load and Y_2 repetitions

$3 \times X_3$ seconds with 50% load and Y_3 repetitions

The variable X represents the time (in seconds) that the individual can maintain maximum movement speed at that load (30%, 40%, or 50% of maximum). For example, in setting up the program, the individual would determine how long maximum movement speed could be maintained at each training load; this would establish X_1, X_2, and X_3. Then in training the goal would be to perform

Table 8.2   Elbow Flexor Strength (P_o), Maximum Angular Velocity (ω_{max}), and Power for Arm-Trained Males and Untrained Males and Females

	Arm-trained males	Untrained males	Untrained females
P_o (N•m)	90.9 ± 15.6	68.5 ± 11.0	42.7 ± 6.9
ω_{max} (rad/s)	17.0 ± 1.6	16.6 ± 1.5	14.9 ± 1.3
Power (W)	253.0 ± 58.0	195.0 ± 46.0	111.0 ± 24.0

Note. Figures are given as x ± = SD.

as many repetitions as possible (Y_1, Y_2, and Y_3) at each of the loads and within each of the durations (X_1, X_2, and X_3).

Despite the appeal of this logic, however, Duchateau and Hainaut (1984) found that the gains in power production were greater with isometric rather than dynamic training. Duchateau and Hainaut had two groups of subjects train a small hand muscle (adductor pollicis) at moderate intensity (10 repetitions) every day for 3 months; one group used maximum isometric contractions, and the other group did rapid dynamic contractions against a load of 30%-40% of maximum. The effects of both training methods on the force-velocity relationship provided further evidence for the principle of specificity; pre- and posttraining measurements revealed a separation of the force-velocity curves in the high-force region for the isometric group and in the high-speed region for the dynamic group (Figure 8.12). Surprisingly, however, the isometric group produced a 51% increase in maximum power compared to 19% for the dynamic group. This observation needs to be verified in subjects after a high-intensity training program because it suggests *the greatest increases in power are obtained with high-force rather than high-velocity training*. Perhaps this study could be duplicated with a higher load for the dynamic training.

Assessment is one of the most difficult aspects associated with the concept of power. In terms of the simple joint system, the measurement of power can be accomplished by either a task performance (e.g., vertical

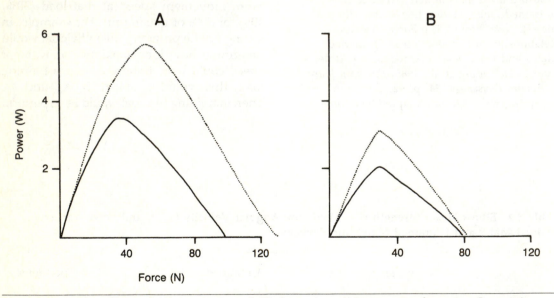

Figure 8.14. The effects of (A) isometric and (B) dynamic training on muscle power. Isometric training involved a 5-s maximum isometric contraction each minute for 10 min, every day for 3 months. Dynamic training involved the same number of repetitions and length of training, but the exercise comprised a rapid concentric movement. Isometric training produced a greater increase in the maximum power and a shift in the force at which the maximum occurred. Solid line = pretraining, dotted line = posttraining. *Note*. From ''Isometric or Dynamic Training: Differential Effects on Mechanical Properties of a Human Muscle'' by J. Duchateau and K. Hainaut, 1984, *Journal of Applied Physiology*, **56**, p. 298. Copyright 1984 by the American Physiological Society. Adapted by permission.

jump, weight-lifting event) or derivation from a set of force-velocity data. The latter approach is illustrated in Figure 8.2 where it is shown that a force-velocity relationship actually comprises a set of individual data points. Each data point (a cross in Figure 8.2) is defined by a force and a velocity value. The power associated with each point is simply obtained by multiplying the force and velocity values (power = force × velocity). The product of force and velocity (i.e., power) can then be plotted against velocity (Figure 6.13) or force (Figure 8.14). The most common way to obtain the force-velocity (torque-angle) data is with an isokinetic device (Froese & Houston, 1985).

The calculation of a power value from a task such as a vertical jump again requires the multiplication of appropriate force and velocity values. This can be done by recording the ground reaction force (e.g., Figure 8.15) during the vertical jump and using this information to determine the average force ($\overline{F}$) applied to the ground and the average velocity ($\overline{v}$) of the center of gravity (Bosco & Komi, 1980). The subjects should be confined to a squat jump (chapter 7), which involves only a concentric and not an eccentric-concentric sequence. $\overline{F}$ is obtained by dividing the impulse (Figure 8.15; area of the ground reaction force time curve above the body-weight line) by the duration of the impulse. From Figure 8.15, these values are approximately as follows:

$$impulse = 179 \text{ N·s}$$
$$time = 0.29 \text{ s}$$
$$force = 617 \text{ N}$$

To get an approximate value of the average velocity during the jump, we can resort to the equations of chapter 1. From Equation 1.3, we can determine final velocity—that is, velocity at the end of the takeoff phase:

$$v_f = at$$

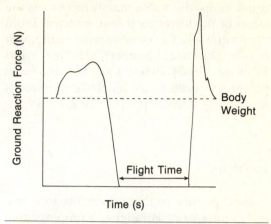

Figure 8.15. Vertical component of the ground reaction force during a squat jump.

where a = acceleration due to gravity = 9.81 m/s² and t = one-half flight time = 0.20 s.

$$v_f = 9.81 \times 0.20$$
$$= 1.96 \text{ m/s}$$

The average velocity during the takeoff phase is then determined as the average of the initial and final velocities:

$$\overline{v} = \frac{v_f + v_i}{2}$$
$$= \frac{1.96 + 0}{2}$$
$$= 0.98 \text{ m/s}$$

Finally, the *average* power produced by the jumper is determined as the product of the average force and the average velocity.

$$power = \overline{F} \times \overline{v}$$
$$= 617 \times 0.98 \text{ (N} \times \text{m/s)}$$
$$= 605 \text{ W (1 W} = 1 \text{ J/s} = 1 \text{ N·m/s)}$$

This approach indicates that the average power produced by the jumper during the squat jump shown in Figure 8.15 has a value of 605 W. Since the arms are not used in the squat jump, this value mainly represents the effect of the lower extremity muscles. From the torque-angular velocity relationship, van Ingen Schenau, Bobbert, Huijing, and Woittiez (1985) determined the *maximum* power produced by the plantarflexor muscles during the vertical jump to be 2,499 W.

Fatigue

A third parameter that we can use to evaluate performance is fatigue, a property that characterizes the performance of the system during sustained efforts. Although this term is probably used as frequently as both strength and power as an index of performance, we are still far from agreement on what we mean by the term. Whenever the simple joint system is activated and that activity is sustained, the interactions among the elements (i.e., rigid link, joint, muscle, neuron, and sensory receptor) change over time. For example, when we want a motor unit to exert a particular force, we excite the motoneuron to discharge a certain number of action potentials at some rate. It seems, however, that when an activity is sustained for a period of time the relationship between action-potential rate and force changes; that is, we may get more or less force for the same discharge rate. Similar adaptations occur in the interactions between all elements of the simple joint system. We normally attribute these adaptations to a variety of changes, such as those associated with temperature, ionic distribution, energy (ATP) availability, and fatigue.

Consider some hypothetical task, such as carrying a heavy suitcase, that you wish to sustain for a long period. From the time you lift the suitcase, adaptations occur in the interactions among the elements of the simple joint system. At some point it will be-come more difficult to hold the suitcase and you will have to try harder to do so. Eventually, however, no matter how hard you try, you will be unable to hold the suitcase any longer, and you will have to either set it down or change hands. It is these two conditions (i.e., the increased difficulty and the impossibility) that we ascribe to the concept of fatigue. That is, fatigue is not a single event in time but rather a series of adaptations that occur during sustained effort. Within this framework, fatigue is an index of performance that encompasses both subjective (i.e., the difficulty) and objective (i.e., the impossibility) capabilities.

Based on this perspective, we have defined fatigue ''as a progressive increase in the effort required to exert a desired force and the progressive inability to maintain this force in sustained or repeated contractions'' (Enoka & Stuart, 1985, p. 2281). As just described, this definition suggests that *there are two parts to fatigue, increased effort and force failure*. Assessment of the difficulty of a task is accomplished by the psychophysical phenomenon known as *sense of effort*, a relative, subjective measure of the effort required to perform a given task. Several such measures can be obtained over the course of a performance. In contrast, the force-failure component of fatigue is more straightforward and may be detected as an inability to exert a desired, normally attainable, force.

Throughout the state of fatigue—the increased effort and the force failure—the adaptations that began at the onset of the activity continue. From at least the beginning of the increased-effort phase, the object of these adaptations must be to optimize the output of the simple joint system. Thus, fatigue represents the state of the simple joint system as a product of a host of physiological adaptations. Accordingly, fatigue is a consequence and not a by-product of the operation of the simple joint system.

Given this extended definition of fatigue, it should be apparent that there are many processes that may contribute to fatigue (Figure 8.16). Researchers working in this area have tended to lump different processes together (e.g., central vs. peripheral, muscular vs. neural) so that it might be easier to understand fatigue. From the perspective of our simple joint system, it should be apparent that the cause of fatigue may reside in either the muscular or the neural components. The neural mechanisms might be quite complex, however, beyond a simple account of motor-unit recruitment and rate coding. To take this possibility into account we shall invoke the tripartite model (Figure 8.1), which conceptualizes the neuromuscular processes associated with movement as belonging to one of three compartments (Feldman & Grillner, 1983; Hasan et al., 1985). These compartments represent general functions that the nervous system performs during movement.

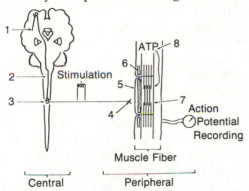

Figure 8.16. The major potential sites associated with the force-failure aspect of fatigue: (1) input to supraspinal centers, (2) excitatory drive to motoneurons, (3) motoneuron excitability, (4) neuromuscular transmission, (5) sarcolemmal excitability, (6) excitation-contraction coupling, (7) contractile machinery, (8) energy metabolism. *Note.* From ''Muscle Fatigue and The Influence of Changing Neural Drive'' by B. Bigland-Ritchie, 1984, *Clinics in Chest Medicine*, **5**, p. 24. Copyright 1984 by W.B. Saunders Co. Reprinted by permission.

Low-Level Controller and Muscle

It is apparent from Figure 8.16 that there are a number of sites at this level that can contribute to the force-failure aspect of fatigue. In contrast, there are no mechanisms at this level that affect the effort involved in an activity. The potential force-failure mechanisms known to exist at this level include *motoneuron excitability, neuromuscular transmission, sarcolemma excitability, excitation-contraction coupling, contractile machinery,* and *energy metabolism.* Sustained use is known to affect these processes such that the force declines over time (i.e., the force-failure aspect of fatigue). The relative importance of these failure mechanisms, however, is difficult to assess because their respective roles vary with the type of activity, and also because the dominance of a particular failure mechanism depends on motor-unit type. For example, we tend to think that slow-contracting motor units (Type S) are more susceptible to energy-metabolism mechanisms whereas fast-contracting units (Type FF, FR) are more sensitive to mechanisms related to discharge rate. Consequently, before we can address the issue of the relative significance of these different failure mechanisms, we need to have a reasonable idea of the pattern (types recruited, activation rates and duration of activity) of motor-unit use in different activities. Unfortunately, not enough is known about motor-unit usage in different tasks, and so we can only speculate on the causes of force reduction in different conditions.

Let us turn our attention then to a brief review of what is known about these fatigue mechanisms at this level. In terms of the simple joint system, movement is accomplished by the following sequence: The motoneuron receives input and decides whether or not to issue a command (action potential); if a command is issued, it is propagated along the axon and across the neuromuscular junction; the action potential is propagated along the sarcolemma; Ca^{++} is released from the lateral sacs due to the muscle action potential; and Ca^{++}-based disinhibition and crossbridge cycling occur. The issue of fatigue mechanisms concerns the question of which of these processes can be caused to fail by sustained use. Under the right conditions, they can all be affected. For example, during a 60-s maximum isometric contraction, motoneuron excitability changes and the rate at which motoneurons discharge action potentials decreases (Bigland-Ritchie, Johansson, Lippold, Smith, & Woods, 1983; Marsden, Meadows, & Merton, 1983). Similarly, once an action potential has been initiated, it may not be transmitted across the neuromuscular junction; this condition is referred to as neuromuscular block. The research evidence in support of this mechanism has largely come from substantially reduced animal preparations (i.e., the physiological state is less than or reduced from normal), and hence it may not occur in normal intact humans (Bigland-Ritchie, 1984). Consequently, the role of the potential neural fatigue mechanisms at the low-level controller remains to be determined.

On the muscular side of this story, the neural excitation becomes transformed into muscle excitation (action potential). It is known that the sarcolemma can become less excitable with fatigue, which results in a reduction in the size of the action potential. The effect of this action-potential reduction on muscle force, however, depends on the safety factor. The system is designed so that there is a margin of safety within which the action-potential size can vary before it will affect excitation-contraction coupling. The size of the safety factor is unknown; furthermore, it probably varies among the different muscle-fiber types. Should the variation in action-potential size be within the range of the safety factor, then the final step in

delivering the neural command would involve the process of excitation-contraction coupling. As with the other mechanisms listed above, it has also been demonstrated that under certain conditions fatigue can affect this coupling process. It appears that these excitation-contraction coupling effects are limited to Type FF and FR motor units (Edwards, Hill, Jones, & Merton, 1977; Jami, Murthy, Petit, & Zytnicki, 1983).

The contraction of muscle depends upon the delivery of a neural command and an available supply of energy (ATP). Previously it was mentioned that the ATP binds to myosin during the detachment phase of the attach-rotate-detach crossbridge cycle. Consequently, any delay in the supply of ATP should affect the relaxation of muscle. Indeed, of the muscle-contraction characteristics (peak force, contraction time, one-half relaxation time; Figure 5.2), the measurement of relaxation is the first to reveal the effects of sustained activity; (i.e., one-half relaxation time increases). The question has been raised, however, as to whether the change in relaxation time reflects changes in energy metabolism (less than adequate ATP) or the effect of an accumulation of metabolites on the contractile machinery.

Despite the uncertainty surrounding the significance of many of these mechanisms, there is substantial evidence to indicate that *fatigue can definitely be due to the failure of the rate of energy supply to meet demand*. This mechanism applies particularly to longer duration events, such as aerobic activities. The energy necessary for muscle contraction is derived from the body's stores, principally stores of glycogen. Hultman, Sjöholm, Sahlin, and Edström (1981), among others, have emphasized that glycogen stores in muscle are used during exercise and that depletion of these stores is closely related to fatigue and exhaustion. Consequently, it appears well documented that fatigue at the low-level controller can be due to an insufficient supply of ATP.

In summary, there is no doubt that the site of fatigue depends upon the type of activity. To date it has been demonstrated that there are a number of potential sites at this level (low-level controller and muscle) that could contribute to fatigue, but we know with any certainty only about the role of one mechanism (i.e., energy metabolism) during this process.

High-Level Controller

In contrast to what is known about the previous level, far less is known about the relationship between the high-level controller and fatigue. We do know, however, that the high-level controller is involved with both the increased-effort and force-failure aspects of fatigue. When the appropriate supraspinal center sends a signal to sustain and activate the low-level controller, a copy of the signal is sent to other supraspinal centers. This copy is referred to as efference copy. It appears that we judge the effort involved in a particular activity on the basis of this efference copy. Our monitoring of the efference copy for this purpose is known as the *sense of effort*. Experimenters typically measure EMG as an index of the efference copy. It has been found that when a subject maintains a submaximal force, there is an increase in the EMG required to maintain the force, and the subject reports an increase in the sense of effort (Figure 8.17). This increased sense of effort occurs before any force failure and represents an increase in the output of the high-level controller to the low-level controller.

Part of the reason for the need to increase the signal from the high-level controller may be related to a second potential fatigue mechanism at this level. There is some evidence to indicate that the excitatory drive to

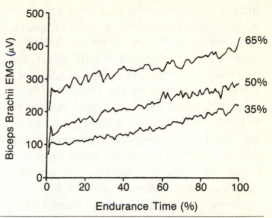

Figure 8.17. Increase in biceps brachii EMG during a constant-force contraction. Subjects are asked to maintain a certain force (35%, 50%, or 65% of maximum) for as long as possible. To maintain the constant force (hence no force failure), subjects increase muscle activity (EMG) and report an increase in the sense of effort. *Note.* From "Role of Central and Peripheral Signals in Force Sensation During Fatigue" by L.A. Jones, 1983, *Experimental Neurology,* **81**, p. 500. Copyright 1983 by Academic Press, Inc. Adapted by permission.

lower motoneurons declines with sustained activation (Kernell & Monster, 1981). Consequently, to maintain the same output from the low-level controller would necessitate an increased effort (supraspinal signal) over time. If the supraspinal drive did not increase then the output from the low-level controller would decline and probably lead to force failure.

Peripheral Receptors

In the tripartite model for the neural control of movement, the low-level controller was depicted as interacting with the compartments containing the high-level controller and the peripheral receptors. In general, muscle receptors serve a variety of functions, which include motor-control, kinesthetic, ergoreceptive, thermoreceptive, and nocioceptive input. Fatigue might affect these functions in three ways: (a) the sensing of the different variables by the receptors, (b) the transmission of the signal from the receptor to the central nervous system (i.e., high- vs. low-level controller), and (c) the response of central structures (e.g., motoneurons) to the input. Of these possibilities, we are aware only that fatigue affects feedback onto motoneurons. During a sustained isometric contraction, feedback has been shown to affect both the range and the rate of motor-unit discharge (Hannerz & Grimby, 1979). In addition, it appears that the response of tendon organs is depressed (Hutton & Nelson, 1986) whereas that of muscle spindles is enhanced (Christakos & Windhorst, 1986; Nelson & Hutton, 1985) in fatigued muscle. This is not meant to imply that this is the only effect of fatigue at this level, but rather we want to emphasize that the issue has received little attention.

There is no doubt that sensory mechanisms play an important role in the physiological adaptations that underscore the increased effort-force failure scheme of fatigue. Let us consider two observations that emphasize these interactions: modulation of motor-unit discharge and variation in muscle-spindle sensitivity. Several investigators have reported that the rate of motor-unit discharge decreases during a sustained effort (Bigland-Ritchie et al., 1983; Dietz, 1978). Since the twitch profile becomes elongated at the same time (especially one-half relaxation time), the decreased discharge appears to match the mechanical conditions in the muscle such that the twitches continue to summate appropriately to produce the necessary tetanic forces. That is, modulation of motor-unit discharge seems to be a well-regulated response; several mechanisms probably contribute to this adaptation, including motoneuron adaptation (Kernell & Monster, 1982) and afferent feedback from the active muscle (Bigland-Ritchie, Dawson, Johansson, & Lippold, 1986). The afferent information may originate from receptors that monitor metabolite accumulation and pain-related effects.

Secondly, we know from our discussion of neural circuitry (chapter 5) that stretch of a muscle may elicit a response known as the stretch reflex. This response involves excitation of the muscle spindles and subsequent activation of the appropriate motor units. Muscle spindles are thought to signal changes in muscle length and to provide the afferent feedback necessary to correct for unexpected changes. As a muscle experiences the force-failure aspect of fatigue, the force that individual motor units can exert decreases. One consequence of this force decline is that for a given muscle-spindle input to the motoneurons, the force exerted by the motor units will be less. To obtain a larger force output, it is necessary to provide a greater muscle-spindle input. Indeed, one of the adaptations associated with fatigue seems to be increased muscle-spindle gain; that is, there is greater response of the muscle spindle to a given change in muscle length.

These examples emphasize the close association between the motor and sensory elements of the simple joint system during fatigue. Their interactions undoubtedly occur during both the increased-effort and force-failure components of fatigue.

Problems

8.1.   Often in the study of human movement we are interested in knowing whether a particular response is mediated by a descending command from the high-level controller or by afferent feedback from peripheral receptors. One way investigators have attempted to monitor the descending command is to record an EMG from a test muscle. With reference to Figure 8.1, comment on the shortcomings of this procedure.

8.2.   How are the base units of performance (strength, power, fatigue) different from one another?

8.3.   What is the relationship between a reflex and a motor program?

8.4.   What is efference copy?
   a. A copy of the strategy encoded in the motor program.
   b. Feedback from peripheral receptors.
   c. Output of the low-level controller.
   d. Copy of the descending command.
   e. Interaction among the elements of the high-level controller.

8.5.   Identify the correct statement(s) (a-e) about the force-velocity relationship. Both parts (i-v) of a-e have to be correct for the statement to be correct.
   i. P_o refers to the force value when velocity is zero.
   ii. The value v_{max} refers to the steepest part of the curve.
   iii. The point at which force = 0 never occurs in the simple joint system.
   iv. The data for a force-velocity graph are obtained from isometric measurements.
   v.   Peak power does not occur at P_o because force is high at that point.
   a. i, iii
   b. ii, iv
   c. iii, v
   d. iv, ii
   e. v, ii

8.6.   Why is it unwise to describe strength with such terms as *dynamic strength, isokinetic strength,* and *static strength*?

8.7.   Strength is influenced by neural, mechanical, and muscular effects. The muscular effects are length and cross-sectional area. How do length and cross-sectional area affect strength?

8.8.   Strength was defined as a complex variable. Identify the incorrect statements about this ability.

a. Strength cannot be measured during movement.
b. Hyperplasia refers to the increase in myofibrils within each muscle fiber.
c. The greatest strength gains do not occur when the heaviest loads are used.
d. An isokinetic contraction is described as static because of the zero acceleration.
e. The cross-sectional area of slow-twitch fibers does not increase with strength training.

8.9.   Given the SI units of measurement for the simple joint system, answer the following:

a. What units are used to measure strength?
b. In a certain sense, power is a measure of strength rate and is expressed in watts (W). This relationship can be illustrated by showing how W is derived from the measure of strength. Show how this can be done.
c. Recall from Part I that velocity was defined as the slope of a position-time graph. What are the units of measurement given by the slope of the force-velocity graph? What mechanical variable does this represent?

8.10.   The terms *isometric, concentric, eccentric* were defined as the quotient of the load and the resultant muscle torques. Where does the term *isotonic* fit into this scheme?

8.11.   In order to compare the relative merits of different strength-training programs, it is necessary to control or account for the many factors that will affect the comparison. Make a list of the factors that will affect the results obtained with a strength-training program. How would you design a study to account for these different issues?

8.12.   According to Newton's laws of motion, isokinetic exercises represent a mechanically static state. Draw a velocity-time graph to illustrate this condition and explain why it is considered static.

8.13.   Draw a diagram of the neural circuitry underlying the stretch reflex, and explain how the stretch reflex might play a role in plyometric exercises.

8.14.   Identify the correct statements about electromyostimulation:

a. It represents an artificial means of activating muscle fibers.
b. It has been demonstrated to produce substantial gains in strength.
c. Action potentials are generated in the axon branches within the muscle and then propagated along the muscle fibers.
d. The activation of muscle fibers occurs in the same order as that achieved naturally by orderly recruitment.
e. Type FF motor units cannot be activated with electromyostimulation.

8.15. Consider the individual performing a bent-knee sit-up in Figure 8.6B. Suppose the parameters have the following dimensions:

F_i = 1,200 N
F_j = 1,570 N
W = 487 N
Angle of push for F_i = 0.67 rad
Distance from H to point of application for F_i = 27 cm
Angle of pull for F_m = 0.45 rad
Distance from H to point of application for F_m = 8 cm

Also, the moment-arm length (dotted line) for the weight vector depends on the position of the arms. In the top position (arms at the side), this distance (dotted line) is 12 cm; in the bottom position (arms overhead) the distance is 18 cm. Calculate the value of F_m for these two positions (top and bottom in Figure 8.6B).

8.16. Qualitatively draw a graph to show how the moment arms for the load relative to the axis of rotation in a constant- and a variable-load exercise vary over the range of motion. Imagine that the exercise is for the knee extensors and requires the person to be seated. The moment arm in question is the distance from the point of application of the load to the knee joint.

8.17. The quantity of EMG has been found to increase in maximal efforts after strength training. The three mechanisms postulated to account for this increase in EMG are central command, motoneuron excitability, and motor-unit synchronization. Explain how each of these mechanisms might contribute to an increased EMG.

8.18. There are a number of controversies in the literature concerning the effects of strength training on muscle. Which of the following statements (a-e) about strength training are incorrect? Just one part (i-v) of a-e has to be incorrect for the statement to be incorrect.

  i. Hyperplasia and hypertrophy both involve an increase in the number of myofibrils.
  ii. If the average muscle-fiber cross-sectional area for a body builder were the same as for control subjects, then the larger muscles of the body builder would be due to hypertrophy.
  iii. There is no evidence of fiber-type conversions with training.
  iv. Type SO muscle fibers do not hypertrophy with strength training.
  v. The specific tension of fast-twitch muscle fibers is approximately 30 kN/cm².

a. ii, v
b. iv, ii
c. iii, i
d. v, i
e. iv, iii

8.19. Researchers have found that the speed at which a muscle action potential travels along the sarcolemma is greater for body builders than it is for control subjects.

a. Is this difference due to the fact that the muscles of body builders are able to attach Ca^{++} to TN-C more quickly?

b. Does this observation tell us whether or not the body builders are stronger? Explain your answer.

c. Does the principle of specificity suggest that, because the body builders have this ability, they must be stressing the mechanisms associated with action-potential propagation during training?

8.20. Figure 8.14 shows data that indicate that the greatest increases in power are obtained with high-force rather than high-velocity training. What reservations might you have about the study on which this conclusion is based?

8.21. What are the conceptual differences between the power-calculation examples in the section on power compared to Figure 8.15? If we had used the latter approach (force × velocity) for the weight-lifting examples, what values would we obtain for the clean, squat, and bench press? Why are these values different from what is reported?

8.22. Suppose that, after a vigorous warm-up (in which muscle temperature was increased), an individual was able to increase her vertical-jump height by 15 cm. Would the ground reaction force associated with the post-warm-up jump be any different to the pre-warm-up jump? Explain your answer.

8.23. Identify the correct statement(s) about fatigue:

a. The increased-effort component of fatigue occurs within the low-level controller.

b. The fatigue mechanisms appear to be similar for the three motor-unit types.

c. The depletion of glycogen stores in muscle is a major cause of fatigue in short-duration events.

d. Since an action potential is an all-or-none event, its amplitude does not change.

e. As force decreases, the sensitivity of muscle spindles appears to increase.

f. The cause of fatigue is probably similar for most human activities.

Summary—Part III

The goal of Part III has been to examine the mechanical interaction between the simple joint system and its surrounding environment. At the beginning of Part III we identified a number of specific objectives. Now that we have completed the section you should be familiar with the following major concepts:

- The motor unit is the functional unit of neuromuscular interaction. The nervous system modulates muscle force by varying both the number of motor units that are active and the rate at which each active motoneuron discharges action potentials.
- The force that the force-generating units of muscle can exert depends on the length of the muscle and the rate at which this length changes.
- The conditions isometric, concentric, and eccentric refer to the quotient of muscle torque to load torque.
- A warm-up alters the temperature of muscle, which has an affect on its contractile speed and hence the power (force × velocity) it can produce.
- The force exerted by the force-generating units is influenced by their arrangement within the muscle, that is, whether they are arranged end to end, side by side, or at an angle to the line of action of the muscle-force vector.
- The characteristics of muscle are affected by the location of the points of attachment and the proportion of whole-muscle length that contains contractile protein.
- There are at least six different features of movement control (set, hold, drive, punch, catch, throw), and they probably each require a different sequence of nervous-system commands.
- A minimum of one pair (agonist-antagonist set) of muscles is necessary to control each degree of freedom at a joint.
- The actual force associated with bone-on-bone contact has a much greater magnitude than that deduced by the net-activity technique of determining joint reaction force.
- Movement speed is critical in the deduction of the patterns of net muscle activity from the kinematic and kinetic features of a movement. As movement speed increases, the mechanical coupling between segments becomes a significant factor in the control of movement.
- A muscle can perform more positive work if it is first stretched (eccentric contraction) before being allowed to shorten (concentric contraction). This enhanced work performance is probably supported by increased energy from chemical and elastic sources.
- It has been proposed that the state of the simple joint system can be evaluated by the measurement of strength, power, and fatigability. These measurements are taken to represent reasonably independent features of the simple joint system.
- Strength is defined as the force output capability of the system as revealed in an isometric torque measurement. As such, the strength of the system includes neural, mechanical, and muscular effects.
- A second feature of the system, the rate of energy use, can be measured as power production. In short-duration events, the critical characteristic appears to be the

maximum power that the system can produce, where power production is limited by either the rate of ATP supply or the rate at which chemical energy is converted into mechanical work. In longer-duration events, it is the average power output for the duration of the event rather than the maximum that is more important.

- A third feature, the performance of the simple joint system during sustained efforts, can be assessed by how well the system resists fatigue. As a complex phenomenon, fatigue may be induced by an increase in the effort necessary to sustain a force or by failure of the neuromuscular apparatus at a variety of sites.

Furthermore, the failure site(s) is (are) not the same for different movements. As a consequence, a complete characterization of the fatigability of the system should involve two or three tests that represent the continuum of movement possibilities.

- From these base parameters (strength, power, fatigue) it should be possible to construct appropriate combinations of base and derived parameters that might predict performance. Although we are far from being able to assess these parameters adequately (particularly power and fatigue), this conceptual construct provides a framework toward which researchers are directing their efforts.

APPENDIX

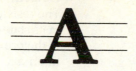

A

SI Units

The abbreviation SI is derived from *Le Systeme International d'Unites*, which represents the modern metric system. There are seven base units in this measurement system from which other units of measurement are derived.

Base

1. **length** meter (m)
Defined as 1,650,763.73 wavelengths of an isotope of the element krypton (Kr-86).
$$1 \text{ m} = 3.28 \text{ ft} = 39.37 \text{ in.}$$
$$1 \text{ in.} = 2.54 \text{ cm}$$
$$1 \text{ km} = 0.6214 \text{ mile}$$

2. **mass** kilogram (kg)
Defined as the mass of a platinum iridium cylinder preserved in Sevres, France.
$$1 \text{ kg} = 2.2 \text{ lb}$$

Derived

area (m²)
Two-dimensional measure of length.
$$1 \text{ m}^2 = 1 \text{ centare (ca)} = 10.76 \text{ ft}^2$$
$$1 \text{ hectare (10,000 ca)} = 2.471 \text{ acres}$$

volume (m³)
Three-dimensional measure of length. Although not an SI unit of measurement, volume is often measured in liters (L) where
$$1 \text{ mL H}_2\text{O} = 1 \text{ cm}^3$$
$$1 \text{ L} = 1.057 \text{ qt}$$

density (kg/m³)
Mass per unit volume.

force newton (N)
One newton is a force that accelerates a 1-kg mass at a rate of $1 \text{ m} \cdot \text{s}^{-2}$.
$$1 \text{ N} = 1 \text{ kg} \cdot \text{m} \cdot \text{s}^{-2}$$
$$1 \text{ kg} = 9.81 \text{ N}$$
$$1 \text{ lb} = 4.45 \text{ N}$$

impulse (N·s)
The application of a force over a period of time; the area under a force-time curve.

moment of inertia ($kg \cdot m^2$)
The resistance of an object to a change in its state of angular motion; a measure of the proximity of the mass of an object to an axis of rotation.

power watt (W)
The rate of performing work.
$$1 \text{ W} = 1 \text{ J} \cdot s^{-1}$$

pressure pascal (Pa)
The force applied per unit area.
$$1 \text{ Pa} = 1 \text{ N} \cdot m^{-2}$$

torque ($N \cdot m$)
The rotary effect of a force; synonymous with moment of force.

work, energy joule (J)
Work refers to the application of a force over a distance, and energy denotes the capacity to perform work.
$$1 \text{ J} = 1 \text{ N} \cdot m$$

3. **time** second (s)
Defined in terms of one characteristic frequency of a *cesium clock* (9,192,631,770 cycles of the radiation associated with a specified transition of the cesium-133 atom).

acceleration ($m \cdot s^{-2}$)
Time rate of change in velocity.

frequency hertz (Hz)
The number of cycles per second.
$$1 \text{ Hz} = 1 \text{ cycle} \cdot s^{-1}$$

momentum ($kg \cdot m \cdot s^{-1}$)
Quantity of motion.

speed, velocity ($m \cdot s^{-1}$)
Time rate of change in position, where speed refers to the size of the change and velocity indicates its size and direction.

4. **electric current** ampere (A)
Rate of flow of charged particles.

capacitance farad (F)
The property of an electrical system of conductors and insulators that enables it to store electric charge when a potential difference exists between the conductors.

conductance mho (℧)
The reciprocal of resistance, thus the ease with which charged particles move through an object.

resistance ohm (Ω)
The difficulty with which charged particles flow through an object.

voltage volt (V)
The difference in net distribution of charged particles between two locations.

5. **temperature** kelvin (K)
A measure of the velocity of vibration of the molecules of a body. 100 K from ice point to steam point.
0 K = absolute zero

celsius (°C)
$$0 \text{ °C} = 273.15 \text{ K}$$
Fahrenheit (°F)
$$32 \text{ °F} = 0 \text{ °C} = 273.15 \text{ K}$$
$$\text{°F} = 9/5 \text{ °C} + 32$$

6. **amount of substance** mole (mol)
That amount of a substance containing the same number of particles as there are in 12 g (1 mol) of the nuclide ^{12}C.

concentration (mol•m^{-3})
Amount of substance per unit volume.

7. **luminous intensity** candela (cd)
The luminous intensity of 1/600,00 of 1 m^2 of a blackbody at the temperature of freezing platinum (2,045 K).

lumen (lm)
Measure of light flux.

Supplementary unit

8. **angle** radian (rad)
Measurement of an angle in a plane (i.e., two-dimensional angle).
$$1 \text{ rad} = 57.3 \text{ degrees}$$
Theta (θ) equals one radian when the radius (r) and arc (a) are equal.

steradian (sr)
Three-dimensional angle, also known as a solid angle.

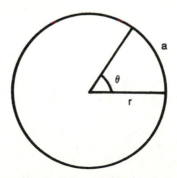

Figure A.1. Definition of a radian.

It is preferable for numbers to range from 0.1 to 9,999. Prefixes (Table A.1) can be attached to the units of measurement to represent a smaller or larger amount of the unit. For example, as indicated above, the SI unit for length is the meter (m). The average height of U.S. adult males is about 1.73 m. To express large distances (e.g., marathon—26 mi, 385 yd), it is more convenient to refer to thousands of meters. The prefix kilo (k) represents 1,000; thus, 1 km = 1,000 m. A marathon race, therefore, covers a distance of approximately 42.2 km. Similarly, prefixes referring to parts of a meter can be used for small distances. For example, there are 1,000 millimeters (mm) in one meter (1 mm = 0.001 m).

Table A.1 Common Prefixes Used With SI Units of Measurement

Prefix	Abbreviation	Multiplication factor
tera	T	$1,000,000,000,000 = 10^{12}$
giga	G	$1,000,000,000 = 10^{9}$
mega	M	$1,000,000 = 10^{6}$
kilo	k	$1,000 = 10^{3}$
hecto	h	$100 = 10^{2}$
deci	d	$0.1 = 10^{-1}$
centi	c	$0.01 = 10^{-2}$
milli	m	$0.001 = 10^{-3}$
micro	μ	$0.000,001 = 10^{-6}$
nano	n	$0.000,000,001 = 10^{-9}$
pico	p	$0.000,000,000,001 = 10^{-12}$

Problems

Convert the following measurements to SI units as indicated:

	SI Unit
1. The weight of a 143-lb individual.	newton
2. A 1,300-sq-ft house on a quarter-acre lot.	square meter, hectare
3. One quart of milk.	liter
4. The mass of a 2-ton truck.	kilogram
5. A gap of 5 Å (angstroms).	meter
6. The highway speed limit of 65 mph.	meters/second
7. A 1-1/2 twisting, double forward somersault.	radian
8. The 186,281 mi/s for the speed of light.	meters/second
9. An athlete generating 1/4 hp (horsepower).	watt
10. A creature traveling at 2.5 furlongs/fortnight.	meters/second

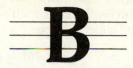

Basic Mathematics

Arithmetic

A. Fractions

A ratio between two quantities, such as 3/4, in which the numerator (3) is divided by the denominator (4), is referred to as a *fraction*. A similar result would be obtained by multiplying the numerator by the inverse of the denominator, the expression becoming

$$3/4 = 3 \times 4^{-1} = 0.75$$

1. Multiplication: Multiply both the number and units of measurement of all numerators together, and place the product over the result obtained with the denominators.

$$60 \text{ kg} \times \frac{16 \text{ m}}{2 \text{ s}} = \frac{60 \times 16 \text{ kg} \cdot \text{m}}{2 \text{ s}}$$
$$= 480 \frac{\text{kg} \cdot \text{m}}{\text{s}}$$
$$= 480 \text{ kg} \cdot \text{m} \cdot \text{s}^{-1} \quad (\text{kg} \cdot \text{m/s})$$

2. Division: Invert the dividing fraction and multiply as above.

$$480 \frac{\text{kg} \cdot \text{m}}{\text{s}} \times \frac{16 \text{ m}}{2 \text{ s}} = 480 \frac{\text{kg} \cdot \text{m}}{\text{s}} \times \frac{2 \text{ s}}{16 \text{ m}}$$
$$= \frac{480 \times 2 \text{ kg} \cdot \text{m} \cdot \text{s}}{16 \text{ m} \cdot \text{s}}$$
$$= 60 \text{ kg}$$

3. Addition and subtraction: Establish a common denominator into which the denomintor of all fractions will divide, multiply the numerator for each fraction by the appropriate factor, then perform the addition and subtraction.

$$\frac{76 \text{ N}}{1 \text{ s}} - \frac{12 \text{ N}}{0.5 \text{ s}} + \frac{3 \text{ N}}{3 \text{ s}} = \frac{(3 \times 76) - (12 \times 6) + (3 \times 1)}{3 \text{ s}} \text{ N}$$

$$= \frac{228 - 72 + 3}{3} \frac{\text{N}}{\text{s}}$$

$$= \frac{159}{3} \frac{\text{N}}{\text{s}}$$

$$= 53 \frac{\text{N}}{\text{s}}$$

$$= 53 \text{ N} \cdot \text{s}^{-1} \quad (\text{N/s})$$

4. Percent: To convert fractions to percentages, divide the numerator by the denominator and multiply by 100.

$$\frac{0.4 \text{ m}}{1.3 \text{ m}} = 0.4 \times 1.3^{-1} \times 100$$

$$= 31\%$$

In this procedure, the units of measurement cancel and the result (31%) is described as dimensionless (i.e., unitless).

B. Equations

An expression of the equality of two sets of relationships is known as an equation. Often the relations will include one or several quantities whose values are unknown. To determine these values, it is necessary to rearrange the equation to isolate the unknown quantity on one side of the equation. For example, to find d:

$$(100 \times d) - (50/2.5) + 37 = (16 \times 9)$$
$$(100 \times d) - (50/2.5) + (50/2.5) + 37 = (16 \times 9) + (50/2.5)$$
$$(100 \times d) + 37 = (16 \times 9) + (50/2.5)$$
$$(100 \times d) + 37 - 37 = (16 \times 9) + (50/2.5) - 37$$
$$(100 \times d) = (16 \times 9) + (50/2.5) - 37$$
$$(100 \times d)/100 = (16 \times 9) + (50/2.5) - 37 \,/100$$
$$d = (16 \times 9) + (50/2.5) - 37 \,/100$$

Circles

a = arc length
r = radius

$$D = \text{diameter} = 2\,r$$
$$\pi = \text{pi} = \text{ratio of circumference to diameter}$$
$$= 3.1415926 \ldots$$
$$C = \text{circumference} = 2\,\pi\,r$$
$$A = \text{area} = C^2/4\,\pi = \pi\,r^2$$
$$\theta = \text{angle}$$

When $a = r$, $\theta = 1$ rad (57.3 degrees); $2\,\pi$ rad = 360 degrees. Since a radian is defined as a ratio, it is dimensionless.

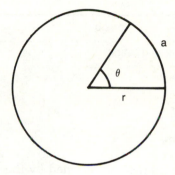

Figure B.1. Characteristics of a circle.

Trigonometry

Trigonometry is a branch of mathematics dealing primarily with relations among the sides and angles of a triangle (*tri* = three, *gonia* = angle, *metria* = measure).

A. Right Triangle

Most problems in motion analysis involve the use of right triangles, which are triangles containing internal right angles (1.57 rad, 90 degrees).

$$A = \text{right angle}$$
$$a = \text{hypotenuse (longest side; opposite right angle)}$$
$$B + C = A = 1.57 \text{ rad (90 degrees)}$$
$$a^2 = b^2 + c^2 \text{ (Pythagorean relationship)}$$
$$\text{area} = 1/2\,bc$$
$$h = \frac{bc}{a} \qquad m = \frac{c^2}{a} \qquad n = \frac{b^2}{a}$$

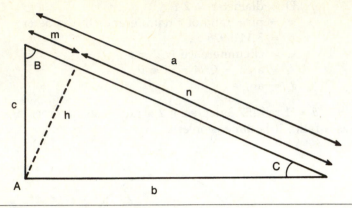

Figure B.2. Features of a right triangle.

B. Trigonometric Functions

The angles within a right triangle are defined by the ratios of the sides of the triangle. That is,

$$\text{sine} = \frac{\text{opposite side}}{\text{hypotenuse}} \qquad \sin B = \frac{b}{a} \qquad \sin C = \frac{c}{a}$$

$$\text{cosine} = \frac{\text{adjacent side}}{\text{hypotenuse}} \qquad \cos B = \frac{c}{a} \qquad \cos C = \frac{b}{a}$$

$$\text{tangent} = \frac{\text{opposite side}}{\text{adjacent side}} \qquad \tan B = \frac{b}{c} \qquad \tan C = \frac{c}{b}$$

where B and C represent the angles and a, b, and c the sides of the triangle (above).

C. Examples

1. Find θ:

$$\theta = 3.14 - (1.57 + 0.90)$$
$$\theta = 0.67 \text{ rad}$$

Find b:

$$\sin 0.9 = b/5 \qquad\qquad \cos \theta = b/5$$
$$b = 5 \sin 0.9 \qquad\qquad b = 5 \cos 0.67$$
$$= 3.92 \text{ cm} \qquad\qquad = 3.92 \text{ cm}$$

Find a:

$$\sin \theta = a/5 \qquad\qquad \cos 0.9 = a/5$$
$$a = 5 \sin 0.67 \qquad\qquad a = 5 \cos 0.9$$
$$= 3.11 \text{ cm} \qquad\qquad\qquad = 3.11 \text{ cm}$$

Check:

$$\text{hypotenuse} = \sqrt{a^2 + b^2}$$
$$= \sqrt{3.92^2 + 3.11^2}$$
$$= \sqrt{15.37 + 9.67}$$
$$= \sqrt{25.04}$$
$$= 5 \text{ cm}$$

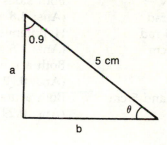

Figure B.3. Example C.1.

2. Find θ:

$$\cos \theta = 3/7$$
$$\theta = \cos^{-1} 3/7 \qquad (\cos^{-1} = \text{arc cos} = \text{angle whose cosine is . . .})$$
$$= \cos^{-1} 0.4286$$
$$\theta = 1.13 \text{ rad}$$

Find d:

$$d^2 = 7^2 - 3^2 \qquad\qquad \sin \theta = d/7$$
$$= 49 - 9 \qquad\qquad\qquad d = 7 \sin 1.13$$
$$d^2 = 40 \qquad\qquad\qquad\qquad = 7 \times 0.9035$$
$$d = 6.32 \text{ N} \qquad\qquad\qquad\quad = 6.32 \text{ N}$$

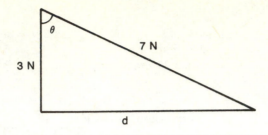

Figure B.4. Example C.2.

D. Problems

Given	Find
1. Hypotenuse = 10 N	Both sides of the triangle
One angle = 0.5 rad	(Ans: 4.8 and 8.8 N)
2. One angle = 0.95 rad	Hypotenuse and adjacent side
Opposite side = 3.5 cm	(Ans: 2.5 and 4.3 cm)
3. Hypotenuse = 4 N	Both acute (less than 1.57 rad) angles
One side = 3 N	(Ans: 0.72 rad, 2.7 N)
4. Sides = 1.5 and 5 cm	Both acute angles and hypotenuse
	(Ans: 0.29 and 1.28 rad, 5.2 cm)

Vectors

A. Characteristics

Quantities that convey both magnitude and direction are called *vectors* (e.g., velocity, acceleration, force, momentum). Those variables that are defined by a magnitude only are called *scalars* (e.g., mass, length, speed, time, temperature). Vectors can be represented graphically as a directed line segment (i.e., as arrows). The length of the arrow specifies the magnitude of the vector, and its direction is indicated by a line of action and a sense (direction of arrowhead).

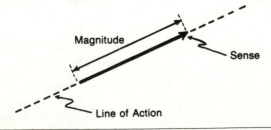

Figure B.5. Features of a vector.

B. Force Parallelogram Law

Two forces (F_p and F_q) acting on an object can be replaced by their resultant (F_r), which is obtained as the diagonal on the parallelogram having F_p and F_q as sides. By definition, the opposite sides of a parallelogram are parallel to one another and, therefore, have the same length.

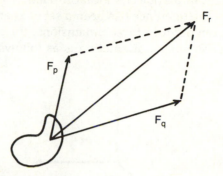

Figure B.6. A force parallelogram.

The replacement of a force system (two or more forces) by a single resultant force is called the **composition** of a force system. Alternatively, the term **resolution** refers to the substitution of a given force by two or more components.

As an example of these procedures, suppose the runner depicted in Figure 2.3C experiences the following ground reaction force components:

vertical (R_z)	812 N	(positive = upward)
forward-backward (R_y)	−286 N	(positive = forward)
side to side (R_x)	61 N	(positive = lateral)

a. Draw a diagram of the two components and the resultant force in each of the sagittal (divides body into left and right), frontal (divides body into front and back), and horizontal (divides body into upper and lower) planes.
b. Calculate the magnitude and direction for each of these resultants. (Ans: sagittal = 861 N, frontal = 814 N, horizontal = 292 N)
c. Use the Pythagorean relationship to determine the magnitude of the resultant (R_g) ground reaction force ($R_g = \sqrt{R_x + R_y + R_z}$). (Ans: R_g = 863 N)

C. Vector Algebra

In the analysis of biomechanical systems, there are usually many vector quantities that need to be considered. To be able to do this, it is necessary to manipulate vectors with rigorous techniques. This section on vector algebra introduces some of the more basic elements of these procedures.

1. Right-hand coordinate system
   Throughout the text, it has been emphasized that movement and its associated mechanics are relative phenomena. For example, changes in position are noted as a shift in an object's location relative to some reference. In the simplest case, the reference has been a set of x- and y-axes. However, since movement can occur in three dimensions, the standard reference is a set of xyz-axes. The usual orientation is as follows:

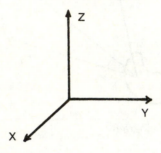

Figure B.7.   Right-hand coordinate system.

If you take your right hand and curl your fingers in the direction of rotating the positive x-axis onto the positive y-axis, then the direction of your extended thumb indicates the positive z-axis. For this reason, this configuration of the xyz-axes is known as the right-hand coordinate system.

Vector quantities can be related to the right-hand coordinate system by saying that the direction of a specific vector quantity is so many units in the x-direction, so many in the y-direction, and so many in the z-direction. This idea has been abbreviated with the use of the terminology **i**, **j**, and **k**. These are known as unit vectors; **i** represents the x-direction, **j** refers to the y-direction, and **k** indicates the z-direction.

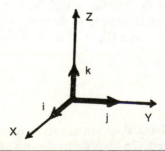

Figure B.8.   Relationship between unit vectors and the right-hand coordinate system.

Suppose a vector were described by the expression $61\mathbf{i} - 286\mathbf{j} + 812\mathbf{k}$. This would mean its direction would be 61 units in the x-direction, 286 units in the negative y-direction, and 812 units in the z-direction. The magnitude of the vector could be determined with the Pythagorean theorem:

$$\mathbf{R}_g = \sqrt{61^2 + (-286)^2 + 812^2}$$

You should recognize this as the resultant ground reaction force discussed under "vectors" (B.) above.

2. Scalar product

When describing physical systems and the interaction of their various components, we often have to manipulate vector quantities in algebraic expressions. The addition and subtraction of vectors is a simple procedure in that we add or subtract the $\mathbf{i}$, $\mathbf{j}$, and $\mathbf{k}$ terms separately. For example, consider the addition of

$$\mathbf{F}_p = 10\mathbf{i} + 28\mathbf{j} + 92\mathbf{k} \text{ and } \mathbf{F}_q = 3\mathbf{i} - 11\mathbf{j} + 46\mathbf{k}$$
$$\mathbf{F}_p + \mathbf{F}_q = (10 + 3)\mathbf{i} + (28 - 11)\mathbf{j} + (92 + 46)\mathbf{k}$$
$$= 13\mathbf{i} + 17\mathbf{j} + 138\mathbf{k}$$

Multiplication, however, is a more involved procedure. In fact, there are two procedures, scalar products and vector products. (Actually the procedures are more commonly known as dot and cross products, but the terms *scalar* and *vector* seem more appropriate for an overview of these techniques.) The distinction between the two procedures, scalar (dot) and vector (cross) products, has to do with the character of the result, that is, whether it is a scalar or a vector quantity.

The definition of a scalar product is given by the expression

$$\mathbf{d} \cdot \mathbf{F} = dF \cos \theta$$

The dot product (notice the dot between $\mathbf{d}$ and $\mathbf{F}$) of the two vectors $\mathbf{d}$ and $\mathbf{F}$ is calculated as the magnitude of $\mathbf{d}$ (d) times the magnitude of $\mathbf{F}$ (F) times the cosine of the angle (θ) between the two vectors. Pictorially, this appears as in Figure B.9A.

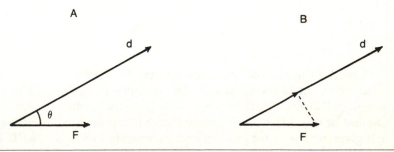

Figure B.9. The scalar product. The product involves determining how much of $\mathbf{F}$ (A) acts in the same direction as $\mathbf{d}$ (B).

This gives the magnitude of **F** that is directed along **d** multiplied by the magnitude of d. The magnitude of **F** directed along d is shown in Figure B.9B as the base of the right triangle (i.e., the side that equals **F** cos θ). Thus the scalar product is just **d** times **F** cos θ.

The multiplication of vectors with the scalar product is appropriate for the calculation of scalar quantities. One example is the calculation of work, where work is defined as the product of force and displacement (distance). Both force and displacement are vectors. The rigorous definition of work (a scalar quantity derived by the scalar product) is that it equals the component of force in the direction of the displacement times the displacement.

3. Vector product

Alternatively, when the result of vector multiplication is a vector quantity, then it is appropriate to use the technique for determining the vector (cross) product. In other words, when we are interested in multiplying two vectors together and we want to consider both magnitude and direction, then we use the vector product. This is given by the expression

$$\mathbf{r} \times \mathbf{F} = rF \sin \theta$$

which reads as **r** cross **F** is equal to the magnitude of **r** (r) times the magnitude of **F** (F) times the sine of the angle (θ) between the two vectors. In this instance, the direction of the product is perpendicular to the plane that contains the other two vectors. This relationship is illustrated in Figure B.10.

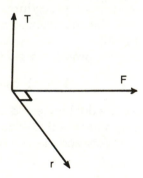

Figure B.10.   The vector product of **r** and **F** is the vector **T**.

Consider the example in which a force (**F**) acts on a system that is constrained to rotate about an axis. The distance from this axis to the line of action of **F** is given by the vector **r**—we have called the perpendicular component of this distance the moment arm (chapter 2). The product of **r** and **F** is given by the vector product and is shown in Figure B.10 as **T**. We recognize this product as the torque. That is, torque is equal to the product of force and moment arm. What is important here, however, is that the product (torque, **T**) is a vector whose direction is perpendicular to the plane in which **r** and **F** lie. For example, if a net muscle force and the moment arm from the force vector to the joint were located in the plane of this page, then the direction of the net muscle torque vector would be perpendicular to the page. The actual sense of the vector (Figure B.5) could be either toward or away from you and would depend on the directions of **r** and **F**.

There are several ways to determine the direction, including the sense, of a vector product. The most rigorous approach is to manipulate vectors in terms of their **i**, **j**, and **k** components. These procedures are beyond the scope of this text but are explained simply and well by Miller and Nelson (1973; Appendix B). Alternatively, we have opted for a more qualitative procedure that is commonly known as the right-hand thumb rule. As described in chapter 2 for determining the direction of torque vectors, the fingers of the right hand are curled in the direction of the rotation that the force produces about the axis, and the extended thumb indicates the direction of the associated torque vector.

APPENDIX
C

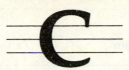

Natural Trigonometric Functions

Angle (rad)	Angle (deg)	Sin	Tan	Cot	Cos
.00	.0	.0000	.0000	—	1.0000
.01	.6	.0100	.0100	99.997	.9999
.02	1.1	.0200	.0200	49.993	.9998
.03	1.7	.0300	.0300	33.323	.9995
.04	2.3	.0399	.0400	24.987	.9992
.05	2.9	.0499	.0500	19.983	.9987
.06	3.4	.0599	.0600	16.647	.9982
.07	4.0	.0699	.0700	14.262	.9975
.08	4.6	.0799	.0801	12.473	.9968
.09	5.2	.0898	.0902	11.081	.9959
.10	5.7	.0998	.1003	9.966	.9950
.11	6.3	.1097	.1104	9.054	.9939
.12	6.9	.1197	.1205	8.293	.9928
.13	7.4	.1296	.1307	7.648	.9915
.14	8.0	.1395	.1409	7.096	.9902
.15	8.6	.1494	.1511	6.616	.9887
.16	9.2	.1593	.1613	6.196	.9872
.17	9.7	.1691	.1716	5.825	.9855

Angle (rad)	Angle (deg)	Sin	Tan	Cot	Cos

Angle (rad)	(deg)	Sin	Tan	Cot	Cos
.18	10.3	.1790	.1819	5.495	.9838
.19	10.9	.1888	.1923	5.199	.9820
.20	11.5	.1986	.2027	4.933	.9800
.21	12.0	.2084	.2131	4.691	.9780
.22	12.6	.2182	.2236	4.471	.9759
.23	13.2	.2279	.2341	4.270	.9736
.24	13.8	.2377	.2447	4.086	.9713
.25	14.3	.2474	.2553	3.916	.9689
.26	14.9	.2570	.2660	3.759	.9663
.27	15.5	.2667	.2767	3.613	.9637
.28	16.0	.2763	.2875	3.477	.9610
.29	16.6	.2859	.2984	3.351	.9582
.30	17.2	.2955	.3093	3.232	.9553
.31	17.8	.3050	.3203	3.121	.9523
.32	18.3	.3145	.3313	3.017	.9492
.33	18.9	.3240	.3425	2.919	.9460
.34	19.5	.3334	.3537	2.827	.9427
.35	20.1	.3429	.3650	2.739	.9393
.36	20.6	.3522	.3764	2.656	.9359
.37	21.2	.3616	.3878	2.578	.9323
.38	21.8	.3709	.3994	2.503	.9286
.39	22.3	.3801	.4110	2.432	.9249
.40	22.9	.3894	.4227	2.365	.9210
.41	23.5	.3986	.4346	2.300	.9171
.42	24.1	.4077	.4465	2.239	.9130
.43	24.6	.4168	.4586	2.180	.9089
.44	25.2	.4259	.4707	2.124	.9047
.45	25.8	.4349	.4830	2.070	.9004
.46	26.4	.4439	.4954	2.018	.8960
.47	26.9	.4528	.5079	1.968	.8915
.48	27.5	.4617	.5206	1.920	.8869
.49	28.1	.4706	.5333	1.874	.8823
.50	28.6	.4794	.5463	1.830	.8775
.51	29.2	.4881	.5593	1.787	.8727
.52	29.8	.4968	.5725	1.746	.8678
.53	30.4	.5055	.5859	1.706	.8628

Angle (rad)	(deg)	Sin	Tan	Cot	Cos

Angle (rad)	Angle (deg)	Sin	Tan	Cot	Cos
.54	30.9	.5141	.5994	1.668	.8577
.55	31.5	.5226	.6131	1.631	.8525
.56	32.1	.5311	.6269	1.595	.8472
.57	32.7	.5396	.6409	1.560	.8419
.58	33.2	.5480	.6551	1.526	.8364
.59	33.8	.5563	.6695	1.493	.8309
.60	34.4	.5646	.6841	1.461	.8253
.61	35.0	.5728	.6989	1.430	.8196
.62	35.5	.5810	.7139	1.400	.8138
.63	36.1	.5891	.7291	1.371	.8080
.64	36.7	.5972	.7445	1.343	.8021
.65	37.2	.6051	.7602	1.315	.7960
.66	37.8	.6131	.7761	1.288	.7899
.67	38.4	.6209	.7922	1.262	.7838
.68	39.0	.6287	.8086	1.236	.7775
.69	39.5	.6365	.8253	1.211	.7712
.70	40.1	.6442	.8422	1.187	.7648
.71	40.7	.6518	.8595	1.163	.7583
.72	41.3	.6593	.8770	1.140	.7518
.73	41.8	.6668	.8949	1.117	.7451
.74	42.4	.6742	.9130	1.095	.7384
.75	43.0	.6816	.9316	1.073	.7316
.76	43.5	.6889	.9504	1.052	.7248
.77	44.1	.6961	.9696	1.031	.7179
.78	44.7	.7032	.9892	1.010	.7109
.79	45.3	.7103	1.0092	.9908	.7038
.80	45.8	.7173	1.0296	.9712	.6967
.81	46.4	.7242	1.0505	.9519	.6895
.82	47.0	.7311	1.0717	.9330	.6822
.83	47.6	.7379	1.0934	.9145	.6748
.84	48.1	.7446	1.1156	.8963	.6674
.85	48.7	.7512	1.1383	.8784	.6599
.86	49.3	.7578	1.1616	.8609	.6524
.87	49.8	.7643	1.1853	.8436	.6448
.88	50.4	.7707	1.2097	.8266	.6371
.89	51.0	.7770	1.2346	.8099	.6294

Angle (rad)	Angle (deg)	Sin	Tan	Cot	Cos

Angle (rad)	(deg)	Sin	Tan	Cot	Cos
.90	51.6	.7833	1.2602	.7935	.6216
.91	52.1	.7895	1.2864	.7773	.6137
.92	52.7	.7956	1.3133	.7614	.6058
.93	53.3	.8016	1.3409	.7457	.5978
.94	53.9	.8075	1.3692	.7303	.5897
.95	54.4	.8134	1.3984	.7151	.5816
.96	55.0	.8191	1.4284	.7001	.5735
.97	55.6	.8248	1.4592	.6853	.5653
.98	56.1	.8305	1.4910	.6707	.5570
.99	56.7	.8360	1.5237	.6563	.5486
1.00	57.3	.8414	1.5574	.6420	.5403
1.01	57.9	.8468	1.5922	.6280	.5318
1.02	58.4	.8521	1.6281	.6142	.5233
1.03	59.0	.8573	1.6652	.6005	.5148
1.04	59.6	.8624	1.7036	.5869	.5062
1.05	60.2	.8674	1.7433	.5736	.4975
1.06	60.7	.8723	1.7844	.5604	.4888
1.07	61.3	.8772	1.8270	.5473	.4801
1.08	61.9	.8819	1.8712	.5344	.4713
1.09	62.5	.8866	1.9171	.5216	.4624
1.10	63.0	.8912	1.9648	.5089	.4536
1.11	63.6	.8957	2.0143	.4964	.4446
1.12	64.2	.9001	2.0660	.4840	.4356
1.13	64.7	.9044	2.1198	.4717	.4266
1.14	65.3	.9086	2.1759	.4595	.4175
1.15	65.9	.9127	2.2345	.4475	.4084
1.16	66.5	.9168	2.2958	.4355	.3993
1.17	67.0	.9207	2.3600	.4237	.3901
1.18	67.6	.9246	2.4273	.4119	.3809
1.19	68.2	.9283	2.4979	.4003	.3716
1.20	68.8	.9320	2.5722	.3887	.3623
1.21	69.3	.9356	2.6503	.3773	.3530
1.22	69.9	.9391	2.7328	.3659	.3436
1.23	70.5	.9424	2.8198	.3546	.3342

Angle (rad)	(deg)	Sin	Tan	Cot	Cos

Angle (rad)	Angle (deg)	Sin	Tan	Cot	Cos
1.24	71.0	.9457	2.9110	.3434	.3248
1.25	71.6	.9489	3.0096	.3322	.3153
1.26	72.2	.9520	3.1133	.3212	.3058
1.27	72.8	.9551	3.2236	.3102	.2962
1.28	73.3	.9580	3.3413	.2992	.2867
1.29	73.9	.9608	3.4672	.2884	.2771
1.30	74.5	.9635	3.6021	.2776	.2675
1.31	75.1	.9661	3.7471	.2668	.2578
1.32	75.6	.9687	3.9033	.2561	.2481
1.33	76.2	.9711	4.0723	.2455	.2384
1.34	76.8	.9734	4.2556	.2349	.2287
1.35	77.3	.9757	4.4552	.2244	.2109
1.36	77.9	.9778	4.6734	.2139	.2092
1.37	78.5	.9799	4.9131	.2035	.1994
1.38	79.1	.9818	5.1774	.1931	.1896
1.39	79.6	.9837	5.4707	.1827	.1798
1.40	80.2	.9854	5.7979	.1724	.1699
1.41	80.8	.9871	6.1654	.1622	.1601
1.42	81.4	.9886	6.5811	.1519	.1502
1.43	81.9	.9901	7.0555	.1417	.1403
1.44	82.5	.9914	7.6018	.1315	.1304
1.45	83.1	.9927	8.2381	.1213	.1205
1.46	83.7	.9938	8.9886	.1112	.1105
1.47	84.2	.9949	9.8874	.1011	.1006
1.48	84.8	.9958	10.983	.0910	.0906
1.49	85.4	.9967	12.350	.0809	.0807
1.50	85.9	.9974	14.101	.0709	.0707
1.51	86.5	.9981	16.428	.0608	.0607
1.52	87.1	.9987	19.670	.0508	.0507
1.53	87.7	.9991	24.498	.0408	.0407
1.54	88.2	.9995	32.461	.0308	.0307
1.55	88.8	.9997	48.078	.0208	.0207
1.56	89.4	.9999	92.620	.0108	.0108
1.57	90.0	1.0000	1255.8	.0008	.0008
Angle (rad)	Angle (deg)	Sin	Tan	Cot	Cos

APPENDIX

D

Body Segments

The distinction between the 14 body segments as used by Chandler et al. (1975): head, trunk, upper arm, forearm, hand, thigh, shank (or leg), foot (see Figure D.1).

The distinction between the 16 body segments used by Zatsiorsky and Seluyanov (1983): head, upper torso, middle torso, lower torso, upper arm, forearm, hand, thigh, shank, foot (see Figure D.2).

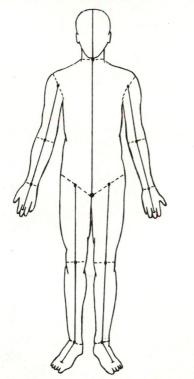

Figure D.1. The body-segment organization used by Chandler et al. (1975).

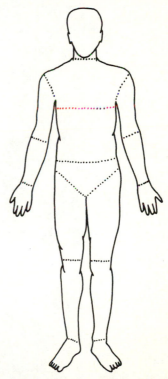

Figure D.2. The body-segment organization used by Zatsiorsky and Seluyanov (1983).

APPENDIX E

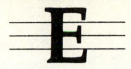

Abbreviations

a	acceleration	F_a	air resistance force
A	projected area; ampere	F actin	fibrous actin
A band	anisotropic	FBD	free-body diagram
ACh	acetylcholine	F_c	centripetal force
AHP	afterhyperpolarization	F_d	drag force
alpha GPD	alpha-glycerophosphate dehydrogenase	F_f	fluid resistance force
		F_g	ground reaction force
AP	action potential	F_i	intraabdominal pressure
ATP	adenosine triphosphate	F_J	joint reaction force
		F_l	lift force
BW	body weight	F_m	muscle force
		F_n	normal component of force
c	centi		
C	chemical energy	F_p	propulsive force
Ca^{++}	calcium ion	FS	footstrike
CC	contractile component	F_t	tangential component of force
cd	candela		
CFS	contralateral footstrike	F_x	force in the x-direction
CG	center of gravity	F_y	force in the y-direction
Cl^-	chloride ion		
cm	centimeter	g	conductance; gram
CT	contraction time	g_{Ca}	calcium conductance
CTO	contralateral takeoff	g_k	potassium conductance
		g_{Na}	sodium conductance
d	deci	G	giga
EMG	electromyogram	G actin	globular actin
EPP	end-plate potential	Group Ia	muscle-spindle afferent
EPSP	excitatory postsynaptic potential	Group Ib	tendon-organ afferent
		h	hecto
F	force; farad	H	heat or thermal energy
$\bar{F}$	average force		

273

H band	Hellerscheibe	PE	potential energy
HMM	heavy meromyosin	PEC	parallel-elastic component
HR	hold-relax		
HR-AC	hold-relax agonist-contraction	PNF	Proprioceptive Neuromuscular Facilitation
Hz	hertz	P_o	isometric force
I	moment of inertia	r	position
I band	isotropic	r_f	final position
IFS	ipsilateral footstrike	r_i	initial position
I_g	moment of inertia about the center of gravity	R	resultant; Renshaw cell
		rad	radian
ITO	ipsilateral takeoff	RCP	Renshaw-cell pool
		Rh	rheobase
J	joule	RM	repetition maximum
k	proportionality constant; kilo	RMP	resting membrane potential
K	Kelvin	R_N	input resistance
K^+	potassium ion	RT	relaxation time
KE	kinetic energy	R_x	side-to-side component of the ground reaction force
kg	kilogram		
L	angular momentum; liter	R_y	forward-backward component of the ground reaction force
lm	lumen		
l_o	resting muscle length		
LMM	light meromyosin	R_z	vertical component of the ground reaction force
LS	lumbosacral joint		
m	meter; mass; milli	s	second
M	moment of force; mega	S1	subfragment 1
MAD	mass-acceleration diagram	S2	subfragment 2
		SDH	succinic dehydrogenase
M band	Mittelscheibe	SEC	series-elastic component
mm	millimeter	SI units	*Le Systeme Internationale d'Unites*
M_o	moment of force about point o		
mol	mole	spII	Group II afferent from a muscle spindle
n	nano		
N	newton	sr	steradian
Na^+	sodium ion	SW	segment weight
NADH-TR	nicotinamide adenine dinucleotide-tetrazolium reductase	t	time
		T	torque; tera
		T_l	load torque
NMJ	neuromuscular junction	T_m	muscle torque
p	momentum; pico	TM	tropomyosin
Pa	pascal	TN	troponin

TN-C	Ca^{++}-binding component of troponin	v_f	final velocity
TN-I	inhibitory component of troponin	v_i	initial velocity
TN-T	tropomyosin-binding component of troponin	V_m	membrane voltage
		v_{max}	maximum velocity of muscle shortening
TO	takeoff		
T tubule	transverse tubule	W	weight; watt
T_w	weight torque	x	side-to-side direction
Type FF	fast-twitch, fatigable motor unit	XB	crossbridge
Type FG	fast-twitch, glycolytic muscle fiber	y	forward-backward direction
Type FOG	fast-twitch, oxidative-glycolytic muscle fiber	z	vertical direction
Type FR	fast-twitch, fatigue-resistant motor unit	Z band	Zwischenscheibe
Type I	slow-twitch muscle fiber	α (alpha)	angular acceleration; skeletomotor neuron
Type II	fast-twitch muscle fiber	β (beta)	angle of pinnation; skeletofusimotor neuron
Type S	slow-contracting motor unit		
Type SO	slow-twitch, oxidative muscle fiber	γ (gamma)	fusimotor motoneuron
		δ (delta)	change in
v	velocity	θ (theta)	angular position
$\bar{v}$	average velocity	μ (mu)	micro
V	volt	π (pi)	3.14 rad
		Σ (sigma)	sum of
		ω (omega)	angular velocity

Problem Answers

To assist students in working some of the problems on their own, selected answers are listed here.

Chapter 1

1.1. 1.73 m

1.2. d

1.3. b

1.4.

Distance	Women m/s	Men m/s
100 m	9.29	10.17
200 m	9.21	10.14
400 m	8.40	9.12
800 m	7.06	7.86
1,500 m	6.45	7.16
1 mi	6.27	7.11
3,000 m	5.97	6.64
5,000 m	5.70	6.42
10,000 m	5.51	6.12
Marathon	4.89	5.53

1.7. d

1.8. b,e

1.9. a. 1.43 s
c. -14.0 m•s^{-1}

1.10. 2.01 m•s^{-2}

1.11. -0.13 m•s^{-2}

1.12. 21.2 m•s^{-1}

1.14. a. -2.46 m•s^{-1}

1.17. a. 6.06 m•s^{-1}
b. -2.08 m•s^{-2}
c. 2.90 m•s^{-2}

1.18. c, e

1.19. B

1.21. horizontal = 16.0 m/s
vertical = 15.8 m/s

1.22. a. 0.43 m
b. 0.18 m

1.23. b. shooter = 1.96 s
defender = 2.49 s

1.24. a. 6.26 m/s
b. 0.64 s
c. 0.32 s
d. 1.5 m

1.25. 192 m/s

Chapter 2

2.1. a,c,d,e

2.2. e

2.3. d

2.4. 678 N, up the midline

2.5. 802.9 N, 0.39 rad

2.6. area, velocity

2.7. 618 N, 0.03 rad to the left of vertical

2.8. normal 165 N
tangential 451 N

2.9.   d

2.12.   271 N, 52%

2.13.   furthest: leg 14.9 cm
closest: forearm 10.4 cm

2.14.   a. 393 N
b. 30 N/cm²
c. 30 N/cm²

2.18.   a. 50 N•m
b. 48 N•m
c. 0
d. −48.3 N•m
e. 0
f. −24.5 N•m

2.19.   569 N•m

Chapter 3

3.1.   a. E = 4 N   F = 9 N
b. H = 100 N   J = 65 N
c. M = 19.1 N   L = 10.9 N
d. S = 1.15 N   T = 3.85 N

3.3.   c

3.4.   185 N and 1.46 kN

3.5.   156 N and normal = 88 N
tangential = 129 N

3.6.   197 N

3.7.   a. 5.6 N•m
b. normal 112 N
tangential 361 N
c. 13.8 cm

3.8.   c,e

3.9.   b,e

3.10.   a. 103.6 N•m
b. knee extensors, less than
103.6 N•m
c. 105 N•m

3.11.   a. 2.76 kg•m•s⁻¹
b. 5.52 kN
c. 14.2 m•s⁻¹

3.12.   43.4 J

3.13.   42.0 m•s⁻¹

3.15.   382 N

3.16.   5069 N

Chapter 4

4.1.   b. rigid link, synovial joint, neuron,
muscle, sensory receptor

4.2.   a. pressure
b. 5.8 kN/cm²

4.4.   b

4.6.   cross-sectional area

4.9.   a

4.14.   c,f

4.16.   b

4.17.   c

4.18.   2,880

4.19.   a

4.20.   a

4.21.   two

4.22.   two

4.23.   d,e

4.24.   c,d

4.25.   a

4.27.   d

4.30.   a. gamma motoneurons
b. Group Ia and II

4.31.   Their cross-sectional area is small
compared to skeletomotor fibers.

4.32.   a. Relationship between magnitudes
of input and output signals.
b. The gain can be changed.
d. No

4.33.   b,e

4.34.   a. 40,000

Chapter 5

5.3.   One-half relaxation time is easier to
measure.

5.4.   121.6 mN

5.5.   Contraction time and fatigability.

5.6.   d

5.7.   0.017 mN

5.8.   FR

5.10. 7.3 mN

5.11. e

5.14. a

5.15. a

5.16. Not in humans

5.21. Ca^{++}, because it inhibits the effect of an inhibitor.

5.22. c

5.24. c

5.27. a

5.30. a

Chapter 6

6.1.   a,c,d,e

6.2.   b,d,e

6.5.   b,d,e

6.7   b. maximum = 5.71 cm
           minimum = 2.86 cm

6.8.   b. No
           c. Muscle force probably does not remain constant due to moment-arm and synergist effects.

6.10. a,c,d

6.11. a. N•m and J, respectively
           b. Potential and kinetic energy.

6.13. b

6.14. a,b

6.16. d

6.17. 15.6 mm

6.18. 8,430 N

Chapter 7

7.1.   a

7.2.   d

7.4.   b,e

7.5.   c. 54.9 N•m

7.6.   b. greatest torque at Position 3
           least torque at Position 1
           c. 69.1 N•m

7.8.   a,b,c,d

7.9.   a. storage and utilization of elastic energy
           preload
           stretch reflex

7.11. d

Chapter 8

8.4.   d

8.5.   a

8.8.   b, e

8.9.   a. N•m
           b. Strength = torque (N•m)
           Rate of torque = $\dfrac{N•m}{s}$ = rate of doing work = power
           c. $\dfrac{N}{m/s} = \dfrac{N•s}{m}$

8.10. Isotonic is a special case of concentric or eccentric (i.e., unequal load and muscle torques) where the muscle force remains constant.

8.14. a,c

8.15. arms by side (12 cm), F_m = 7.42 kN
           arms overhead (18 cm), F_m = 8.25 kN

8.18. a, b, c, d, e

8.19. a. False
           b. No, strength is defined as isometric torque.
           c. Yes

8.23. e

Glossary

A band—anisotropic or dark striation in skeletal muscle due to the double refraction of light rays from a single source.

acceleration—rate of change in velocity with respect to time.

accommodating resistance—a device that can vary the load encountered by a subject to match the torque exerted by the subject.

acetylcholine—a neurotransmitter that is used, among other locations, at the neuromuscular junction.

action potential—an all-or-none, propagated signal of neurons and muscle fibers. Physically, it represents a patch of membrane that contains a transient reversal of the Na+ and K+ ionic distribution.

afferent—sensory.

afterhyperpolarization—a period of hyperpolarization that follows an action potential.

agonist—muscle(s) whose activity causes the movement under consideration.

agonist contract stretch—a stretching technique that involves submaximal activation of a muscle while stretching its antagonist (e.g., contract the quadriceps femoris muscle group while stretching the hamstrings).

alpha motoneuron—a neuron whose axon innervates skeletomotor muscle fibers.

angle-angle diagram—a graph that shows the changes in one angle (y-axis) as a function of another angle (x-axis).

anisometric—the mechanical condition in which the load and muscle torques are not equal.

anode—an attractor of anions, or negatively charged particles, in an electronic circuit. Frequently used to refer to the positive electrode of a stimulating pair.

antagonist—muscle(s) whose action opposes that of the agonist.

anthropometric—measurements of the human body.

articular cartilage—a visoelastic gel reinforced with collagen.

axon—a tubular process that arises from the soma of a neuron and functions as a cable for transmitting the signals generated by the neuron.

ballistic—describes a movement or part of a movement in which the motion of the system is the result of its own momentum and is not due to external forces. Ballistic is often used as a synonym for rapid, but this is incorrect.

Bell-Magendie law—states that axons exiting the spinal cord via the ventral root serve a motor function whereas those entering through the dorsal root perform a sensory function.

beta motoneuron—a neuron whose axon innervates both fusimotor and skeletomotor muscle fibers.

biomechanics—the application of the principles of mechanics to the study of biological systems.

Ca^{++} disinhibition—the inhibition of an inhibitor by Ca^{++}; the mechanism that links a muscle action potential to crossbridge activity.

catch property of muscle—the substantial increase in force (motor-unit or whole-muscle) due to a doublet.

cathode—an attractor of cations, or positively charged particles, in an electronic circuit. Frequently used to refer to the negative electrode of a stimulating pair.

center of gravity—a balance point, a location about which all the particles of the object are evenly distributed based on their mass.

center of pressure—the point of application of the ground reaction force.

central command—the motor output of the high-level controller.

centripetal force—an inward-directed force (toward the axis of rotation) that is responsible for changing linear motion into angular motion.

closed-loop control—the use of sensory feedback signals to provide continuous guidance of a movement.

cocontraction—concurrent activity in an agonist-antagonist set of muscles.

collagen—a molecule that consists of three intertwined polypeptide chains. Each polypeptide chain consists of about 1,000 amino acids (known as an alpha chain) and is found in connective tissue, including skin, bone, ligament, and cartilage.

composition—the process of determining the resultant of several forces.

compressive force—a pushing force.

concentric—the mechanical condition in which the load torque is less than the muscle torque; this is not a type of contraction.

conductance—a property of a membrane that depends on the permeability to an ion and the availability of the ion.

conservation of momentum—a concept stating that when a system is not subjected to an impulse its momentum remains constant.

constant load—a condition during which the load experienced by a system remains constant, both over time and over a range of motion.

contraction—the internal state in which muscle actively exerts a force, regardless of whether it shortens its length.

contraction time—the time from force onset to the peak value of a twitch response.

contralateral—opposite side.

coplanar—confined to the same plane.

crossbridge—the subfragment 1 extension of the myosin molecule. Subfragment 1 represents the globular component of the heavy meromyosin fragment.

cross-sectional area—the area of the end-on view of an object (e.g., muscle) when it has been sectioned (cut) at right angles to its long axis.

degree of freedom of a joint—the number of axes about which a joint can rotate.

demineralization—the excessive loss of salts from the skeleton.

dendrite—a process, other than the axon, that extends from the soma of a neuron.

depolarization—a reduction in the polarity (potential) across the membrane.

derecruitment—the inactivation of a motor unit.

dipole—a pair, consisting of an anode and a cathode, separated by some specified physical distance across which current flows.

displacement—a change in position.

doublet—a sequential pair of action potentials separated by an interval of about 10 ms.

drag—the component of the fluid-resistance vector that acts parallel to the direction of fluid flow.

dynamic—a mechanical state in which a system experiences an acceleration.

eccentric—the mechanical condition in which the load torque is greater than the muscle torque; this is not a type of contraction.

economy—the minimum use of energy to perform a task.

efference copy—a copy of the central command issued by the high-level controller that is routed back to various elements of the high-level controller (supraspinal centers).

efferent—motor.

efficiency—the relationship between work output and energy input; often confused with economy.

elastic force—the passive property of a stretched material that tends to return it toward its original length.

electrical potential—voltage.

electromyogram—an extracellular record of changes in sarcolemmal voltage that are associated with the propagation of muscle action potentials.

electromyostimulation—the stimulation of muscle with an electric current, generally in a rehabilitation setting.

endomysium—connective tissue that surrounds individual muscle fibers.

energy—the capacity to do work.

epimysium—the outer layer of connective tissue that ensheathes an entire muscle.

excitation-contraction coupling—the electrochemical processes involved in converting a muscle action potential into crossbridge activity.

exocytosis—the process of vesicular fusion and subsequent release of neurotransmitter.

exteroreceptor—a sensory receptor that detects selected external stimuli that impinge on the system.

F actin—fibrous actin; a strand of a few hundred G-actin molecules.

fatigue—a progressive increase in the effort required to exert a desired force and the progressive inability to maintain this force during sustained or repeated contractions (i.e., increased effort and force failure).

feedback—signals emanating from various peripheral receptors that serve to report to the nervous system the mechanical events in muscles, joints, and associated tissues.

fibril—the basic load-bearing unit of tendon and ligament that consists of bundles of microfibrils held together by cross-links. The number and state of the cross-links are thought to determine the strength of connective tissue.

final common pathway—an expression characterizing the function of motoneurons as the route by which the nervous system controls muscle activity.

fluid resistance—the resistance that a fluid offers to any object that passes through it. The magnitude of the resistance depends on the physical characteristics of the fluid and the extent to which the motion of the object disturbs the fluid.

force—a mechanical interaction between an object and its surroundings.

free-body diagram—a graphic-analysis technique that defines a system and indicates how the system interacts with its surroundings. A free-body diagram represents a graphic version of the left-hand side of Newton's law of acceleration.

fusimotor muscle fibers—miniature, striated muscle fibers contained within a muscle spindle; these include chain and bag fibers.

G actin—globular actin molecule.

gamma motoneuron—a neuron whose axon innervates fusimotor muscle fibers.

generator potential—the potential that a sensory receptor generates in response to the stimulus to which it is sensitive.

gravity—the force of attraction between and object and a planet. Gravity causes an acceleration of 9.81 m/s² on Earth.

ground reaction force—the reaction force provided by the supporting horizontal surface.

Group Ia afferent—the larger muscle-spindle afferent.

Group Ib afferent—the tendon-organ afferent.

Group II (spII) afferent—the smaller muscle-spindle afferent.

H band—Hellerscheibe; the region of the A band that is devoid of thin filaments.

heavy meromyosin—one fragment, being the head end, of the myosin molecule. This fragment can be further subdivided into subfragments 1 and 2 (S1 and S2).

heteronymous—an anatomical relation between sensory receptors and motoneurons that serve different muscles.

high-level controller—the controlling capabilities of the supraspinal centers.

hold-relax agonist-contract stretch—a stretching technique that includes the hold-relax maneuver and, in addition, a submaximal contraction of the agonist muscles while the target muscle (antagonist) is being stretched.

hold-relax stretch—a stretching technique in which the stretch of a muscle follows a brief, maximum, isometric contraction of the same muscle.

homonymous—an anatomical relation between sensory receptors and motoneurons that serve the same muscle.

hyperplasia—an increase in the number, rather than the cross-sectional area, of muscle fibers.

hyperpolarization—an increase in the polarity of a membrane, characterized by the inside becoming more negative with respect to the outside.

hypertrophy—an increase in the number of myofibrils per muscle fiber.

hypotrophy—progressive degeneration and functional loss of cells and tissues.

Ia inhibitory interneuron—an interneuron that receives excitatory input from Ia afferents and, in turn, exerts an inhibitory effect on other neurons. This interneuron mediates the response known as reciprocal inhibition.

I band—isotropic or light band of skeletal muscle, named for the single refraction of light rays from a single source.

ideation—the generation of an idea.

impulse—the area under a force-time graph; the force-time integral.

inertia—the resistance an object offers to any change in its motion.

inertia force—the product of mass and acceleration.

inertia torque—the product of moment of inertia and angular acceleration.

innervation ratio—the number of muscle fibers innervated by a single axon.

in parallel—arranged side by side.

input resistance—the electrical resistance of a motoneuron to a current input.

in series—arranged end to end.

interneuron—a neuron whose axon is confined to the limits of the spinal cord.

ipsilateral—same side.

isokinetic—a term describing constant angular velocity about a joint.

isometric—the mechanical condition in which the load and muscle torques are equal; this is not a type of contraction.

isotonic—literally, it means constant tension. This condition does not occur in intact human subjects, only in isolated-muscle preparations.

joint reaction force—a concept that accounts for the forces due to bone-on-bone contact between adjacent body segments.

joint receptor—a class of sensory receptors that sense joint-related events.

kinematic—a description of motion in terms of position, velocity, and acceleration.

kinesiology—the study of movement.

kinetic—a description of motion that includes consideration of force as the cause of movement.

kinetic energy—the capacity of an object to perform work because of its motion.

law of acceleration—$F = ma$.

law of action-reaction—the concept that to every action there is an equal and opposite reaction.

law of gravitation—states that all bodies attract one another with a force proportional to the product of their masses and inversely proportional to the square of the distance between them.

law of inertia—the notion that a force is required to start, stop, or alter motion.

lift—the component of the fluid-resistance vector that acts perpendicular to the direction of fluid flow.

light meromyosin—one fragment, being the tail end, of the myosin molecule.

local-graded potential—a nonpropagated excitatory or inhibitory signal of neurons and muscle fibers.

low-level controller—the task-specific controlling capabilities of the spinal cord and brain stem.

magnitude—size.

mass—a measure of the amount of matter comprising an object.

mass-acceleration diagram—a graphic version of the right hand side of Newton's law of acceleration that indicates the kinematic effect of the forces acting on a system.

maxima—the high points or peaks in a graph (e.g., set of position-time data).

M band—Mittelscheibe; intrasarcomere connection of two sets of thick filaments.

meter—the unit measurement of linear motion.

microfibril—an elongated bundle composed of five parallel rows of three-stranded collagen molecules arranged in series.

minima—the low points or valleys in a graph (e.g., set of position-time data).

moment arm—the shortest distance (perpendicular) from the line of action of a force vector to an axis of rotation.

moment of force—the rotary effect of a force; torque.

moment of inertia—the resistance that an object offers to any change in its angular motion.

momentum—the quantity of motion possessed by an object.

motion—a change in position that occurs over an interval of time.

motoneuron—a neuron whose axon connects directly to muscle fibers. Since it represents the final stage in the output from the nervous system and is the only means by which muscle can be activated, the motoneuron is referred to as the final common pathway.

motoneuron excitability—the responsiveness of a motoneuron to its input.

motoneuron pool—a group of motoneurons serving one muscle.

motor control—the study of the execution phase of movement performance.

motor-control strategy—the organization of a central command that will produce the desired pattern of muscle activity.

motor program—the set of commands sent out by the low-level controller for a particular sequence of muscle activity.

motor unit—the cell body and dendrites of a motoneuron, the multiple branches of its axon, and the muscle fibers that it innervates.

muscle—a tissue that contains contractile cells that convert chemical energy into mechanical energy, and that has the properties of irritability, conductivity, contractility, and a limited growth and regenerative capacity.

muscle architecture—the arrangement of the force-generating units in muscle.

muscle mechanics—the study of the mechanical properties of the force-generating units of muscle.

muscle soreness—the pain and tenderness in muscle that occur 24-48 hr after exercise. This soreness appears to be associated with structural damage.

muscle spindle—an intramuscular sensory receptor arranged in parallel with skeletal muscle fibers that monitors changes in muscle length.

muscle tone—clinically, it is defined as the passive resistance that a joint and its associated structures offer to extension. However, some investigators suggest that muscle tone is due to the low-level activation of the contractile machinery.

myelin—a fatty, insulating sheath that, in peripheral nerves, is provided by Schwann cells.

myofibril—a collection of myofilaments.

myofilaments—the thick and thin filaments of a muscle fiber that contain the contractile machinery.

myosin—the major protein comprising the thick filament of muscle fiber; includes the crossbridge.

Na^+-K^+ pump—a membrane-bound protein that transports Na^+ from the intracellular to the extracellular fluid, and K^+ in the reverse direction.

negative feedback—information flow from sensory receptors back to the central nervous system that tends to reduce the stimulus eliciting the input.

negative work—the work done on the system when the load torque exceeds that exerted by muscle; the surroundings perform work on a system.

neuroglia—one of two cell types in the nervous system. They are primarily thought to provide structural, metabolic, and protective support for the neurons.

neuromuscular junction—a synapse between a motoneuron and a muscle fiber; also known as a motor end plate.

neuromuscular transmission—the transformation of an axonal action potential into a muscle action potential.

neuron—one of two cell types in the nervous system; capable of generating and transmitting an electrical signal.

neurotrophism—the sustaining influence that one biological element exerts directly on another.

normal component—a component at right angles to a surface.

one-half relaxation time—the time of decay in a twitch response from peak force to a value one-half of the peak.

open-loop control—the control of movements or responses entirely by the neural command without reference to feedback signals.

orderly recruitment—the phenomenon that describes the organized sequence of motor-unit activation.

orthogonal—perpendicular.

orthograde—in the normal or forward direction.

overlap of myofilaments—interdigitation of the thick and thin filaments that allows the crossbridges to cycle and to exert a force. The greater the overlap, the greater the number of crossbridges that can be formed, and hence the greater the force.

overload principle—in order to increase the size or functional ability of muscle fibers, they must be stressed toward their present capacity to respond.

perimysium—connective tissue that collects bundles of muscle fibers into fascicles.

physiologic cross-sectional area—the measure of muscle cross-sectional area that takes into account muscle-fiber length and the angle of pinnation.

pinnation—the angle of deviation of a muscle fiber from the line of pull of the muscle.

planar—confined to a single plane.

plastic—a change in length of a material that extends beyond its elastic capabilities and causes structural changes within the material.

plyometric—a training technique that involves eccentric-concentric sequences of muscle activity.

P_o—an expression representing the maximum isometric force; from the Latin *potestas* = power to do something.

position—the location of an object relative to some reference.

positive work—the work done by a system when the muscle torque exceeds that due to the load; work done by a system on its surroundings.

posture—a neuromechanical state that concerns the maintenance of equilibrium.

potential energy—an object possesses potential energy when it has had work done on it to counteract the effect of another force.

power—the rate of doing work; the rate of change in energy; the product of force and velocity.

power absorption—the flow of mechanical energy from the surroundings to the system. A system absorbs power when it does negative work.

power production—the flow of mechanical energy from the system to the surroundings. A system produces power when it performs positive work.

preload effect—the increased initial force exerted by muscle that is associated with the eccentric-concentric pattern of muscle activity.

progressive-resistance exercise—an exercise in which the load is increased over repeated performances (repetitions).

projected area—the silhouette that an object presents as it passes through a fluid.

projectile—an object projected or propelled into space.

propagation—the conduction of an action potential by active, regenerative processes that tend to preserve the quantity of the signal.

Proprioceptive Neuromuscular Facilitation—a rehabilitation program for neurologically impaired patients. Its main constituents include maximal resistance activities, stretch, mass movement patterns, facilitation through reflexes, and reversal of antagonists.

proprioceptor—a sensory receptor (e.g., muscle spindle, tendon organ) that can detect stimuli that the system itself generates.

qualitative—describes the type or kind.

quantitative—describes the quantity or how much.

quasistatic—a mechanical state in which the acceleration experienced by a system is small enough to assume that it is zero.

radian—an angle that is represented as the quotient of a distance on the circumference of the circle relative to its radius.

range of motion—the maximum displacement about a joint that does not cause tissue damage.

rate coding—the discharge frequency of action potentials.

reciprocal inhibition—a reflex in which Ia-afferent feedback results, via the Ia inhibitory interneuron, in the relaxation of intra-limb, antagonist muscles.

recruitment—the process of motor-unit activation.

recurrent inhibition—a reflex in which action potentials generated by a motoneuron activate a Renshaw cell, which, in turn, exerts an inhibitory influence on neurons, including the motoneuron that initiated the Renshaw cell activity.

reflex—a phase- and state-dependent, input-output relationship in which the input is a sensory stimulus and the output a motor response.

regression equation—a mathematical expression that allows us to estimate the value of one parameter based upon values for another parameter.

remodeling—the growth, reinforcement, and resorption experienced by living bone.

Renshaw cell—an interneuron that receives excitatory input from collaterals of moto-neuron axons and that, in turn, exerts an inhibitory effect on other neurons.

repolarization—a return of membrane polarity to steady-state conditions.

resolution—the process of breaking a resultant down into several components.

resting membrane potential—the transmembrane voltage during steady-state conditions.

resultant muscle force—the net force exerted by a group of muscles about a joint.

resultant muscle torque—the net torque about a joint due to muscle activity.

retrograde—in the reverse or backward direction.

reversibility principle—a principle stating that training effects are transient.

rheobase—an index of motoneuron excitability.

right-hand thumb rule—a technique for determining the direction of a torque vector. The fingers of the right hand are curled in the direction that the force will cause the system to rotate, and the extended thumb indicates the direction of the associated torque vector.

rotation—motion in which all parts of the system are not displaced by a similar amount.

run—a mode of human gait that contains an interval (swing) when neither foot is in contact with the ground.

safety factor—the margin of safety before failure occurs.

sag—a decline in unfused-tetanic force after an initial four to eight stimuli.

sarcolemma—the excitable plasma membrane of a muscle fiber.

sarcolemmal excitability—the capability of the sarcolemma to propagate muscle action potentials.

sarcomere—the components of a myofibril contained in the region from one Z band to the next. The sarcomere contains all the contractile machinery necessary to convert chemical energy into force.

sarcoplasm—the fluid enclosed within a muscle fiber by the sarcolemma.

sarcoplasmic reticulum—a hollow membranous system within the muscle fiber that bulges into lateral sacs in the vicinity of the transverse tubules.

sense of effort—the task-related perception of effort that is based on the efference copy.

shear force—a side-to-side force.

simple joint system—a biological model comprising five basic elements (rigid link, synovial joint, muscle, neuron, and sensory receptor), which are necessary for the performance of movement.

size principle—a concept that attributes the mechanism underlying orderly, motor-unit recruitment to variations in motoneuron size.

skeletomotor—the skeletal muscle fibers that exert the force associated with muscle activity.

sliding-filament theory—a concept describing the sliding of thick and thin myofilaments past one another during a contraction.

soma—the cell body of a neuron.

specificity principle—the concept that training adaptations are specific to the cells and their structural and functional elements that are overloaded.

specific tension—a measure of force per unit of cross-sectional area.

stance—the support phase during a stride.

static—a mechanical state in which the system is in equilibrium, either remaining stationary or moving at a constant velocity—the system is not accelerating.

step—a part of the human gait cycle from one event (e.g., footstrike) to the same event on the other foot.

storage and utilization of elastic energy—an attribute of muscle that describes its ability to exploit the passive, elastic properties of its elements.

strain—the change in length of material expressed relative to its original length.

strength—the magnitude of the torque exerted by a muscle (or group of muscles) in a single, maximal, isometric contraction of unrestricted duration.

stress—force per unit area.

stretch reflex—the response of muscle to a sudden change in its length (stretch).

stride—one complete cycle of human gait from an event (e.g., left foot takeoff) to the next appearance of the same event. A stride contains two steps.

swing—the nonsupport phase during a stride.

synapse—a unique structure by which a neuron transfers its signals to a target cell.

synchrony—a greater than normal temporal association between the discharge of motor units.

synovial fluid—a clear, lubricating fluid secreted by the synovial membrane of a joint.

synovial joint—a freely movable, encapsulated joint.

synovial membrane—a vascular membrane that secretes synovial fluid into the joint cavity.

tangential component—a component parallel to a surface.

temporal patterning of motor-unit activity—the relationship, in time, between an action potential and other action potentials generated by the same and other motor units.

tendon organ—an intramuscular sensory receptor located at the junction between skeletomotor muscle fibers and an aponeurosis of attachment; arranged in series with skeletal muscle fibers.

tensile force—a pulling force.

terminal velocity—the speed of an object under free-fall conditions when the weight and air-resistance vectors have equal magnitudes.

tetanus—the force response of muscle (single fiber, motor unit, or whole muscle) to a series of excitatory inputs; represents a summation of twitch responses.

three-burst pattern—sequence of agonist-antagonist muscle activity that is associated with a unidirectional movement to a target.

three-component model of muscle—a model of the mechanical characteristics of muscle. The components include parallel-elastic, series-elastic, and contractile elements.

torque—the rotary effect of a force quantified as the product of force and moment arm.

trajectory—the position-time record of a projectile.

transducer—a device for measuring a particular form of energy (e.g., light, heat, pressure).

transduction—a process by which energy is converted from one form to another.

translation—motion in which all parts of the system are displaced by a similar amount.

transverse tubules—invaginations of the sarcolemma that facilitate a rapid communication between sarcolemmal events and myofilaments located deep within the muscle fiber.

tripartite model—a three-compartment model of the neuromuscular processes associated with movement. The compartments include the high-level controller, the low-level controller and muscle, and the peripheral receptors.

tropomyosin—a thin-filament protein involved in regulating the interaction between actin and myosin.

troponin—a three-component molecule that forms part of the thin filament and is involved in the regulation of the interaction between actin and myosin.

twitch—the force response of muscle (single fiber, motor unit, or whole muscle) to a single excitatory input.

Type FF motor unit—fast-contracting, fast-to-fatigue.

Type FG muscle fiber—fast-twitch, glycolytic.

Type FOG muscle fiber—fast-twitch, oxidative-glycolytic.

Type FR motor unit—fast-contracting, fatigue-resistant.

Type I muscle fiber—slow-twitch; low myosin ATPase.

Type II muscle fiber—fast-twitch; high myosin ATPase.

Type S motor unit—slow-contracting, fatigue resistant.

Type SO muscle fiber—slow-twitch, oxidative.

variable load—a load acting on a system that varies over the system's range of motion.

vector—a variable that possesses both magnitude and direction.

velocity—the rate of change in position with respect to time.

vesicle—a neurotransmitter-containing organelle within the axon enlargement of a synapse.

v_{max}—the maximum rate at which a muscle can shorten against a zero load.

voltage-gated—describes a change in membrane conditions that depends on the potential across the membrane.

volume conductor—the weakly conductive saline of physiological fluid.

walk—a mode of human gait in which at least one foot is always in contact with the ground.

weight—an expression of the amount of gravitational attraction between an object and Earth.

Wolff's law—states that all changes in the function of bone are attended by alterations in its internal structure.

work—the area under a force-distance graph. It equals the component of force in the direction of the displacement times the displacement.

Z band—Zwischenscheibe; intrasarcomere connection of the two sets of thin filaments.

References

Abbott, N.J. (1985). Are glial cells excitable after all? *Trends in Neurosciences*, **8**, 141-142.

Abraham, W.M. (1977). Factors in delayed muscle soreness. *Medicine and Science in Sports*, **9**, 11-20.

Alexander, R.M. (1981). Mechanics of skeleton and tendons. In V.B. Brooks (Ed.), *Handbook of physiology: Sec. I. The nervous system: Vol. II. Motor control. Part 1* (pp. 17-42). Bethesda, MD: American Physiological Society.

Alexander, R.M. (1984a). Optimal strengths for bones liable to fatigue and accidental fracture. *Journal of Theoretical Biology*, **109**, 621-636.

Alexander, R.M. (1984b). Walking and running. *American Scientist*, **72**, 348-354.

Alexander, R.M., & Vernon, A. (1975). The dimensions of knee and ankle muscles and the forces they exert. *Journal of Human Movement Studies*, **1**, 115-123.

Amar, J. (1920). *The human motor*. London: G. Routledge & Sons.

American Society of Biomechanics. (1986.) *American Society of Biomechanics.* (Membership pamphlet).

An, K.N., Hui, F.C., Morrey, B.F., Linscheid, R.L., & Chao, E.Y. (1981). Muscles across the elbow joint: A biomechanical analysis. *Journal of Biomechanics*, **14**, 659-669.

Anderson, S.A., & Cohn, S.H. (1985). Bone demineralization during space flight. *Physiologist*, **28**, 212-217.

Andersson, G.B.J., Örtengren, R., & Nachemson, A. (1977). Intradiskal pressure, intra-abdominal pressure and myoelectric back muscle activity related to posture and loading. *Clinical Orthopaedics and Related Research*, **129**, 156-164.

Andrews, J.G. (1982). On the relationship between resultant joint torques and muscular activity. *Medicine and Science in Sports and Exercise*, **14**, 361-367.

Aristotle. (1968). Movement of animals, progression of animals. In E. Forster (Trans.), *Aristotle in twenty-three volumes* (Vol. 12). Cambridge: Harvard University Press. (Part of the Loeb Classical Library series)

Armstrong, R.B. (1984). Mechanisms of exercise-induced delayed onset muscular soreness: A brief review. *Medicine and Science in Sports and Exercise*, **16**, 529-538.

Armstrong, R.B., Ogilvie, R.W., & Schwane, J.A. (1983). Eccentric exercise-induced injury to rat skeletal muscle. *Journal of Applied Physiology*, **54**, 80-93.

Arsenault, A.B., & Chapman, A.E. (1974). An electromyographic investigation of the individual recruitment of the quadriceps muscles during isometric contraction of the knee extensors in different patterns of movement. *Physiotherapy of Canada*, **26**, 253-261.

Asami, T., & Nolte, V. (1983). Analysis of powerful ball kicking. In H. Matsui & K. Kobayashi (Eds.), *Biomechanics VIII-B* (pp. 695-700). Champaign, IL: Human Kinetics.

Ashmore, C.R., & Summers, P.J. (1981). Stretch-induced growth in chicken muscles: Myofibrillar proliferation. *American Journal of Physiology*, **241**, C93-C97.

Atha, J. (1981). Strengthening muscle. In D.I. Miller (Ed.), *Exercise and sport sciences reviews*, (Vol. 9, pp. 1-73). Philadelphia: Franklin Institute.

Atwater, A.E. (1970, April). *Overarm throwing patterns: A kinematographic analysis*. Paper presented at the National Convention of the American Association for Health, Physical Education and Recreation, Seattle, WA.

Atwater, A.E. (1980). Kinesiology/biomechanics: Perspectives and trends. *Research Quarterly for Exercise and Sport*, **51**, 193-218.

Bailey, A.J., Robins, S.P., & Balian, G. (1974). Biological significance of the intermolecular crosslinks of collagen. *Nature*, **251**, 105-109.

Baldissera, F., Hultborn, H., & Illert, M. (1981). Integration in spinal neuronal systems. In V.B. Brooks (Ed.), *Handbook of physiology: Sec. I. The nervous system. Vol. II. Motor control. Part I* (pp. 509-595). Bethesda, MD: American Physiological Society.

Barnard, R.J., Edgerton, V.R., & Peter, J.B. (1970a). Effect of exercise on skeletal muscle I. Biochemical and histochemical properties. *Journal of Applied Physiology*, **28**, 762-766.

Barnard, R.J., Edgerton, V.R., & Peter, J.B. (1970b). Effect of exercise on skeletal muscle II. Contractile properties. *Journal of Applied Physiology*, **28**, 767-770.

Barnes, W.S. (1980). The relationship between maximum isometric strength and intramuscular circulatory occlusion. *Ergonomics*, **23**, 351-357.

Bartee, H., & Dowell, L. (1982). A cinematographical analysis of twisting about the longitudinal axis when performers are free of support. *Journal of Human Movement Studies*, **8**, 41-54.

Basmajian, J.V., & Latif, A. (1957). Integrated actions and functions of the chief flexors of the elbow. *Journal of Bone and Joint Surgery*, **39-A**, 1106-1118.

Bawa, P., & Calancie, B. (1983). Repetitive doublets in human flexor carpi radialis muscle. *Journal of Physiology* (London), **339**, 123-132.

Belanger, A.Y., & McComas, A.J. (1981). Extent of motor unit activation during effort. *Journal of Applied Physiology*, **51**, 1131-1135.

Belen'kii, V.Ye., Gurfinkel', V.S., & Pal'tsev, Ye.I. (1967). Elements of control of voluntary movements. *Biophysics*, **12**, 154-161.

Bergh, U., & Ekblom, B. (1979). Influence of muscle temperature on maximal muscle strength and power output in human skeletal muscles. *Acta Physiologica Scandinavica*, **107**, 33-37.

Bigland, B., & Lippold, O.C.J. (1954). The relation between force, velocity and integrated electrical activity in human muscles. *Journal of Physiology* (London), **123**, 214-224.

Bigland-Ritchie, B. (1984). Muscle fatigue and the influence of changing neural drive. *Clinics in Chest Medicine*, **5**, 21-34.

Bigland-Ritchie, B., Johansson, R., Lippold, O.C.J., Smith, S., & Woods, J.J. (1983). Changes in motoneurone firing rates during sustained maximal voluntary contractions. *Journal of Physiology* (London), **340**, 335-346.

Bigland-Ritchie, B., Dawson, N.J., Johansson, R.S., & Lippold, O.C.J. (1986). Reflex origin for the slowing of motoneurone firing rates in fatigue of human voluntary contractions. *Journal of Physiology* (London), **379**, 451-459.

Binder, M.D., Houk, J.C., Nichols, T.R., Rymer, W.Z., & Stuart, D.G. (1982). Properties and segmental actions of mammalian muscle receptors: An update. *Federation Proceedings*, **41**, 2907-2918.

Binkhorst, R.A., Hoofd, L., & Vissers, A.C.A. (1977). Temperature and force-velocity relationship of human muscles. *Journal of Applied Physiology*, **42**, 471-475.

Bizzi, E., & Abend, W. (1983). Posture control and trajectory formation in single- and multi-joint arm movements. In J.E. Desmedt (Ed.), *Motor control mechanisms in health and disease* (pp. 31-45). New York: Raven.

Blangé, T., Karemaker, J.M., & Kramer, A.E.J.L. (1972). Elasticity as an expression of cross-bridge activity in rat muscle. *Pflügers Archiv*, **336**, 277-288.

Blattner, S.E., & Noble, L. (1979). Relative effects of isokinetic and plyometric training on vertical jumping performance. *Research Quarterly*, **50**, 583-588.

Bloom, W., & Fawcett, D.W. (1968). *A textbook of histology* (9th ed.). Philadelphia: Saunders.

Bodine, S.C., Roy, R.R., Eldred, E., & Edgerton, V.R. (1985). Innervation ratio, fiber size and specific tension of type-identified motor units in the cat tibialis anterior. *Society for Neuroscience Abstracts*, **11**, 211.

Bosco, C., & Komi, P.V. (1980). Influence of aging on the mechanical behavior of leg extensor muscles. *European Journal of Applied Physiology*, **45**, 209-219.

Botterman, B.R., Binder, M.D., & Stuart, D.G. (1978). Functional anatomy of the association between motor units and muscle receptors. *American Zoologist*, **18**, 135-152.

Brancazio, P.J. (1984). *Sport science: Physical laws and optimum performance*. New York: Simon and Schuster.

Brand, R.A. (1986). Knee ligaments: A new view. *Journal of Biomechanical Engineering*, **108**, 106-110.

Brand, R.A., Crowninshield, R.D., Wittstock, C.E., Pedersen, D.R., Clark, C.R., & van Krieken, F.M. (1982). A model of lower extremity muscular anatomy. *Journal of Biomechanical Engineering*, **104**, 304-310.

Braune, W., & Fischer, O. (1889). Uber den Schwerpunkt des menschlichen Korpers mit Rucksicht auf die Ausrustung des deutschen Infanteristen. *Abhandlungen der Mathematisch-Physischen Klasse der Saecksischen Akademie der Wissenschaften*, **26**, 561-672.

Brooke, M.H., & Kaiser, K.K. (1974). The use and abuse of muscle histochemistry. *Annals of the New York Academy of Sciences*, **228**, 121-144.

Brooks, V.B. (1986). *The neural basis of motor control*. New York: Oxford University.

Burke, R.E. (1981). Motor units: Anatomy, physiology, and functional organization. In V.B. Brooks (Ed.), *Handbook of physiology: Sec. I. The nervous system: Vol. II. Motor control. Part 1* (pp. 345-422). Bethesda, MD: American Physiological Society.

Burke, R.E. (1985). Integration of sensory information and motor commands in the spinal cord. In P.S.G. Stein (Organizer), *Motor control: From movement trajectories to neural mechanisms* (pp. 44-66). Class at the Society for Neuroscience, Washington, DC.

Burke, R.E., & Edgerton, V.R. (1975). Motor unit properties and selective involvement in movement. In J.H. Wilmore & J.F. Koegh (Eds.), *Exercise and sport sciences reviews* (Vol. 3, pp. 31-81). New York: Academic.

Burke, R.E., Levine, D.N., Tsairis, P., & Zajac, F.E., III. (1973). Physiological types and histochemical profiles in motor units of the cat gastrocnemius. *Journal of Physiology* (London), **234**, 723-748.

Burke, R.E., Rudomin, P., & Zajac, F.E. III. (1976). The effect of activation history on tension production by individual muscle units. *Brain Research*, **109**, 515-529.

Burke, R.E., & Tsairis, P. (1973). Anatomy and innervation ratios in motor units of cat gastrocnemius. *Journal of Physiology* (London), **234**, 749-765.

Caiozzo, V.J., Barnes, W.S., Prietto, C.A., & McMaster, W.C. (1981). The effect of isometric precontractions on the slow velocity-high force region of the in vivo force-velocity relationship. *Medicine and Science in Sports and Exercise*, **13**, 128.

Caiozzo, V.J., Laird, T., Chow, K., Prietto, C.A., & McMaster, W.C. (1982). The use of precontractions to enhance the in vivo force-velocity relationship. *Medicine and Science in Sports and Exercise*, **14**, 162.

Caiozzo, V.J., Perrine, J.J., & Edgerton, V.R. (1981). Training-induced alterations of the in vivo force-velocity relationship of human muscle. *Journal of Applied Physiology*, **51**, 750-754.

Cavagna, G.A. (1977) Storage and utilization of elastic energy in skeletal muscle. In R.S. Hutton (Ed.), *Exercise and sport sciences reviews* (Vol. 5, pp. 89-129). Santa Barbara, CA: Journal Publishing Affiliates.

Cavagna, G.A., & Citterio, G. (1974). Effect of stretching on the elastic characteristics and the contractile component of frog striated muscle. *Journal of Physiology* (London), **239**, 1-14.

Cavanagh, P.R., Andrew, G.C., Kram, R., Rodgers, M.M., Sanderson, D.J., & Hennig, E.M. (1985) An approach to biomechanical profiling of elite distance runners. *International Journal of Sport Biomechanics*, **1**, 36-62.

Cavanagh, P.R., & Grieve, D.W. (1973). The graphical display of angular movement of the body. *British Journal of Sports Medicine*, **7**, 129-133.

Cavanagh, P.R., & Lafortune, M.A. (1980). Ground reaction forces in distance running. *Journal of Biomechanics*, **13**, 397-406.

Cavanagh, P.R., Pollock, M.L., & Landa, J. (1977). A biomechanical comparison of elite and good distance runners. *Annals of the New York Academy of Sciences*, **301**, 328-345.

Chandler, R.F., Clauser, C.E., McConville, J.T., Reynolds, H.M., & Young, J.W. (1975). *Investigation of inertial properties of the human body* (AMRL-TR-74-137). Wright-Patterson Air Force Base, OH: Aerospace Medical Research Laboratories, Aerospace Medical Division (NTIS No. AD-A016 485).

Chao, E.Y.S. (1986). Biomechanics of the human gait. In G.W. Schmid-Schönbein, S.L.-Y. Woo, & B.W. Zweifach (Eds.), *Frontiers in biomechanics* (pp. 225-244). New York: Springer.

Cheney, P.D. (1985). Role of cerebral cortex in voluntary movements. A review. *Physical Therapy*, **65**, 624-635.

Christakos, C.N., & Windhorst, U. (1986). Spindle gain increase during muscle unit fatigue. *Brain Research*, **365**, 388-392.

Clark, F.J., Burgess, R.C., Chapin, J.W., & Lipscomb, W.T. (1985). Role of intramuscular receptors in the awareness of limb position. *Journal of Neurophysiology*, **54**, 1529-1540.

Clarke, T.E., Frederick, E.C., & Hamill, C.L. (1983). The effects of shoe design parameters on rearfoot control in running. *Medicine and Science in Sports and Exercise*, **15**, 376-381.

Clarke, T.E., Frederick, E.C., & Hamill, C.L. (1984). The study of rearfoot movement in running. In E.C. Frederick (Ed.), *Sport shoes and playing surfaces* (pp. 166-189). Champaign, IL: Human Kinetics.

Condon, S.M., & Hutton, R.S. (1987). Soleus muscle electromyographic activity and ankle dorsiflexion range of motion during four stretching procedures. *Physical Therapy*, **67**, 24-30.

Cowin, S.C. (1983). The mechanical and stress adaptive properties of bone. *Annals of Biomedical Engineering*, **11**, 263-295.

Coyle, E.F., Feiring, D.C., Rotkis, T.C., Cote, R.W., III, Roby, F.B., Lee, W., & Wilmore, J.H. (1981). Specificity of power improvements through slow and fast isokinetic training. *Journal of Applied Physiology*, **51**, 1437-1442.

Crenna, P., & Frigo, C. (1984). Evidence of phase-dependent nociceptive reflexes during locomotion in man. *Experimental Neurology*, **85**, 336-345.

Crowninshield, R.D., & Brand, R.A. (1981). The prediction of forces in joint structures: Distribution of intersegmental resultants. In D.I. Miller (Ed.), *Exercise and sport sciences reviews* (Vol. 9, pp. 159-181). Philadelphia: Franklin Institute.

Dainis, A. (1981). A model for gymnastics vaulting. *Medicine and Science in Sports and Exercise*, **13**, 34-43.

Dalén, N., & Olsson, K.E. (1974). Bone mineral content and physical activity. *Acta Orthopaedica Scandinavica*, **45**, 170-174.

Davies, C.T.M., Dooley, P., McDonagh, M.J.N., & White, M.J. (1985). Adaptation of mechanical properties of muscle to high force training in man. *Journal of Physiology* (London), **365**, 277-284.

Davies, C.T.M., & Young, K. (1983). Effect of temperature on the contractile properties and muscle power of triceps surae in humans. *Journal of Applied Physiology*, **55**, 191-195.

De Koning, F.L., Binkhorst, R.A., Vissers, A.C.A., & Vos, J.A. (1982). Influence of static strength training on the force-velocity relationship of the arm flexors. *International Journal of Sports Medicine*, **3**, 25-28.

De Koning, F.L., Binkhorst, R.A., Vos, J.A., & van't Hof, M.A. (1985). The force-velocity relationship of arm flexion in untrained males and females and arm-trained athletes. *European Journal of Applied Physiology*, **54**, 89-94.

DeLorme, T.L. (1945). Restoration of muscle power by heavy-resistance exercises. *Journal of Bone and Joint Surgery*, **27**, 645-667.

Dempster, W.T. (1955). *Space requirements of the seated operator* (WADC-TR-55-159). Wright-Patterson Air Force Base, OH: Aerospace Medical Research Laboratory (NTIS No. AD-87892).

Denny-Brown, D. (1949). Interpretation of the electromyogram. *Archives of Neurology and Psychiatry*, **61**, 99-128.

Denny-Brown, D., & Pennybacker, J.B. (1938). Fibrillation and fasciculation in voluntary muscle. *Brain*, **61**, 311-334.

de Vries, H.A. (1966). Quantitative electromyographic investigation of the spasm theory of muscle pain. *American Journal of Physical Medicine*, **45**, 119-134.

Dietz, V. (1978). Analysis of the electrical muscle activity during maximal contraction and the influence of ischaemia. *Journal of the Neurological Sciences*, **37**, 187-197.

Duchateau, J., & Hainaut, K. (1981). Adaptation of human muscle and its motor units to exercise. *Journal de Biophysique & Medecine Nucleaire*, **5**, 249-253.

Duchateau, J., & Hainaut, K. (1984). Isometric or dynamic training: Differential effects on mechanical properties of a human muscle. *Journal of Applied Physiology*, **56**, 296-301.

Edman, K.A.P., Elzinga, G., & Noble, M.I.M. (1978). Enhancement of mechanical performance by stretch during tetanic contractions of vertebrate skeletal muscle fibres. *Journal of Physiology* (London), **281**, 139-155.

Edström, L., & Grimby, L. (1986). Effect of exercise on the motor unit. *Muscle & Nerve*, **9**, 104-126.

Edström, L., & Kugelberg, E. (1968). Histochemical composition, distribution of fibres and fatiguability of single motor units. *Journal of Neurology, Neurosurgery, & Psychiatry*, **31**, 424-433.

Edwards, R.H.T. (1981). Human muscle function and fatigue. In R. Porter & J. Whelan (Eds.), *Human muscle fatigue: Physiological mechanisms* (pp. 1-18). London: Pitman Medical.

Edwards, R.H.T., Hill, D.K., Jones, D.A., & Merton, P.A. (1977). Fatigue of long duration in human skeletal muscle after exercise. *Journal of Physiology* (London), **272**, 769-778.

Eie, N. (1966). Load capacity of the low back. *Journal of the Oslo City Hospitals*, **16**, 73-98.

Elftman, H. (1938). The measurement of the external force in walking. *Science*, **88**, 152-153.

Elftman, H. (1939). Forces and energy changes in the leg during walking. *American Journal of Physiology*, **125**, 339-356.

Elson, P. (1974, December). Strength increases by electrical stimulation. *Track Technique*, p. 1856.

Engelhorn, R. (1983). Agonist and antagonist muscle EMG activity pattern changes with skill acquisition. *Research Quarterly for Exercise and Sport*, **54**, 315-323.

Enoka, R.M. (1979). The pull in Olympic weightlifting. *Medicine and Science in Sports*, **11**, 131-137.

Enoka, R.M. (1983). Muscular control of a learned movement: The speed control system hypothesis. *Experimental Brain Research*, **51**, 135-145.

Enoka, R.M. (in press). Load- and skill-related changes in segmental contributions to a weightlifting movement. *Medicine and Science in Sports and Exercise*.

Enoka, R.M., Miller, D.I., & Burgess, E.M. (1982). Below-knee amputee running gait. *American Journal of Physical Medicine*, **61**, 66-84.

Enoka, R.M., & Stuart, D.G. (1984). Henneman's 'size principle': Current issues. *Trends in Neurosciences*, **7**, 226-228.

Enoka, R.M., & Stuart, D.G. (1985). The contribution of neuroscience to exercise studies. *Federation Proceedings*, **44**, 2279-2285.

Etemadi, A.A., & Hosseini, F. (1968). Frequency and size of muscle fibers in athletic body build. *Anatomical Record*, **162**, 269-274.

Etnyre, B.R., & Abraham, L.D. (1986). Gains in range of ankle dorsiflexion using three popular stretching techniques. *American Journal of Physical Medicine*, **65**, 189-196.

Fahey, T.D., Harvey, M., Schroeder, R.V., & Ferguson, F. (1985). Influence of sex differences and knee joint position on electrical stimulation-modulated strength increases. *Medicine and Science in Sports and Exercise*, **17**, 144-147.

Feldman, J.L., & Grillner, S. (1983). Control of vertebrate respiration and locomotion: A brief account. *Physiologist*, **26**, 310-316.

Fenn, W.O. (1924). The relation between the work performed and the energy liberated in muscular contraction. *Journal of Physiology* (London), **58**, 373-395.

Fenn, W.O. (1930). Work against gravity and work due to velocity changes in running. *American Journal of Physiology*, **93**, 433-462.

Fick, R. (1904). *Handbuch der anatomie des menschen* (Vol. 2). Stuttgart: Gustav Fischer Verlag.

Fletcher, J.G., & Lewis, H.E. (1960). Human power output: The mechanics of pole vaulting. *Ergonomics*, **3**, 30-34.

Frankeny, J.R., Holly, R.G., & Ashmore, C.R. (1983). Effects of graded duration of stretch on normal and dystrophic skeletal muscle. *Muscle & Nerve*, **6**, 269-277.

Froese, E.A., & Houston, M.E. (1985). Torque-velocity characteristics and muscle fiber type in human vastus lateralis. *Journal of Applied Physiology*, **59**, 309-314.

Frohlich, C. (1980, March). The physics of somersaulting and twisting. *Scientific American*, pp. 154-164.

Fujiwara, M., & Basmajian, J.V. (1975). Electromyographic study of two-joint muscles. *American Journal of Physical Medicine*, **54**, 234-242.

Galea, V., & Norman, R.W. (1985). Bone-on-bone forces at the ankle joint during a rapid dynamic movement. In D.A. Winter, R.W. Norman, R.P. Wells, K.C. Hayes, & A.E. Patla (Eds.), *Biomechanics IX-A* (pp. 71-76). Champaign, IL: Human Kinetics.

Gans, C. (1982). Fiber architecture and muscle function. In R.L. Terjung (Ed.), *Exercise and sport sciences reviews* (Vol. 10, pp. 160-207). Philadelphia: Franklin Institute.

Garhammer, J. (1980). Power production by Olympic weightlifters. *Medicine and Science in Sports and Exercise*, **12**, 54-60.

Gergely, J. (1974). Some aspects of the role of the sarcoplasmic reticulum and the tropomyosin-troponin system in the control of muscle contraction by calcium ions. *Circulation Research*, **34**(Suppl. 3), 74-82.

Gollnick, P.D., Parsons, D., Riedy, M., & Moore, R.L. (1983). Fiber number and size in overloaded chicken anterior latissimus dorsi muscle. *Journal of Applied Physiology*, **54**, 1292-1297.

Gonyea, W.J. (1980). Role of exercise in inducing increases in skeletal muscle fiber number. *Journal of Applied Physiology*, **48**, 421-426.

Gonyea, W.J., & Ericson, G.C. (1977). Morphological and histochemical organization of the flexor carpi radialis muscle in the cat. *American Journal of Anatomy*, **148**, 329-344.

Gonyea, W.J., Sale, D.G., Gonyea, F.B., & Mikesky, A. (1986). Exercise induced increases in muscle fiber number. *European Journal of Applied Physiology*, **55**, 137-141.

Gorman, P.H., & Mortimer, J.T. (1983). The effect of stimulus parameters on the recruitment characteristics of direct nerve stimulation. *IEEE Transactions on Biomedical Engineering*, **BME-30**, 407-414.

Green, H.J., Klug, G.A., Reichmann, H., Seedorf, U., Wiehrer, W., & Pette, D. (1984). Exercise-induced fibre type transitions with regard to myosin, parvalbumin, and sarcoplasmic reticulum in muscles of the rat. *Pflügers Archiv*, **400**, 432-438.

Grieve, D.W. (1969, June). Stretching active muscles and leading with the hips. *Coaching Review*, pp. 3-4, 10.

Gross, A.C., Kyle, C.R., & Malewicki, D.J. (1983, December). The aerodynamics of human-powered land vehicles. *Scientific American*, pp. 142-145, 148-152.

Gustafsson, B., & Pinter, M.J. (1985). On factors determining orderly recruitment of motor units: A role for intrinsic membrane properties. *Trends in Neurosciences*, **8**, 431-433.

Gydikov, A., & Kosarov, D. (1973). Physiological characteristics of the tonic and phasic motor units in human muscles. In A.A. Gydikov, N.T. Tankov, & D.S. Kosarov (Eds.), *Motor control* (pp. 75-94). New York: Plenum.

Gydikov, A., & Kosarov, D. (1974). Some features of different motor units in human biceps brachii. *Pflügers Archiv*, **347**, 75-88.

Gydikov, A.A., Kossev, A.R., Kosarov, D.S., & Kostov, K.G. (1987). Investigations of single motor units firing during movements against elastic resistance. In B. Jonsson, (Ed.), *Biomechanics X-A* (pp. 227-232). Champaign, IL: Human Kinetics.

Gydikov, A., Kossev, A., Radicheva, N., & Tankov, N. (1981). Interaction between reflexes and voluntary motor activity in man revealed by discharges of separate motor units. *Experimental Neurology*, **73**, 331-344.

Häkkinen, K. (1985). Research overview: Factors influencing trainability of muscular strength during short term and prolonged training. *National Strength & Conditioning Association Journal*, **7**(2), 32-37.

Häkkinen, K., Alén, M., & Komi, P.V. (1985). Changes in isometric force- and relaxation-time, electromyographic and muscle fibre characteristics of human skeletal muscle during strength training and detraining. *Acta Physiologica Scandinavica*, **125**, 573-585.

Häkkinen, K., & Komi, P.V. (1983). Electromyographic changes during strength training and detraining. *Medicine and Science in Sports and Exercise*, **15**, 455-460.

Häkkinen, K., Komi, P.V., & Alén, M. (1985). Effect of explosive type strength training on isometric force- and relaxation-time, electromyographic and muscle fibre characteristics of leg extensor muscles. *Acta Physiologica Scandinavica*, **125**, 587-600.

Hall, S.J., & DePauw, K.P. (1982). A photogrammetrically based model for predicting total body mass centroid location. *Research Quarterly for Exercise and Sport*, **53**, 37-45.

Hanavan, E.P. (1964). A mathematical model of the human body (AMRL-TR-64-102). Wright-Patterson Air Force Base, OH: Aerospace Medical Research Laboratories (NTIS No. AD-608463).

Hanavan, E.P., Jr. (1966). A personalized mathematical model of the human body. *Journal of Spacecraft and Rockets*, **3**, 446-448.

Hannaford, B., & Stark, L. (1985). Roles of the elements of the triphasic control signal. *Experimental Neurology*, **90**, 619-635.

Hannerz, J., & Grimby, L. (1979). The afferent influence on the voluntary firing range of individual motor units in man. *Muscle & Nerve*, **2**, 414-422.

Harre, D. (Ed.). (1982). *Principles of sports training: Introduction to the theory and methods of training*. East Berlin: Sportverlag.

Harrison, P.J. (1983). The relationship between the distribution of motor unit mechanical properties and the forces due to recruitment and to rate coding for the generation of muscle force. *Brain Research*, **264**, 311-315.

Hasan, Z. (1986). Optimized movement trajectories and joint stiffness in unperturbed, inertially loaded movements. *Biological Cybernetics*, **53**, 373-382.

Hasan, Z., & Enoka, R.M. (1985). Isometric torque-angle relationship and movement-related activity of human elbow flexors: Implications for the equilibrium-point hypothesis. *Experimental Brain Research*, **59**, 441-450.

Hasan, Z., Enoka, R.M., & Stuart, D.G. (1985). The interface between biomechanics and neurophysiology in the study of movement: Some recent approaches. In R.L. Terjung (Ed.), *Exercise and sport sciences reviews* (Vol. 13, pp. 169-234). New York: Macmillan.

Hasan, Z., & Stuart, D.G. (1988). Animal solutions to problems of movement control: The role of proprioceptors. *Annual Review of Neuroscience*, **11**, 199-223.

Hatze, H. (1980). A mathematical model for the computational determination of parameter values of anthropomorphic segments. *Journal of Biomechanics*, **13**, 833-843.

Hatze, H. (1981a). Estimation of myodynamic parameter values from observations on isometrically contracting muscle groups. *European Journal of Applied Physiology*, **46**, 325-338.

Hatze, H. (1981b). *Myocybernetic control models of skeletal muscle. Characteristics and applications*. Pretoria: University of South Africa.

Hay, J.G. (1975). Straddle or flop? *Athletic Journal*, **55**, 8, 83-85.

Hay, J.G. (1978). *The biomechanics of sports techniques*. Englewood Cliffs, NJ: Prentice-Hall.

Hay, J.G., Andrews, J.G., & Vaughan, C.L. (1980). The influence of external load on the joint torques exerted in a squat exercise. In J.M. Cooper & B. Haven (Eds.), *Proceedings of the Biomechanics Symposium* (pp. 286-293). Indiana University: Indiana State Board of Health.

Hay, J.G., Andrews, J.G., Vaughan, C.L., & Ueya, K. (1983). Load, speed and equipment effects in strength-training exercises. In H. Matsui & K. Kobayashi (Eds.), *Biomechanics VIII-B* (pp. 939-950). Champaign, IL: Human Kinetics.

Henneman, E. (1979). Functional organization of motoneuron pools: The size-principle. In H. Asanuma & V.J. Wilson (Eds.), *Integration in the nervous system* (pp. 13-25). Tokyo: Igaku-Shoin.

Henneman, E. (1957). Relation between size of neurons and their susceptibility to discharge. *Science*, **126**, 1345-1347.

Hershler, C., & Milner, M. (1980a). Angle-angle diagrams in above-knee amputee and cerebral palsy gait. *American Journal of Physical Medicine*, **59**, 165-183.

Hershler, C., & Milner, M. (1980b). Angle-angle diagrams in the assessment of locomotion. *American Journal of Physical Medicine*, **59**, 109-125.

Hettinger, T. (1961). *Physiology of strength*. Springfield, IL: Charles C Thomas.

Higgins, S. (1985). Movement as an emergent form: Its structural limits. *Human Movement Science*, **4**, 119-148.

Hill, A.V. (1928). The air-resistance to a runner. *Proceedings of the Royal Society of London*, B, **102**, 380-385.

Hill, A.V. (1938). The heat of shortening and the dynamic constants of muscle. *Proceedings of the Royal Society of London*, B, **126**, 136-195.

Hník, P. (1981). What is muscle tone? *Physiologia Bohemoslovaca*, **30**, 389-395.

Hochmuth, G. (1968). Biomechanische prinzipien. In J. Wartenweiler, E. Jokl, & M. Hebbelinck (Eds.), *Biomechanics I* (pp. 155-160). Basel: S. Karger.

Hof, A.L. (1984). EMG and muscle force: An introduction. *Human Movement Science*, **3**, 119-153.

Hof, A.L., & Van den Berg, J.W. (1981a). EMG to force processing I: An electrical analogue of the Hill muscle model. *Journal of Biomechanics*, **14**, 747-758.

Hof, A.L., & Van den Berg, J.W. (1981b). EMG to force processing II: Estimation of parameters of the Hill muscle model for the human triceps surae by means of a calfergometer. *Journal of Biomechanics*, **14**, 759-770.

Hof, A.L., & Van den Berg, J.W. (1981c). EMG to force processing III: Estimation of model parameters for the human triceps surae muscle and assessment of the accuracy by means of a torque plate. *Journal of Biomechanics*, **14**, 771-785.

Hof, A.L., & Van den Berg, J.W. (1981d). EMG to force processing IV: Eccentric-concentric contractions on a spring-flywheel set up. *Journal of Biomechanics*, **14**, 787-792.

Hofmann, W.W. (1980). Mechanisms of muscular hypertrophy. *Journal of the Neurological Sciences*, **45**, 205-216.

Hoppeler, H. (1986). Exercise-induced ultrastructural changes in skeletal muscle. *International Journal of Sports Medicine*, **7**, 187-204.

Howald, H. (1982). Training-induced morphological and functional changes in skeletal muscle. *International Journal of Sports Medicine*, **3**, 1-12.

Howard, J.D., & Enoka, R.M. (1987). Interlimb interactions during maximal efforts. *Medicine and Science in Sports and Exercise*, **19**, S3.

Howard, J.D., Ritchie, M.R., Gater, D.A., Gater, D.R., & Enoka, R.M. (1985). Determining factors of strength: Physiological foundations. *National Strength &*

Conditioning Association Journal, 7(6), 16-22.

Hoy, M.G., Zernicke, R.F., & Smith, J.L. (1985). Contrasting roles of inertial and muscle moments at knee and ankle during paw-shake response. *Journal of Neurophysiology*, **54**, 1282-1295.

Hoyle, G. (1983). *Muscles and their neural control*. New York: Wiley.

Hubbard, M. (1980). Dynamics of the pole vault. *Journal of Biomechanics*, **13**, 965-976.

Hubley, C.L., & Wells, R.P. (1983). A work-energy approach to determine individual joint contributions to vertical jump performance. *European Journal of Applied Physiology*, **50**, 247-254.

Hultman, E., Sjöholm, H., Sahlin, K., & Edström, L. (1981). Glycolytic and oxidative energy metabolism and contraction characteristics of intact human muscle. In R. Porter & J. Whelan (Eds.), *Human muscle fatigue: Physiological mechanisms* (pp. 19-40). London: Pitman Medical.

Hutton, R.S., & Nelson, D.L. (1986). Stretch sensitivity of Golgi tendon organs in fatigued gastrocnemius muscle. *Medicine and Science in Sports and Exercise*, **18**, 69-74.

Ikai, M., & Fukunaga, T. (1968). Calculation of muscle strength per unit cross-sectional area of human muscle by means of ultrasonic measurement. *Internationale Zeitschrift für angewandte Physiologie einschliesslich Arbeitsphysiologie*, **26**, 26-32.

Ingjer, F., & Strømme, S.B. (1979). Effects of active, passive or no warm-up on the physiological response to heavy exercise. *European Journal of Applied Physiology*, **40**, 273-282.

Jami, L., Murthy, K.S.K., Petit, J., & Zytnicki, D. (1983). After-effects of repetitive stimulation at low frequency on fast-contracting motor units of cat muscle. *Journal of Physiology* (London), **340**, 129-143.

Jankowska, E., & Odutola, A. (1980). Crossed and uncrossed synaptic actions on motoneurones of back muscles in the cat. *Brain Research*, **194**, 65-78.

Jarić, S., Gavrilović, P., & Ivančević, V. (1985). Effects of previous muscle contractions on cyclic movement dynamics. *European Journal of Applied Physiology*, **54**, 216-221.

Johns, R.J., & Wright, V. (1962). Relative importance of various tissues in joint stiffness. *Journal of Applied Physiology*, **17**, 824-828.

Johnson. B.L., Adamczyk, J.W., Tennøe, K.O., & Strømme, S.B. (1976). A comparison of concentric and eccentric muscle training. *Medicine and Science in Sports*, **8**, 35-38.

Jones, L.A. (1983). Role of central and peripheral signals in force sensation during fatigue. *Experimental Neurology*, **81**, 497-503.

Jørgensen, K. (1976). Force-velocity relationship in human elbow flexors and extensors. In P.V. Komi (Ed.), *Biomechanics V-A* (pp. 145-151). Baltimore: University Park Press.

Kabat, H. (1950). Studies on neuromuscular dysfunction XIII: New concepts and techniques of neuromuscular reeducation for paralysis. *Permanente Foundation Medical Bulletin*, **8**, 121-143.

Kanda, K., Burke, R.E., & Walmsley, B. (1977). Differential control of fast and slow twitch motor units in the decerebrate cat. *Experimental Brain Research*, **29**, 57-74.

Kandel, E.R. (1985). Nerve cells and behavior. In E.R. Kandel & J.H. Schwartz (Eds.), *Principles of neural science* (2nd ed., pp. 13-24). New York: Elsevier/North Holland.

Kane, T.R., & Scher, M.P. (1969). A dynamical explanation of the falling cat phenomenon. *International Journal of Solids and Structures*, **5**, 663-670.

Kanehisa, H., & Miyashita, M. (1983). Effect of isometric and isokinetic muscle training on static strength and dynamic power. *European Journal of Applied Physiology*, **50**, 365-371.

Karst, G.M., & Hasan, Z. (1987). Antagonist muscle activity during human forearm movements under varying kinematic and loading conditions. *Experimental Brain Research*, **67**, 391-401.

Kereshi, S., Manzano, G., & McComas, A.J. (1983). Impulse conduction velocities in human biceps brachii muscles. *Experimental Neurology*, **80**, 652-662.

Kernell, D. (1984). The meaning of discharge rate: Excitation-to-frequency transduction as studied in spinal motoneurones. *Archives Italiennes de Biologie*, **122**, 5-15.

Kernell, D., & Monster, A.W. (1981). Threshold current for repetitive impulse firing in motoneurones innervating muscle fibers of different fatigue sensitivity in the cat. *Brain Research*, **229**, 193-196.

Kernell, D., & Monster, A.W. (1982). Time course and properties of late adaptation in spinal motoneurones of the cat. *Experimental Brain Research*, **46**, 191-196.

Knott, M., & Voss, D.E. (1968). *Proprioceptive neuromuscular facilitation: Patterns and techniques*. (2nd ed.). New York: Hoeber Medical Division, Harper & Row.

Koester, J. (1981). Active conductances underlying the action potential. In E.R. Kandel & J.H. Schwartz (Eds.), *Principles of neural science* (pp. 53-62). New York: Elsevier.

Koester, J. (1985a). Functional consequences of passive membrane properties of the neuron. In E.R. Kandel & J.H. Schwartz (Eds.), *Principles of neural science* (2nd ed., pp. 66-74). New York: Elsevier.

Koester, J. (1985b). Resting membrane potential and action potential. In E.R. Kandel & J.H. Schwartz (Eds.), *Principles of neural science* (2nd ed., pp. 49-57). New York: Elsevier.

Komi, P.V. (1979). Neuromuscular performance: Factors influencing force and speed production. *Scandinavian Journal of Sports Science*, **1**, 2-15.

Komi, P.V., & Bosco, C. (1978). Utilization of stored elastic energy in leg extensor muscles by men and women. *Medicine and Science in Sports*, **10**, 261-265.

Komi, P.V., & Buskirk, E.R. (1972). Effect of eccentric and concentric muscle conditioning on tension and electrical activity of human muscle. *Ergonomics*, **15**, 417-434.

Komi, P.V., Viitasalo, J.T., Rauramaa, R., & Vihko, V. (1978). Effect of isometric strength training on mechanical, electrical, and metabolic aspects of muscle function. *European Journal of Applied Physiology*, **40**, 45-55.

Kraemer, W.J. (1983). Exercise prescription in weight training: A needs analysis. *National Strength & Conditioning Association Journal*, **5**(1), 64-65.

Kudina, L.P. (1980). Reflex effects of muscle afferents on antagonist studied on single firing motor units in man. *Electroencephalography and Clinical Neurophysiology*, **50**, 214-221.

Kugelberg, E., & Thornell, L-E. (1983). Contraction time, histochemical type, and terminal cisternae volume of rat motor units. *Muscle & Nerve*, **6**, 149-153.

Kuipers, H., Drukker, J., Frederik, P.M., Geurten, P., & v. Kranenburg, G. (1983). Muscle degeneration after exercise in rats. *International Journal of Sports Medicine*, **4**, 45-51.

Kukulka, C.G., & Clamann, H.P. (1981). Comparison of the recruitment and discharge properties of motor units in human brachial biceps and adductor pollicis during isometric contractions. *Brain Research*, **219**, 45-55.

Kulig, K., Andrews, J.G., & Hay, J.G. (1984). Human strength curves. In R.L. Terjung (Ed.), *Exercise and sport sciences reviews* (Vol. 12, pp. 417-466). New York: Macmillan.

Lagasse, P., Boucher, J., Samson, J., & Jacques, L. (1979). Training effects of functional electrical stimulation in weight-lifting. *Journal of Human Movement Studies*, **5**, 61-67.

Lanyon, L.E., & Rubin, C.T. (1984). Static vs dynamic loads as an influence on bone remodelling. *Journal of Biomechanics*, **17**, 897-905.

Larsson, L., & Tesch, P.A. (1986). Motor unit fibre density in extremely hypertrophied skeletal muscles in man. *European Journal of Applied Physiology*, **55**, 130-136.

Laughman, R.K., Youdas, J.W., Garrett, T.R., & Chao, E.Y.S. (1983). Strength changes in the normal quadriceps femoris muscle as a result of electrical stimulation. *Physical Therapy*, **63**, 494-499.

Lexell, J., Henriksson-Larsén, K., & Sjöström, M. (1983). Distribution of different fibre types in human skeletal muscles: 2. A study of cross-sections of whole m. vastus lateralis. *Acta Physiologica Scandinavica*, **117**, 115-122.

Liberson, W.T., Holmquest, H.J., Scot, D., & Dow, M. (1961). Functional electro-therapy: Stimulation of the peroneal nerve synchronized with the swing phase of the gait of hemiplegic patients. *Archives of Physical Medicine and Rehabilitation*, **42**, 101-105.

Lindh, M. (1979). Increase of muscle strength from isometric quadriceps exercises at different knee angles. *Scandinavian Journal of Rehabilitation Medicine*, **11**, 33-36.

Loeb, G.E., & Gans, C. (1986). *Electromyography for experimentalists*. Chicago: University of Chicago Press.

Lømo, T., Westgaard, R.H., & Engebretsen, L. (1980). Different stimulation patterns affect contractile properties of denervated rat soleus muscles. In D. Pette (Ed.), *Plasticity of muscle* (pp. 297-309). New York: Walter de Gruyter.

Lucas, S.M., Ruff, R.L., & Binder, M.D. (1987). Specific tension measurements in single soleus and medial gastrocnemius muscle fibers of the cat. *Experimental Neurology*, **95**, 142-154.

Luhtanen, P., & Komi, P.V. (1980). Force-, power-, and elasticity-velocity relationships in walking, running, and jumping. *European Journal of Applied Physiology*, **44**, 279-289.

MacDougall, J.D. (1986). Morphological changes in human skeletal muscle following strength training and immobilization. In N.L. Jones, N. McCartney, & A.J. McComas (Eds.), *Human muscle power* (pp. 269-288). Champaign, IL: Human Kinetics.

MacDougall, J.D., Elder, G.C.B., Sale, D.G., Moroz, J.R., & Sutton, J.R. (1980). Effects of strength training and immobilization on human muscle fibres. *European Journal of Applied Physiology*, **43**, 25-34.

MacDougall, J.D., Sale, D.C., Elder, G.C.B., & Sutton, J.R. (1982). Muscle ultrastructural characteristics of elite powerlifters and bodybuilders. *European Journal of Applied Physiology*, **48**, 117-126.

Madsen, N., & McLaughlin, T. (1984). Kinematic factors influencing performance and injury risk in the bench press exercise. *Medicine and Science in Sports and Exercise*, **16**, 376-381.

Magnus, R. (1922). Wie sich die fallende katze in der luft umdreht. *Archives Neerlandaises de Physiologie de l'Homme et des Animaux*, **7**, 218-222.

Mann, R.V. (1981). A kinetic analysis of sprinting. *Medicine and Science in Sports and Exercise*, **13**, 325-328.

Manter, J.T. (1938). The dynamics of quadrupedal walking. *Journal of Experimental Biology*, **15**, 522-540.

Marey, E.-J. (1874). *Animal mechanism: A treatise on terrestial and aerial locomotion*. New York: D. Appleton and Co.

Marey, E.-J. (1894). Des mouvements que certains animaux executent pour retomber sur leurs pieds, lorsqu'ils sont precipites d'un lieu eleve. *Academie des Sciences*, **119**, 714-718.

Marras, W.S., Joynt, R.L., & King, A.I. (1985). The force-velocity relation and intra-abdominal pressure during lifting activities. *Ergonomics*, **28**, 603-613.

Marsden, C.D., Meadows, J.C., & Merton, P.A. (1983). "Muscular wisdom" that minimizes fatigue during prolonged effort in man: Peak rates of motoneuron discharge and slowing of discharge during fatigue. In J.E. Desmedt (Ed.), *Motor control mechanisms in health and disease* (pp. 169-211). New York: Raven.

Martin, J.P. (1977). A short essay on posture and movement. *Journal of Neurology, Neurosurgery, and Psychiatry*, **40**, 25-29.

McCafferty, W.B., & Horvath, S.M. (1977). Specificity of exercise and specificity of training: A subcellular review. *Research Quarterly*, **48**, 358-371.

McCloskey, M. (1983, April). Intuitive physics. *Scientific American*, pp. 122-130.

McDonagh, J.C., Binder, M.D., Reinking, R.M., & Stuart, D.G. (1980). A commentary on muscle unit properties in cat hindlimb muscles. *Journal of Morphology*, **166**, 217-230.

McDonagh, M.J.N., & Davies, C.T.M. (1984). Adaptive response of mammalian skeletal muscle to exercise with high loads. *European Journal of Applied Physiology*, **52**, 139-155.

McLaughlin, T.M., Dillman, C.J., & Lardner, T.J. (1977). A kinematic model of performance in the parallel squat by champion powerlifters. *Medicine and Science in Sports*, **9**, 128-133.

McMahon, T.A. (1984). *Muscles, reflexes, and locomotion*. Princeton, NJ: Princeton University Press.

Miller, D.I. (1976). A biomechanical analysis of the contribution of the trunk to standing vertical jump take-offs. In J. Broekhoff (Ed.), *Physical education, sports and the sciences* (pp. 355-374). Eugene, OR: Microform Publications.

Miller, D.I. (1978). Biomechanics of running—what should the future hold? *Canadian Journal of Applied Sport Sciences*, **3**, 229-236.

Miller, D.I. (1979). Modelling in biomechanics: An overview. *Medicine and Science in Sports*, **11**, 115-122.

Miller, D.I. (1980). Body segment contributions to sport skill performance: Two contrasting approaches. *Research Quarterly for Exercise and Sport*, **51**, 219-233.

Miller, D.I. (1981, June). *Biomechanics of diving*. Paper presented at the meeting of the Canadian Amateur Diving Association, Seattle.

Miller, D.I'., Enoka, R.M., McCulloch, R.G., Burgess, E.M., Hutton, R.S., & Frankel, V.H. (1979). *Biomechanical analysis of lower extremity amputee extra-ambulatory activities* (Contract No. V5244P-1540/VA). New York: Veterans Administration.

Miller, D.I., & Morrison, W.E. (1975). Prediction of segmental parameters using the Hanavan human body model. *Medicine and Science in Sports*, **7**, 207-212.

Miller, D.I., & Munro, C.F. (1985). Joint torque patterns of below-knee amputees during running stance. *Journal of Biomechanics*, **18**, 236.

Miller, D.I., & Nelson, R.C. (1973). *Biomechanics of sport*. London: Henry Kimpton.

Milner-Brown, H.S., Stein, R.B., & Lee, R.G. (1975). Synchronization of human motor units: Possible roles of exercise and supraspinal reflexes. *Electroencephalography and Clinical Neurophysiology*, **38**, 245-254.

Mohr, T., Carlson, B., Sulentic, C., & Landry, R. (1985). Comparison of isometric exercise and high volt galvanic stimulation on quadriceps femoris muscle strength. *Physical Therapy*, **65**, 606-609.

Monster, A.W., & Chan, H. (1977). Isometric force production by motor units of extensor digitorum communis muscle in man. *Journal of Neurophysiology*, **40**, 1432-1443.

Moore, M.A., & Hutton, R.S. (1980). Electromyographic investigation of muscle stretching techniques. *Medicine and Science in Sports and Exercise*, **12**, 322-329.

Moreno-Aranda, J., & Seireg, A. (1981a). Electrical parameters for over-the-skin muscle stimulation. *Journal of Biomechanics*, **14**, 579-585.

Moreno-Aranda, J., & Seireg, A. (1981b). Force response to electrical stimulation of canine skeletal muscles. *Journal of Biomechanics*, **14**, 595-599.

Moreno-Aranda, J., & Seireg, A. (1981c). Investigation of over-the-skin electrical stimulation parameters for different normal muscles and subjects. *Journal of Biomechanics*, **14**, 587-593.

Moritani, T., & de Vries, H.A. (1979). Neural factors versus hypertrophy in the time course of muscle strength gain. *American Journal of Physical Medicine*, **58**, 115-130.

Mussa-Ivaldi, F.A., Hogan, N., & Bizzi, E. (1985). Neural, mechanical and geometric factors subserving arm posture in humans. *Journal of Neuroscience*, **5**, 2732-2743.

Nashner, L.M. (1976). Adapting reflexes controlling the human posture. *Experimental Brain Research*, **26**, 59-72.

Nashner, L.M. (1982). Adaptation of human movement to altered environments. *Trends in Neurosciences*, **5**, 358-361.

Nashner, L.M., & McCollum, G. (1985). The organization of human postural movements: A formal basis and experimental synthesis. *Behavioral and Brain Sciences*, **8**, 135-172.

Nelson, D.L., & Hutton, R.S. (1985). Dynamic and static stretch responses in muscle spindle receptors in fatigued muscle. *Medicine and Science in Sports and Exercise*, **17**, 445-450.

Németh, G., & Ohlsén, H. (1985). *In vivo* moment arm lengths for hip extensor muscles at different angles of hip flexion. *Journal of Biomechanics*, **18**, 129-140.

Nemeth, P.M., & Pette, D. (1981). Succinate dehydrogenase activity in fibres classified by myosin ATPase in three hind limb muscles of rat. *Journal of Physiology* (London), **320**, 73-80.

Nemeth, P., Solanki, L., Gordon, D.A., Hamm, T.M., Reinking, R.M., & Stuart, D.G. (1986). Uniformity of metabolic enzymes within individual motor units. *Journal of Neuroscience*, **6**, 892-898.

Nisell, R., & Ekholm, J. (1985). Patellar forces during knee extension. *Scandinavian Journal of Rehabilitation Medicine*, **17**, 63-74.

Nissinen, M., Preiss, R., & Brüggemann, P. (1985). Simulation of human airborne movements on the horizontal bar. In D.A. Winter, R.W. Norman, R.P. Wells, K.C. Hayes, & A.E. Patla (Eds.), *Biomechanics IX-B* (pp. 373-376). Champaign, IL: Human Kinetics.

Noble, E.G., Dabrowski, B.L., & Ianuzzo, C.D. (1983). Myosin transformation in hypertrophied rat muscle. *Pflügers Archiv*, **396**, 260-262.

Ohtsuki, T. (1983). Decrease in human voluntary isometric arm strength induced by simultaneous bilateral exertion. *Behavioural Brain Research*, **7**, 165-178.

Pedemonte, J. (1983). A new approach in selecting proper loads for power development. *National Strength & Conditioning Association Journal*, **5**(3), 47.

Pepe, F.A., & Drucker, B. (1979). The myosin filament IV: Myosin content. *Journal of Molecular Biology*, **130**, 379-393.

Perry, J., & Bekey, G.A. (1981). EMG-force relationships in skeletal muscle. *CRC Critical Reviews in Biomedical Engineering*, **7**, 1-22.

Person, R.S. (1958). An electromyographic investigation on co-ordination of the activity of antagonist muscles in man during the development of a motor habit. *Pavlov Journal of Higher Nervous Activity*, **8**, 13-23.

Person, R.S. (1963). Problems in the interpretation of electromyograms. 1. Comparison of electromyograms on recording with skin and needle electrodes. *Biophysics*, **8**, 89-97.

Person, R.S., & Kudina, L.P. (1972). Discharge frequency and discharge pattern of human motor units during voluntary contraction of muscle. *Electroencephalography and Clinical Neurophysiology*, **32**, 471-483.

Phillips, S.J., & Roberts,E.M. (1980). Muscular and non-muscular moments of force in the swing limb of Masters runners. In J.M. Cooper & B. Haven (Eds.), *Proceedings of the biomechanics symposium* (pp. 256-274). Bloomington, IN: Indiana State Board of Health.

Phillips, S.J., Roberts, E.M., & Huang, T.C. (1983). Quantification of intersegmental reactions during rapid swing motion. *Journal of Biomechanics*, **16**, 411-417.

Pollack, G.H. (1983). The cross-bridge theory. *Physiological Reviews*, **63**, 1049-1113.

Powers, R.K., & Binder, M.D. (1985a). Determination of afferent fibers mediating oligosynaptic group I input to cat medial gastrocnemius motoneurons. *Journal of Neurophysiology*, **53**, 518-529.

Powers, R.K., & Binder, M.D. (1985b). Distribution of oligosynaptic group I input to the cat medial gastrocnemius motoneuron pool. *Journal of Neurophysiology*, **53**, 497-517.

Prince, F.P., Hikida, R.S., & Hagerman, F.C. (1976). Human muscle fiber types in power lifters, distance runners and untrained subjects. *Pflügers Archiv*, **363**, 19-26.

Putnam, C.A. (1983). Interaction between segments during a kicking motion. In H. Matsui & K. Kobayashi (Eds.), *Bio-mechanics VIII-B* (pp. 688-694). Champaign, IL: Human Kinetics.

Rab, G.T., Chao, E.Y.S., & Stauffer, R.N. (1977). Muscle force analysis of the lumbar spine. *Orthopedic Clinics of North America*, **8**, 193-199.

Rack, P.M.H., & Westbury, D.R. (1969). The effects of length and stimulus rate on tension in the isometric cat soleus muscle. *Journal of Physiology* (London), **204**, 443-460.

Rack, P.M.H., & Westbury, D.R. (1974). The short range stiffness of active mammalian muscle and its effect on mechanical properties. *Journal of Physiology* (London), **240**, 331-350.

Ralston, H.J., Inman, V.T., Strait, L.A., & Shaffrath, M.D. (1947). Mechanics of human isolated voluntary muscle. *American Journal of Physiology*, **151**, 612-620.

Records Section. (1988, January). *Track & Field News*, pp. 14-17.

Roberts, T.D.M. (1976). The role of vestibular and neck receptors in locomotion. In R.M. Herman, S. Grillner, P.S.G. Stein, & D.G. Stuart (Eds.), *Neural control of locomotion* (pp. 539-560). New York: Plenum.

Romero, J.A., Sanford, T.L., Schroeder, R.V., & Fahey, T.D. (1982). The effects of electrical stimulation of normal quadriceps on strength and girth. *Medicine and Science in Sports and Exercise*, **14**, 194-197.

Rossignol, S., Julien, C., & Gauthier, L. (1981). Stimulus-response relationships during locomotion. *Canadian Journal of Physiology and Pharmacology*, **59**, 667-674.

Rüegg, J.C. (1983). Muscle. In R.F. Schmidt & F. Thews (Eds.), *Human physiology* (pp. 32-50). Berlin: Springer-Verlag.

Saito, M., Kobayashi, K., Miyashita, M., & Hoshikawa, T. (1974). Temporal patterns in running. In R.C. Nelson & C.A. Morehouse (Eds.), *Biomechanics IV* (pp. 106-111). Baltimore: University Park Press.

Sale, D.G. (1986). Neural adaptation in strength and power training. In N.L. Jones, N. McCartney, & A.J. McComas (Eds.), *Human muscle power* (pp. 289-307). Champaign, IL: Human Kinetics.

Sale, D.G. (1987). Influence of exercise and training on motor unit activation. In K.B. Pandolf (Ed.), *Exercise and sport sciences reviews* (Vol. 15, pp. 95-151). New York: Macmillan.

Sale, D.G., & MacDougall, J.D. (1981). Specificity in strength training: A review for the coach and athlete. *Canadian Journal of Applied Sport Sciences*, **6**, 87-92.

Sale, D.G., MacDougall, D., Upton, A.R.M., & McComas, A.J. (1983). Effect of strength training upon motoneuron excitability in man. *Medicine and Science in Sports and Exercise*, **15**, 57-62.

Sale, D.G., McComas, A.J., MacDougall, J.D., & Upton, A.R.M. (1982). Neuromuscular adaptation in human thenar muscles following strength training and immobilization. *Journal of Applied Physiology*, **53**, 419-424.

Saltin, B., & Gollnick, P.D. (1983). Skeletal muscle adaptability: Significance for metabolism and performance. In L.D. Peachey (Ed.), *Handbook of physiology: Sec. 10. Skeletal muscle* (pp. 555-631). Bethesda, MD: American Physiological Society.

Sanes, J.N., & Evarts, E.V. (1984). Motor psychophysics. *Human Neurobiology*, **2**, 217-225.

Sapega, A.A., Quedenfeld, T.C., Moyer, R.A., & Butler, R.A. (1981). Biophysical factors in range-of-motion exercise. *Physician and Sportsmedicine*, **9**(12), 57-65.

Sargeant, A.J. (1983). Effect of muscle temperature on maximal short-term power output in man. *Journal of Physiology* (London), **341**, 35P.

Sargeant, A.J., & Boreham, A. (1981). Measurement of maximal short-term (anaerobic) power output during cycling. In J.

Borms, M. Hebbelinck, & A. Venerando (Eds.), *Women and sport* (pp. 119-124). Basel: S. Karger.

Schantz, P., Fox, E.R., Norgren, P., & Tydén, A. (1981). The relationship between mean muscle fibre area and the muscle cross-sectional area of the thigh in subjects with large differences in thigh girth. *Acta Physiologica Scandinavica*, **113**, 537-539.

Schleihauf, R.E., Jr. (1979). A hydrodynamic analysis of swimming propulsion. In J. Terauds & E.W. Bedingfield (Eds.), *Swimming III* (pp. 70-109). Baltimore: University Park Press.

Schmidtbleicher, D., & Haralambie, G. (1981). Changes in contractile properties of muscle after strength training in man. *European Journal of Applied Physiology*, **46**, 221-228.

Schwartz, J.H. (1981). Biochemical control mechanisms in synaptic transmission. In E.R. Kandel & J.H. Schwartz (Eds.), *Principles of neural science* (pp. 121-131). New York: Elsevier.

Seals, D.R., Washburn, R.A., Hanson, P.G., Painter, P.L., & Nagle, F.J. (1983). Increased cardiovascular response to static contraction of larger muscle groups. *Journal of Applied Physiology*, **54**, 434-437.

Secher, N.H. (1975). Isometric rowing strength of experienced and inexperienced oarsmen. *Medicine and Science in Sports*, **7**, 280-283.

Selkowitz, D.M. (1985). Improvement in isometric strength of the quadriceps femoris muscle after training with electrical stimulation. *Physical Therapy*, **65**, 186-196.

Shanebrook, J.R., & Jaszczak, R.D. (1976). Aerodynamic drag analysis of runners. *Medicine and Science in Sports*, **8**, 43-45.

Shellock, F.G. (1986). Physiological, psychological, and injury prevention aspects of warm-up. *National Strength & Conditioning Association Journal*, **8**(5), 24-27.

Shellock F.G., & Prentice, W.E. (1985). Warming-up and stretching for improved physical performance and prevention of sports-related injuries. *Sports Medicine*, **2**, 267-278.

Sherrington, C.S. (1931). Quantitative management of contraction in lowest level co-ordination. *Brain*, **54**, 1-28.

Shumskii, V.V., Merten, A.A., & Dzenis, V.V. (1978). Effect of the type of physical stress on the state of the tibial bones of highly trained athletes as measured by ultrasound techniques. *Mekhanika Polimerov*, **5**, 884-888.

Sjöström, M., Ängquist, K.-A., Bylund, A.-C., Fridén, J., Gustavsson, L., & Scherstén, T. (1982). Morphometric analyses of human muscle fiber types. *Muscle & Nerve*, **5**, 538-553.

Sjöström, M., Kidman, S., Larsén, K.H., & Ängquist, K.-A. (1982). Z- and M-band appearance in different histochemically defined types of human skeletal muscle fibers. *Journal of Histochemistry and Cytochemistry*, **30**, 1-11.

Smith, F. (1982). Dynamic variable resistance and the Universal system. *National Strength & Conditioning Association Journal*, **4**(4), 14-19.

Stevenson, J.M. (1985). The impact force of entry in diving from a ten-meter tower. In D.A. Winter, R.W. Norman, R.P. Wells, K.C. Hayes, & A.E. Patla (Eds.), *Biomechanics IX-B* (pp. 106-111). Champaign, IL: Human Kinetics.

Stroup, F., & Bushnell, D.L. (1970). Rotation, translation, and trajectory in diving. *Research Quarterly*, **40**, 812-817.

Stuart, D.G. (1987a). Muscle receptors, mammalian. In G. Adelman (Ed.), *Encyclopedia of neuroscience* (Vol. II, pp. 716-718). Boston: Birkhäuser.

Stuart, D.G. (1987b). Muscle receptors, mammalian, spinal actions. In G. Adelman (Ed.), *Encyclopedia of neuroscience* (Vol. II, pp. 718-719). Boston: Birkhäuser.

Stuart, D.G., & Enoka, R.M. (1983). Motoneurons, motor units and the size principle. In W.D. Willis, Jr. (Ed.), *The clinical neurosciences: Sec. 5. Neurobiology* (pp. 471-517). New York: Churchill Livingstone.

Suzuki, S., & Sugi, H. (1983). Extensibility of the myofilaments in vertebrate skeletal muscle as revealed by stretching rigor muscle fibers. *Journal of General Physiology*, **81**, 531-546.

Taylor, N.A.S., & Wilkinson, J.G. (1986). Exercise-induced skeletal muscle growth: Hypertrophy or hyperplasia? *Sports Medicine*, **3**, 190-200.

Tesch, P.A., & Larsson, L. (1982). Muscle hypertrophy in bodybuilders. *European Journal of Applied Physiology*, **49**, 301-306.

Thigpen, L.K., Moritani, T., Thiebaud, R., & Hargis, J.L. (1985). The acute effects of static stretching on alpha motoneuron excitability. In D.A. Winter, R.W. Norman, R.P. Wells, K.C. Hayes, & A.E. Patla (Eds.), *Biomechanics IX-A* (pp. 352-357). Champaign, IL: Human Kinetics.

Thorstensson, A. (1977). Observations on strength training and detraining. *Acta Physiologica Scandinavica*, **100**, 491-493.

Vailas, A.C., Tipton, C.M., Matthes, R.D., & Gart, M. (1981). Physical activity and its influence on the repair process of medial collateral ligaments. *Connective Tissue Research*, **9**, 25-31.

Vandervoort, A.A., Sale, D.G., & Moroz, J. (1984). Comparison of motor unit activation during unilateral and bilateral leg extension. *Journal of Applied Physiology*, **56**, 46-51.

van Ingen Schenau, G.J. (1984). An alternative view of the concept of utilisation of elastic energy in human movement. *Human Movement Science*, **3**, 301-336.

van Ingen Schenau, G.J., Bobbert, M.F., Huijing, P.A., & Woittiez, R.D. (1985). The instantaneous torque-angular velocity relation in plantar flexion during jumping. *Medicine and Science in Sports and Exercise*, **17**, 422-426.

van Mameren, H., & Drukker, J. (1979). Attachment and composition of skeletal muscles in relation to their function. *Journal of Biomechanics*, **12**, 859-867.

Vaughan, C.L. (1980). A kinetic analysis of basic trampoline stunts. *Journal of Human Movement Studies*, **6**, 236-251.

Vaughan, C.L. (1985). Biomechanics of running gait. *CRC Critical Reviews of Biomedical Engineering*, **12**, 1-48.

Wachholder, K., & Altenburger, H. (1926). Beiträge zur Physiologie der willkürlichen Bewegung: X. Mitteilung, Einzelbewegungen. *Pflügers Archiv für die Physiologie*, **214**, 642-661.

Wallin, D., Ekblom, B., Grahn, R., & Nordenborg, T. (1985). Improvement of muscle flexibility. A comparison between two techniques. *American Journal of Sports Medicine*, **13**, 263-268.

Ward-Smith, A.J. (1983). The influence of aerodynamic and biomechanical factors on long jump performance. *Journal of Biomechanics*, **16**, 655-658.

Ward-Smith, A.J. (1984). Air resistance and its influence on the biomechanics and energetics of sprinting at sea level and at altitude. *Journal of Biomechanics*, **17**, 339-347.

Ward-Smith, A.J. (1985). A mathematical analysis of the influence of adverse and favourable winds on sprinting. *Journal of Biomechanics*, **18**, 351-357.

Weis-Fogh, T., & Alexander, R.M. (1977). The sustained power output from striated muscle. In T.J. Pedley (Ed.), *Scale effects in animal locomotion* (pp. 511-525). London: Academic Press.

Wetzel, M.C., & Stuart, D.G. (1977). Activation and co-ordination of vertebrate locomotion. In R.M. Alexander & G. Goldspink (Eds.), *Mechanics and energetics of animal locomotion* (pp. 115-152). London: Chapman and Hall.

Wickiewicz, T.L., Roy, R.R., Powell, P.L., & Edgerton, V.R. (1983). Muscle architecture of the human lower limb. *Clinical Orthopaedics and Related Research*, **179**, 275-283.

Williams, K.R., & Cavanagh, P.R. (1983). A model for the calculation of mechanical power during distance running. *Journal of Biomechanics*, **16**, 115-128.

Williams, P.L., & Warwick, R. (Eds.) (1980). *Gray's anatomy* (36th edition). Edinburgh: Churchill Livingstone.

Wilson, B.D. (1977). Toppling techniques in diving. *Research Quarterly*, **48**, 800-804.

Winter, D.A., Wells, R.P., & Orr, G.W. (1981). Errors in the use of isokinetic dynamometers. *European Journal of Applied Physiology*, **46**, 397-408.

Woittiez, R.D., Rozendal, R.H., & Huijing, P.A. (1985). The functional significance of architecture of the human triceps surae muscle. In D.A. Winter, R.W. Norman, R.P. Wells, K.C. Hayes, & A.E. Patla (Eds.), *Biomechanics IX-A* (pp. 21-26). Champaign, IL: Human Kinetics.

Woo, S.L.-Y., Ritter, M.A., Amiel, D., Sanders, T.M., Gomez, M.A., Kuei, S.C., Garfin, S.R., & Akeson, W.H. (1980). The biomechanical and biochemical properties of swine tendons—long term effects of exercise on the digital extensors. *Connective Tissue Research*, **7**, 177-183.

Wunder, C.C., Matthes, R.D., & Tipton, C.M. (1982a). Knee-ligament loading properties as influenced by gravity: 1. Junction with bone of 3-G rodents. *Aviation, Space, and Environmental Medicine*, **53**, 1098-1104.

Wunder, C.C., Matthes, R.D., & Tipton, C.M. (1982b). Knee-ligament loading properties as influenced by gravity: 2. Junctional capacity vs femur length. *Aviation, Space, and Environmental Medicine*, **53**, 1105-1111.

Zatsiorsky, V., & Seluyanov, V. (1983). The mass and inertia characteristics of the main segments of the human body. In H. Matsui & K. Kobayashi (Eds.), *Biomechanics VIII-B* (pp. 1152-1159). Champaign, IL: Human Kinetics.

Zinovieff, A.N. (1951). Heavy-resistance exercise, the Oxford Technique. *British Journal of Physical Medicine, 14*, 159-162.

Author Index

Subject Index